AYURVEDIC CLINICAL MEDICINE

Indian Medical Science Series No.: 60

Source for Students Practitioners and Student - II

AYURVEDIC CLINICAL MEDICINE

By
ATMAKURI VINAYA KUMAR
M.B.B.S., M.D., M.M.N., Ph.D., D.Sc.

SRI SATGURU PUBLICATIONS
A Division of
INDIAN BOOKS CENTRE
Delhi • India

Published by:

Sri Satguru Publications
A Division of

Indian Books Centre
Indological and Oriental Publishers
40/5, Shakti Nagar,
Delhi-110007
(INDIA)

ISBN : 81-7030-560-8

First Edition : Delhi, 1997

Published by Sunil Gupta for Sri Satguru Publications, a division of Indian Books Centre, 40/5, Shakti Nagar, Delhi-110007, India and printed at Mudran Bharti, Delhi-110007

Contents

Preface xv

Acknowledgments xvii

Ch. 1. Skin Diseases (Kustha) 1-88

General Considerations

Etymology; Definition; Etiology; Pathogenesis; Classification; Symptomology; Management; Treatment; Rasa Aushadhis, Compound Drugs.

Clinical Reports: Mahakustha, Pama, Dadru, Vicarcika (Scabies, Pruritus, Eczema): Management of Ksudra Kustha (Pama, Dadru and Vicarcika) with relation to Female Genital Organs—Swain M; Mistry IU.

Sidmakustha

Study of Anti-Sidmakustha actions of Nimba in accordance with pathogenesis of Kustha—Mirani KJ; Mistry IU: Shastry MS.

Vicarcika (Eczema)

A Clinical evaluation of the effect of Tuvaraka (Hydnocarpus castanea) taila in Vicarcika—Biswas TK. The Aetiopathological study of Vicarcika and its management with special reference to Nimbadi quath—Andharia MJ; Kasavan M; Mistry IU; Shastry MS. Efficacy of Rasakarpura in Kudra Kustha with special reference to Vicarcika—Gandhi DB; Chhaya MK; Yeriswamy H; Sharma HS.

Ksudra Kustha

A Clinical study of the role of Vaman and Virechan in the management of Ksudra Kustha—Vyas PP; Mistry IU; Desai KR.

Dermatophytosis

Preliminary invitro study of Asvatha and Udumbara in certain skin pathogenic microorganisms—Unnikrishnann TM; Sharma JM. Therapeutic effect of coconut shell extract in Dermatophytosis—Nair PKS; Pillai NGK; Kurup PB; Nair CPR. Effect of Resottamadilepa on Dermatophytosis—Nair PKS et al. Action of Patolakaturobinyadi Kwatham and Gopatmajadi Keram on skin diseases—A Clinical trial—Geeta A; Pillai KGS; Kurup PB; Nair CPR.

Filariasis (Sleepada)

Essential Features; Ayurvedic Concept

Clinical Reports: Therapeutic assessment of Shakotaka ghana vati on Slipada (Filariasis)—Pandey PN; Das UK. Prevention of Sleepada (elephantiasis) with Ayurvedic compounds—Venkataraghavan S; Bowri N; Sitaraman R; Srinivasan K; Janaki K. Clinical trial of Ayush-64 in Sleepada—Seshagiri Rao T; Rao PV; Kumari KK; Netaji BB; Nisteswa K; Sharma CRR. Clinical evaluation of certain Herbal preparations in the treatment of Chronic Slipada (Filariasis)—Kishore P; Chaturvedi MK. Clinical Assessment of the effect of Ayush-64 in the Acute cases of Slipada (Filariasis)—Kishore P; Chaturvedi MK;. Evaluation of the effect of Ayurvedic drugs (Internal and External in the Treatment of Slipada (Filariasis)—A pilot study—Seshagiri Rao T; Sharma CRR; Kumari KK; Bikshapathi T. Epidemiological studies and therapeutic trials on Slipada—in the village Malipada (Puri District of Orissa)—Padhi MM; Kishore P.

Leprosy (Kustha)

Essential features; Ayurvedic management.

Clinical Reports: Multi drug (New) with indigenous drugs and Diapason in the treatment of Lepromatous leprosy—Chaudary; Hajra SK; Saha B; Mazumdar V. Traditional treatment of Leprosy and Leucoderma by the tribals of Bundelkhand in Uttar Pradesh—Saxena AP; Vyas KM.

Acne Vulgaris (Tarunya Pidika)

Essential features; Ayurvedic Treatment.

Clinical Reports: Clinical Evaluation of Mahamanjishthadi quath and Sookshma Triphala in the management of Acne Vulgaris—A single blind study—Parnajpe P.

Alopecia Areata (Khalitya)

Essential Features; Ayurvedic concept.

Clinical Reports: Critical Appraisal of Khalitya vis-a-vis Alopecia Areata—Kumar P; Ojha D. A simple Siddha Ready for Puzhuvettu (Alopecia Areata)—A Pilot study—Ponniachamy G; Rajalakshmi S; Saroja PR; Sundaram M; Veluchamy G.

Vitiligo (Shvitra)

Etiology; Pathogenesis; Classification; Clinical features; Differential Diagnosis; Complications; Prognosis; Treatment.

Clinical Reports: A clinical study of Vitiligo with Ayush-57—Seshagiri Rao T.; Kuppurajan K; Rajagopalan V; Janaki K. Clinical Evaluation of Ayurvedic preparation in Vitiligo—Nair PR; Namboodiri MNS; Madhavikutty P; Prabhakaran VA. Traditional treatment of Leprosy and Leucoderma by the tribals of Bundelkhand in Uttar Pradesh—Saxena AP; Vyas KM.

Psoriasis (Ekakustha)

Essential features; Ayurvedic concept of Psoriasis; Treatment.

Clinical Reports: Ksudra Kustha—Clinical Research with special reference to Psoriasis—Sankar Babu; Jinde J; Sankaran Kutty P. Clinical study of Vetpalai 'Wrightia tinctoria Linoil in the treatment of Kalanjaga Padai (Psoriasis)—Krishnamurthy JR; Kalaimani S; Veluchamy G.

References and Notes

Ch. 2. Neurology and Rheumatology **89-303**

Rheumatic Diseases

Introduction; Etiopathogenesis; Management

Rheumatoid Arthritis (Aama Vaat)

Essential Features; Management

Clinical Reports: Role of Sunthi-Guduchi in the Treatment of Amavata—Rheumatoid Arthritis—Kishore P; Pandey PN; Ruhil SD. Clinical Studies on the Treatment of Amavata—Rheumatoid Arthritis with Sunthi—Guggulu—Kishore P; Devi Das KV; Banerjee S. Further Clinical Evaluation of Sunthi-Guggulu in the Treatment of Amavata—Rheumatoid Arthritis—Kishore P; Padhi MN. Clinical Evaluation of Rasonadi Kwath in the Treatment of Amavata—Rheumatoid Arthritis—Kishore P; Banerjee SN. Clinical Study on the Treatment of Amavata with Compound Ayurvedic Preparation—Namboodiri MNS; Sethu KS; Madhavakutty P; Vijaya NP; Namboodiri PKN.

Osteoarthritis (Sandhigata Vata)

Essential Features; Management

Clinical Report: A Preliminary Clinical Trial of Trikustha Guggulu in the Treatment of Sandhigata vata (Osteoarthritis)—Sannd BN; Kumari K.

Ankylosing Spondylitis
Essential Features; Management.

Fibromyalgia (Mamsagatvaat)
General Considerations; Management.

Vatavyadhis
Concept of Vatavyadhis and their Management—ARV Murthy; Introduction—General and specific; Definition; Number; Etiology; Pathogenesis; Premonitory symptoms; Classification; Complications and Prognosis; Principles of Management.

Vatavyadhis Viv-a-vis Vatananktmaja Vyadhi—A Critical Conceptual Analysis

Introduction; Vatavyadhi; Nanatmaja Vatavyadhi

Clinical Reports: Preliminary Clinical Trial of Hingutriguna Taila in Vatavyadhis—Padhi MM; Tewari NS; Kishore P.

Headache

General Considerations

Tension Headache

General considerations; Management.

Clinical Reports: Controlled study on Role of Ksheerabala taila in Psychogenic Headache (Vataj Sirah shoola)—Ramu MG et al.

Apasmara (Epilepsies or Convulsive Diseases)

Definition; General considerations; Pathogenesis; Aetiological factors; Classification; Clinical Manifestations; Diagnosis; Differential Diagnosis; Management; Prognosis.

Clinical Reports: Medhya Rasayana Therapy in the Management of Apasmara vis-a-vis Epilepsies—Murthy ARV; Singh RH.

Sciatica (Gridrasi)

A Critical Analysis of the Ayurvedic Concept of Gridrasi; Abstact; Introduction; Definition; Etiology; Classification; Symptomotology; Management; Conclusion.

Low Backache Syndrome (Katishula)

General considerations; Differential Diagnosis.

Clinical Reports: The role of Shodhana Therapy in Gridhrasi—Nair PR et al.

Facial Palsy (Ardita)

A Critical Analysis of the Ayurvedic Concept of Ardita; Abstract; Introduction; Chronology; Etymology; Etiopathogenensis; Symptomotology; Ckassification; Prognosis; Management; Summary.

Poliomyelitis (Baala Pakshaghat)

Synonyms; Relationship; Definition; General Considerations; Pathogenesis; Diagnositc features; Clinical manifestations; Course of the disease; residual paralysis and sequalae; Diagnosis; Differential Diagnosis; Complications; Prognosis; Management; Prevention; Clinical Reserach Reports.

Clinical Reports: Treatment of Chronic cases of Sasaveeya Vata (Poliomyelitis)—Nair PR. et al.; Effect of Bhadradarvadi Taila and Sahacharadi taila in Poliomylitis—Short Reserach Communication.

Hemiplegia (Pakshagat)

Pakshagat and its Principles of Treatment in Ayurveda—Sarma BP; Upadhyay BN.

Clinical Reports: Effect of Panchakarma treatment with Masadiyoga on Pakshavadha—Pillai SM et al.;

Management of Pakshavadha—A Clinical Study of 109 cases—Namboodiri PKN et al.; Role of Hingutriguna taila in the Treatment of Pakshaghata—Hemiplegia—Kishore P; Padhi MN.; Effect of Bhadradarvadi taila and Sahacharadi taila in Khanja and Pangu (Monoplegia and Paraplegia)—Nair PR et al.

Muscular Dystrophy

General considerations; Ayurvedic concept of Muscular Dystrophies

Clinical Reports: Pseudohy pertrophic Muscular Dystrophy—An Ayurvedic Approach—Nair PR et al.

Ch. 3. Endocrinology **304-376**

Obseity (Sthaulya)

General Considerations; Aetiology; Complications; Prognosis; Treatment; The concept of Obesity in Ayurveda—Nirmal AB; Nirmal BM; Etiology; Samprapti (Pathogenesis); Rupa or manifestations; Management; Clinical Report.

Hyperlipidemia and Obesity

General considerations; Ayurvedic concept.

Clinical Reports: A Clinical Evaluation of Arogyavardhini as a Hypocholesteraemic agent with special reference to Obesity/Corpulence—Tewari NS; Jain PC; A Double Blind Clinical Trial with Ayush-55—An Ayurvedic compound preparation in Obese cases—Kuppurajan K et al.

References

Madhumeha (Diabetes Mellitus)

Prameha with special reference to Madhumeha vis-a-vis Diabetes Mellitus—Mrs Bharti; Relationship; Definition; Gereral considerations; Pathogenesis; Diagnostic features; Clinical Manifestations; Course of the Disease; Diagnosis; Differential Diagnosis; Complications; Management; Clinical Reports; Clinical Experiences; References;

Madhumeha

General considerations; Classification of Madhumeha; Samprapti; Ama; Agni; Srotas; Prodromal symptoms; signs and Symptoms; Complications; Treatment.

Clinical Reports: Diagnosis of 20 subtypes of Prameha based on Physical and Chemical Examination of urine in proved cases of Diabetes Mellitus—Chandola HM; Tripathi SN; Clinical and Biochemical Correlation of Different stages of Diabetes Mellitus with Different Doshic Types of Prameha—Chandola HM; Tripathi SN; Effect of C. tamala (Tej-patra) on Plasma Insulin vis-a-vis Blood Sugar in patients of Diabetes Mellitus—Chandola HM; Tripathi SN; Correlations between Blood Sugar levels and some Biochemical as well as Ayurvedic Phenomena in the patients of Madhumeha (Diabetes Mellitus)—Gupta SN; Misra SK; Singh G.; Clinical studies of Abrage (Mica) Chendooram in the Management of Diabetes Mellitus (Neerazhivu)—Shanker VR; Aggarwal MP.

References.

Ch. 4. Nutritional Disorders **377-395**

Therapeutic Nutrition in Ayurveda

Introduction; Food; Food—Human Body and Disease; Balancing Diet/Wholesome diet (Hitaahara); Unbalancing Diet (Ahita/Viruddha Ahara); Factors responsible for unbalancing diet; diet—Treatment.

References.

Clinical Reports: Effect of Aswagandha (Withania somniferalunal) on the process of Ageing in Human Volunteers—Kuppurajan K; Rajagopalan SS; Sitaraman R; Rajagopalan V; Janaki K; Revathi R; Venkataraghavan S.; The Comparative Effect of Milk Fortified with Aswagandha, Aswagandha and Punarnava in Children—A Double Blind Study—Venkataraghavan S; Seshadri C; Sundareshan TP; Revthi R; Rajagopalan V; Janaki K.; Effect of Chyavanaprasha on Malnutrition—Tersia TL; Sridhar BN; Pillai BKR; Vijayan NP; Namboodiri PKN;.

Drugs (Dravyas) and Their Equivalents 396

Therapeutic Index 400

Index 405

Preface

This is the Second Volume in the series authored by me. The first volume titled 'Principles of Ayurvedic Therapeutics' has already been published by the renowned Sri Satguru Publications of Indian Books Centre, New Delhi, in 1995.

In this book four topics on Clinical Medicine have been dealt with. These are: Skin Diseases (*Tvak Rog*); Neurological and Rheumatic Disorders (*Vaat Rog*), Endocrinology (*Antahsraav Rog*), and Nutritional Disorders (*Poshakjany Rog*).

Under each chapter, only certain important diseases have been considered, paying attention mostly to the essential features of Etiology (*Nidana*), Pathogenesis (*Samprapti*) and detailed description of the management (*Chikitsa*) of each disease concerned. As far as possible, each disease description is followed by Clinical reports from Researchers carried in renowned institutions and Ayurvedic Research Centres from all over the country. These reports have been well authenticated and published in reputed journals in India such as the *Journal of Central Council for Research in Ayurveda* and *Siddha*, New Delhi. These reports have become essential in view of the divergent opinions expressed and the efficacy of the Drugs (*Dravyas*) used in the management (*Chikitsa*) of the diseases, as described in the past in the Ayurvedic Classics and their relevance to the present times. Also, some of the diseases described in the Ayurvedic classics do not find their equivalents in the modern texts of Clinical Medicine and vice versa. Because of these problems, many research studies have been carried out under the patronage of Central Council of Research in Ayurveda and Siddha in designated Research Centres all over the country for the past two decades. Encouraging results have been obtained and new combinations of drugs (*Yoga*) have been formulated, tested on humans and animals based on Ayurvedic descriptions in classics and are being marketed.

I hope that such a way of presentation of the subject matter helps in laying a strong foundation for Ayurvedic Medicine on modern scientific parlance which will be acceptable to everyone concerned in the medical profession.

I am very much grateful to Sri Murthy (Statistics Department) and Dr. K. Srinivasa Rao, LB Nagar, Hyderabad for their financial contribution towards the project. I am very much thankful to the various authors, institutions, Research Centres and Health Care Organisations for utilising their papers, publications and personal communications while preparing the manuscript.

I am very much grateful to the publishers for kindly accepting the script and publishing it neatly and in time.

Hyderabad
June, 1997

ATMAKURI VINAYA KUMAR

Acknowledgements

Authors

Prof. P. Yadaiah. MD, Ph.D.—Prof. and Head of Deptt. of Kayachikitsa, R.T. Ayurvedic College and Hospital, Akola, Maharashtra.

Prof. C.P. Shukla—Ex. Head of the Kayachikitsa Deptt. Institute of PGT&R, and Emeritus Professor, Jamnagar (Gujarat).

Prof. S. N. Tripathi—Prof. of Kayachikitsa, Institute of Medical Sciences, B.H.U. Varanasi.

M. Paramkush Rao, MD—Asst. Prof. Deptt. Dravyaguna & R.S.S.V. Ayurvedic College, Triupati (AP).

A.R.V. Murthy, MD, D.Yoga, Ph.D.—Asst. Prof. Deptt. of Kayachikitsa, S.V. Ayurvedic College & Hospital, Tirupati (AP).

Mrs. Bharti, MD, D.Yoga, Ph.D.—Clinical Registrar, Deptt. of Kayachikitsa, Institute of Medical Sciences, BHU, Varanasi.

B. Sitaram, MD—Asst. Prof. S.V. Ayurvedic College, Tirupati (AP).

Prof. K.N. Udupa—Prof. Emeritus, IMS, B.H.U. Varanasi.

Institutions and Health Care Organizations

Banaras Hindu University, Varanasi.

Institute of P.G.T.&R., Jamnagar.

Dr. A. Lakshmipathi Unit for Research in Indian Medicine (Adyar, Madras), V.H.S. (CCRAS).

Ayurvedic Research Unit, NIMHANS, Bangalore.

Indian Institute of Panchkarma, Cheruthuruthy, Kerala.

Department of Botany, University of Saugar, Sagar-470003.

Central Research Institute (Ayu) Unit I, Bhubaneshwar, Orissa.

Clinical Research Unit (Siddha), Safdarjung Hospital, New Delhi.
Central Research Institute (Siddha), Madras.
Regional Research Institute (DR), SCRAS, Trivandrum.
Central Research Institute for Siddha, Arumbakkam, Madras.
Central Council for Research in Ayurveda and Siddha, New Delhi (CCRAS).
Dravya guna, Deptt. IPGT&R, Jamnagar.
Institute of Post Graduate Education and Research in Ayurveda, Calcutta.
Department of Rasa Shastra, IMS, BHU.
Department of Kayachikitsa, Trivandrum.
Gujarat Ayurveda University, Jamnagar (Gujarat).
Deptt. of Leprology, School of Tropical Medicine, Calcutta-700073.
R.S.&B.K. Deptt. IPGT&R, Jamnagar.
Indian Council of Medical Research, New Delhi.
World Health Organization (WHO), Geneva.
Swami Prakashanand Ayurveda Research Centre, Juhu, Mumbai-400049.
National Integrated Medical Association (NIMA), Mumbai-400014.
Ayurveda Samachar Printing and Publication, Calcutta-700012.

1

SKIN DISEASES (KUSTHA)

GENERAL CONSIDERATIONS

Nirukti (Etymology of Kustha)

The word Kustha is derived from Kus Dhatu which means that whatever comes to the outer side from inner side of the body.

Definition of Kustha

When the provoked three doshas (vata, pitta and kapha) and vitiated four dushyas: Tvak (skin), Mamsa (flesh), Rakta (blood), and Lasika (lymph) and all these seven dravyas become imbalanced, results in kustha. If it is not treated in time, the disease is formed inside the body and manifests itself on the skin making it Kutsita or diseased and the whole body is disturbed. It is called kustham wherever there is loss of function of sparsha (touch) and depends upon tvak, mamsa, rakta and lasika. In Ayurvedic purview, kustha is called also as skin disease.

According to Ayurveda leprosy as well as all obstinate skin diseases come under the heading of Kustha. Sushruta has defined kustha as Oupasargik disease. Vijay Rakshit says that if any one or both of the parents are suffering from kustha, their offspring become a sufferer, either genetically or congenitally.

Etiology (Nidana)

The etiological factors mentioned for kustha particularly, produce vitiation and imbalancing in three doshas and four dushyas viz. tvak, rakta, mamsa and ambu. As it is well-known in Ayurveda that kustha is a blood-borne disease, so all the factors that vitiate blood are also responsible for kustha. In Charaka Samhita, following etiological factors are described.

Viruddhahara

1. Heavy, liquid and fat prominent food.
2. Constant intake of either honey or pendium or fish or lakucha, mulaka, kakamachi or their combination in large quantity in the condition of indigestion;
3. intake of food, mostly hayanaka, yavaka, along with milk, curd, kola, atasi, kusumbha and snigdha substances.
4. Excessive use of flesh grams and tila, saltish or acidic substances.
5. Masa, pastry, milk and jaggery.

Krama Viruddha Ahara

1. Intake of chilichim type of fish with milk.
2. Vidahi anna.
3. Ajirna bhojana.

Viharajanya Nidana

1. Entering into cold water immediately after one is afflicted with fear, exhaustion and grief.
2. Improper regimen of Panchakarma.
3. Suppression of the urge of emesis.
4. Day sleep.
5. Insulting Brahmins and teachers.
6. Sinful acts.

Achara

1. Disobeying of father, mother, teachers, etc.
2. Performing unsacred works.
3. Misbehaving with women, Brahmin and good people.
4. Taking others property by evil means.

Pathogenesis

Pathogenesis of all skin disorders had been explained in general as:

1. Tridosha Prakopa.

2. Prakupita Tridosha.
3. Doshas causing Saithilya in Dushyas.
4. Sthana Samsraya of Doshas in Sithila Dushya.
5. After Sthana Samsraya in Dushyas again vitiating them thus causing Kusthas.

Samprapti Ghataka

Dosha—Tridosha
Dushya—Tvak, Mamsa and Ambu
Agnimandya—Jatharagnimandya
Srotas—Rasa, Rakta, Mamsa
Ama—Amavisa
Uddhava Sthana—Amapakvashaya
Sanchara—Tvak, Lasika, Rakta, and Mamsa
Avayava—Sarvasarira.

Thus, the above said ahara and vihara with achara, if taken or performed causes vitiation of tridoshas. These vitiated doshas take the help of Dushyas as tvak, mamsa, rakta and lasika and thus causing Kustha (Charaka Ni. 5). In Sushruta Nidana Fifth chapter, it is said that the above said nidanas causes the vitiation of vata. This vitiated vata together with pitta and kapha moves to the siras, causing obstruction of rakta, lasika, tvacha and mamsa. Here the Sthanasamsraya takes place resulting in patches. If these patches are not treated properly gradual vitiation of dhatus goes on. With the above said process, symptoms and signs of disease appear.

Classification of Kustha

Charaka has described kustha as seven types; whereas, Sushruta classified it primarily into two and then into 18 types. Thus, though the kusthas are quoted as innumerable, however, on the basis of etiology, pathogenesis, prognosis and treatment, they are graded as Mahakusthas and Ksudra Kusthas. They are 18; out of which, Ksudra Kustha are 11 and 7 are Mahakusthas. These are summarised below.

Table 1.1: *Classification of Kustha* (Joshi et al)

Name	*Classification*		*Dosha*	
	Charaka	*Sushruta*	*Charaka*	*Sushruta*
1. Aruna	–	Maha	–	Vata
2. Udumbara	–	Maha	Pitta	Pitta
3. Rishyajihwa	–	Maha	Vata + Pitta	Pitta
4. Kapala	–	Maha	Vata	Pitta
5. Kakanaka	–	Maha	Vata + Pitta + Kapha	Pitta
6. Pundarika	–	Maha	Pitta + Kapha	Kapha
7. Dadru	–	Maha	–	Kapha
8. Parisarpa	–	Ksudra	–	Vata
9. Charmadala	–	Ksudra	–	Pitta
10. Visarpa	–	Ksudra	–	Pitta
11. Vicharchika	–	Ksudra	–	Pitta
12. Kitibha	–	Ksudra	–	Pitta
13. Pama	–	Ksudra	–	Pitta
14. Sthularuska	–	Ksudra	–	Kapha
15. Mahakustha	–	Ksudra	–	Kapha
16. Ekakustha	–	Ksudra	–	Kapha
17. Sidhma	–	Ksudra	Vata + Kapha	Kapha
18. Raksha	–	Ksudra	–	Kapha

Symptomology of Kustha in General

After the above said process, symptoms are observed as follows:

1. Stiffness of skin—it may be smooth/dry with discolouration.
2. Romaharsha.
3. Itching and burning sensation.
4. Excess or no sweating.
5. Blood becoming of black colour.
6. The wounds are divergent with pain and durability.
7. Loss of sensation, pin-pricking sense is felt.
8. Vertigo.
9. The wounds even after healing creates roughness of skin.

According to Doshas

A. Vataja symptoms: 1. Aruna Varnata. 2. Ayama. 3. Bheda. 4. Harsha. 5. Kharatva. 6. Parushata. 7. Rouksya. 8. Sankocha. 9. Shosha. 10. Stambha. 11. Shoola. 12. Suti. 13. Syava Varnata. 14. Toda.

B. Pittaja symptoms: 1. Anga Patana. 2. Daha. 3. Kleda. 4. Paka. 5. Parisrava. 6. Raga. 7. Visragandha.

C. Kaphaja symptoms: 1. Gaurava. 2. Kandu. 3. Kleda. 4. Saitya. 5. Sthairya. 6. Svaitya. 7. Upasneha. 8. Utsedha.

If we analyse these factors of nidana, unwholesome diet may cause the allergy, which in turn, produce different skin diseases. It is an accepted fact that the immunity of the body may be decreased due to such type of unwholesome diet and regimen, so that bacterial organisms can easily attack.

According to Ashtanga Hridaya, Raktaja krimi is predominant causative factor of kustha. According to Sushruta, Krimis are also enumerated in the causative factors. The term krimi refers to microscopic and macroscopic organisms like bacteria, fungi and maggots. The Dosa-Dushya-Adhistan of kustha is—Dosa-Tridosa+krimi; Dushya—tvak, rakta, mamsa and ambu (lymph); Adhistan—Bahyaroga marga (specially tvak).

Table 1.2: *Kustha Equivalents (Das and Joshi)*

Mahakustha (7)		
1. Kapala Kustha	:	Non-lepromatous leprosy (tuberculoid L. etc).
2. Audumbara	:	Lepromatous leprosy
3. Mandala	:	Non-lepromatous leprosy
4. Rishyajihwa	:	Non-lepromatous leprosy
5. Pundarika	:	Lepromatous leprosy
6. Sidma	:	Pityriasis versicolour
7. Kakanak	:	Lepromatous leprosy
Kshudrakushtha (11)		
1. Eka Kustha	:	Psoriasis
2. Charma Kustha	:	Xeroderma
3. Kitibh	:	Keloi or Psoriasis
4. Vipadika	:	Rhagades
5. Alasaka	:	Lichen
6. Dadru	:	Ringworm
7. Carmadala	:	Impetigo or infective dermatitis
8. Pama	:	Scabies
9. Vispota	:	Exanthemata
10. Sataru	:	Erythema induratum
11. Vicarcika	:	Eczema
Others		
1. Svitra	:	Vitiligo
2. Kilasa	:	Leucoderma

Management of Kustha

Principles of Treatment

Thus, the main factors in kustha are—Tridosha prakopa, Shaithilya in Dushyas, Ama, and Khavaigunya. So, in the treatment, important things to be followed are Dipana, Pachana, Rakta shodhana and use of Tridosha shamaka dravyas. Drugs causing nourishment to tvak, rakta, mamsa and lasika are essential. Therefore, and since, all kusthas are tridoshajanya, it should be treated according to the bala-bala of the predominance of dosha. If it is vata predominant administration of ghrita; if it is pitta predominant virechana and Raktamokshan; and if it is kapha predominant vamana should be done.

Treatment

1. Nidana Paribarjan.
2. Samshodhana: According to predominance of dosha.
3. Samshamana:
   (a) Antah Parimarjan—specially in Mahakustha
   (b) Bahya parimarjan—specially in Ksudra kustha.

Medicinal Treatment: Following single herbs are recommended: 1. Khadira, 2. Apamarga, 3. Chakramarda, 4. Kutki, 5. Nimba, 6. Haridra, 7. Bidanga, 8. Chitrak, 9. Bakuchi, 10. Aragvadh, 11. Sariva, 12. Karanja, 13. Chirayata, 14. Vasa, 15. Patel, 16. Trifala, 17. Bringaraj. 18. Amalta etc.

Rasa Aushadhis: Rasa Aushadhi has a great role for the management of kustha. Following Rasa Aushadhis are effective for different kinds of Kusthas.

(i) *Rasa Aushadhis for all kinds of kusthas*

1. Administration of lelitaka (sulphur) with the juice of jati (Amlaki) together with honey. It is claimed to cure for 17 kinds of kustha (Ch. Chi. 7/70).
2. Makshika dhatu (copper pyrite) taken together with cow's urine is also effective (Ch. Chi. 7/70).
3. Rasa (mercury) mixed with sulphur or swarna makshika. It is claimed to be remedy for curing all ailments of kustha. In this way mercury processed with diamond and silajatu or yogaraja cures all skin ailments (Ch. Chi. 7/71-72).
4. Application of the paste of ela, kustha, darvi, satapuspa, chitraka, vidanga, rasanjana and abhaya (Ch. Chi. 7/84).
5. The paste of the seeds of Prapunnada, rock-salt, rasanjana, kapittha, lodhra, root of white karavira, fruits of kutaja and karanja and the bark of daruharidra along with the tender leaves of jati (Ch. Chi. 7/93, 94).

6. Decoction of rasanjana, nimba and patala, khadira, aragvadha, and kutaja, triphala, saptaparni is used as alepana and internal use.
7. Medicated oil prepared from kustha, arka, tuttha, katphala, seeds of mulaka, rohini, katuka, fruit of kutaja, utpala, musta, brihati, karavira, kasisa, nimba, patha, duralabha, chitraka, vidanga, seeds of liktalabu, kampillaka, sarsapa, vacha, and daruharidra.
8. Paste of chitraka and sobhanjana, guduchi, apamarga and devadaru, khadira, dhava, syama, danti, and dravanti and laksa, rasanjana etc. and punarnava by adding butter milk (Ch. Chi. 7/124).
9. Local application of paste prepared from mom, gandhak, and chalmoogra (V.R.).

Compound Drugs

1. Vijoyras (R?R.5/20)
2. Suptakusthari ras
3. Kusthajidras
4. Taleswar ras
5. Mahataleswar ras
6. Kanaksundar ras
7. Haribolankush ras
8. Tripurantak ras
9. Viswahita ras
10. Vyoshadi gutika
11. Kusthakuthar ras
12. Bajrasekhar ras
13. Manikyatilak ras
14. Parahita ras
15. Talakeswar ras
16. Khageswar ras
17. Kusthanasan ras
18. Arogyavardhani ras
19. Narayan ras
20. Bajradhar ras
21. Mahatalakeswar ras
22. Kusthakuthar ras
23. Chandranan ras (RSS)
24. Kustha kalanal ras
25. Chandrakanti ras
26. Manikya ras
27. Vijoy Bhairabi ras
28. Vijoynandi ras
29. Gandhak rasayan.

(ii) Mahakustha

1. Kapala Kustha
   (i) Dhanwantari ras
   (ii) Uday Bhaskar ras
   (iii) Bhallatak gur

(iv) Kustha kalanal tailam

2. Audumbar Kustha

(i) Sankosh ras

(ii) Bhallatak gur

(iii) Kustha Rakshas tailam

3. Mandala Kustha

(i) Application of powder of trapu (Tin), sisa (Lead) and ayas (Iron).

(ii) Application of powder of Phalgu, Chitraka, Brihati together with Rock-salt, Devadaru and cow's urine.

(iii) Kanakaksiri taila (Manahsila, Hartal, Kankutha, Tuttha, Kasis).

(iv) Uday Bhaskar ras

(v) Arkeswar ras

(vi) Talakeswar ras

(vii) Rasamanikya

(viii) Rajrajeswar ras

(ix) Brahmaras

(x) Sarbeswar ras

(xi) Bhallatak gur.

4. Rishwajihwaba Kustha

Bhallatak gur (1/2 tola).

5. Pundarika Kustha

(i) Rasa manikya,

(ii) Bhallatak gur.

6. Sidhma Kustha

(i) The paste of Kustha, Tamalapatra, Maricha, Manahsila, Ankasis should be mixed with oil and stored for seven days in a copper vessel. This paste should be applied and the patient should expose himself to the heat of the Sun. This is claimed to cure Sidhma within a week. This recipe also cures freshly occurring kilsa within a month provided the patient does not take bath (Ch. Chi. 7).

(ii) Local application of paste prepared from yabaksar, Suddha Gandhak, and Mustard oil (V.R.).

(iii) Local application of paste prepared from kasamarda vij, mulivij, suddha gandhak, and kanji.

7. Kakanak Kustha

Bhallatak gur.

(iii) Ksudra Kustha

1. Charma Kustha.
2. Eka Kustha.
3. Alasaka Kustha.
   (i) Medicated ghee and oil should be prepared by boiling ghee and or/oil with the paste of Jivanti, Manjistha, Daruharidra, Kampillaka, Payas, and Tuttha. When cooking of this is over, Sarjarasa and Madhuchista (Bee's wax) should be added and massage should be done.
   (ii) Rasamanikya
   (iii) Bhallatak gur.
4. Kitibh Kustha
   (i) Taleswar ras.
   (ii) Rajrajeswar ras.
   (iii) Somraji tailam (Brihat).
5. Vipadika Kustha
   (i) Local application of paste prepared from Rai, Saindhav lavana, Gur, Sahad, Guggul, Gairik, Ghreeta and mom.
   (ii) Bhallatak gur (V.R.)
6. Dadru Kustha
   (i) Tikteksvakvadi taila (Ch. Chi.).
   (ii) Kanakaksiri taila.
   (iii) Paribhadra ras.
   (iv) Rajrajeswar ras.
   (v) Bhallatak gur.
   (vi) Marichadya tailam.
7. Pama Kustha
   (i) Bajravali ras (R.S.S.).
   (ii) Local application of paste prepared from Sindur, Kalimaris and butter (V.R.).

(iii) External application of Gandhak with mustard oil and internal application of Gandhak with milk.
(iv) Bajra Bati.
(v) Bhallatak Gur.
(vi) Kacchurakshak taila (Bh. Pr.).
(vii) Sindhuradya tailam (Cha.D.).
(viii) Jeerakadya tailam.
(ix) Arkamamahshila tailam.
(x) Adityapaka tailam.

8. Vipadika Kustha
(i) Local application of paste prepared from Rai, Saindhav lavan, Gur, Sahad, Guggul, Gairik, Ghreeta and mom.
(ii) Bhallatak Gur (V.R.).

9. Vispotaka Kustha
(i) Rajtakeswar ras (R.S.S.).
(ii) Svatridadripotala lepa (Ch. Chi).
(iii) Rasa manikya.
(iv) Bhallatak Gur.

10. Vicarika Kustha
(i) Local application of paste prepared from Parad, Sankha Bhasma, Gandhak, Manahsila, Chakramarda Veej, Chitrak, Bhallatak, Nimba patra, Gur, Sahad, and Bakuchi mixed with gomutra or kanjee.
(ii) Uday Bhaskar ras.
(iii) Rasa manikya.
(iv) Sinduradya tailam.
(v) Kustha Raashsam tailam.
(vi) Sadvindu tailam.
(vii) Marichya tailam.
(viii) Vicharchika tailam.

11. Svitra Kustha
(i) Local application of: The paste prepared from Manahsila, Vidanga, Kasis, Gorochana, Kanakapuspi (Svarnaksiri) and rock-salt, should be used for external application.
(ii) Manahsila made to a paste by adding peacock bile.

(iii) Seeds of Avalguja, Laksa, cow's bile, both the type of anjana (Sauviranjana and Rasanjana), Pippali and the powder of kalaloha (black iron).
(iv) Medinisar ras (RSS).
(v) Svetari ras.
(vi) Svitrahara lepa.
(vii) Mukha svitrahara lepa.
(viii) Local application of paste prepared from Bakuchi and hartal (V.R.).
(ix) Local application of paste prepared from Gunjaphal, bark of Chitrak and Manahsila mixed with cow's urine.
(x) Local application of paste prepared from Gandhak, Rakta Chitrak mul, Kasis Hartal, Triphala, mixed with water.
(xi) Bhallatak gur.
(xii) Panchana taila.
(xiii) Aragbadhyadam taila.
(xiv) Marichadya tailam.

Alongwith above medicines, some asav, arishta, churna, taila etc. are also effective for the management of kustha.

(*References*: Das B., Joshi D., Pathogenesis and Management of Kustha [with special reference to Rasousadhi, Ayu. Samachar, 13:12:1991]—Bhatt K., Anadjat H., Study of Ksudra Kustha with Its Management by Rasamanikya. Ayu. Sam. 14:9:1992).

Clinical Reports

Management of Ksudra Kustha (Pama, Dadru and Vicarcika) with Relation to Female Genital Organ (Swain M., Mistry I., Management of Kshudra Kustha [Pama, Dadru, Vicarcika] with relation to Female Genital Organ: *Ayu. Samachar:* 14:2:1991).

A total of 15 female patients were divided into two groups—Group A consisting of 8 patients and Group B consisting of 7 patients. These were treated for the complaints of Pama, Dadru and Vicarcika.

Drug Administration

Internal Administration—Group A

Gandhak Rasayan 2 Rati

Vanga Bhasma 2 Rati Administered twice daily with milk.

External Administration—Group B

Nimba, argbadha, haridra mixed churna one gm two times per day.

External Application Group A and B

Local affected part was cleaned by Khadir Kwath and after drying, khadir powder dusting was done in both the groups A and B.

Duration of treatment

15 days.

Diet

During the course of treatment, patients were advised not to take oily things, potato, excessive salt, sour and pungent substances, soap baths. Only black gram and green gram powder was advised for bathing. Easily digestible substances were suggested.

Selection of Patients

Selection of patients based on clinical symptomotology were taken of Pama, Dadru and Vicarcika. The cardinal signs and symptoms noted were—Kandu, Pidaka, Daha, Srava, Paka, Toda, Sopha, Syavatvak, Purusha, Tvak etc.

Dravya Properties

Nimba: Nimba is tikta kashaya rasa, sita veerya, laghu guna, and due to katu vipaka it can do samana of kapha-pitta doshas. Due to kashaya rasa and sita veerya, it acts as sthambana. Due to tikta rasa, laghu guna, it is antibacterial, antipruritic, putihar and vrana sodhana and due to sita veerya it is daha prasamana.

Haridra: Due to tikta katu rasa, it act on leprosy and all types of skin diseases.

Gandhak Rasayan: Due to tikta rasa it is blood purifier, kandughna and twakdoshahara. Due to rasayan, it is vataja and vrusya.

Vanga Bhasma: Due to ushna veerya tikta rasa it is deepana, pachana and blood purifier, krimighna and destroy skin diseases. Due to madhur vipaka it is aphrodisiac.

Aragbadha: Sushruta described Aragbadha as Kanduhara. Due to laxative guna, it can destroy the disease from the body.

Duration of the Disease

More than 2 months (Group A) and less than 2 months in Group B.

Table 1.3: *Table Showing Degree of Improvement*

Result	*Group A*		*Group B*	
	No. of Pts.	*Percentage*	*No. of Pts.*	*Percentage*
Cured	5	62.50	4	57.14
Marked relief	2	25.00	3	42.86
Mild relief	1	12.50	–	–

Mirani K.J., Vaidya A.R., Mistry I.U., Shastry M.S.: *A Study of Anti-Sidhmakustha Actions of Nimba in Accordance with Pathogenesis of Kustha, Ay. Samachar:* 14:4:1991.

A total of 20 patients suffering from Sidhma (Tinea versicolour) were treated with Nimba for a period of 21 days and the results were assessed clinically and microbiologically.

The Nimbavati was selected for trial which was prepared from the bark of the Nimba tree. The patients were prescribed with the Nimbavati 4 tablets twice a day with water and Nimba oil was to be applied once in a day on the Sidhma lesions. The patients were advised to avoid sour things, excessive use of salt, chillies, condiments from the diet. Similarly the patients were adviced to have the bath with gram powder instead of soap of any kind and to wear cotton cloths.

Observations

1. Out of 8 cases, 5 cases (62.5 per cent) were relieved of itching and itching was found diminished in 2 patients (25 per cent). Acharya Charaka has also confirmed its antipruritic action of Nimba by including it in Kandughna Maha Kashaya.
   Similarly burning sensation was also found disappeared in all cases.
2. In 10 out of 16 patients (62.5 per cent) desquamation was found disappeared, while in 4 patients (25 per cent) it was found improving.
3. Out of 20 cases, in 16 cases (80 per cent) the discolouration was found diminished.
4. Antifungal action: Out of 18 cases who were having positive mycological tests, 10 patients (55.6 per cent) were found having diminished fungus.

The overall results show that there was clinical improvement in 12 patients (60 per cent) while there was no change in 8 patients. There was not complete cure at all in the due course of 21 days. Thus Nimba shows encouraging results and may give complete cure if the treatment is prolonged for a longer time, with adjustment of dosage.

(*Drug Action:* Generally tikta rasa diminishes the kapha and pitta doshas. Suppression of pitta has direct effect on sweat. The oil applied externally coats the superficial layer of the skin, penetrates the vitiation and remove the favourable conditions for the fungus, by its bitterness and eradicates them by germicidal activity; due to the presence of sulphur which is also a strong germicide).

Biswas T.K.: *A Clinical Evaluation of the Effect of Tuvaraka (Hydnocarpus castanea) Taila in Vicarcika (Eczema), Ayu. Samachar:* 14:4:1991).

With the textual reference, Tuvaraka (Hydnocarpus castanea) was selected for clinical trial. For the study 11 patients of Vicarcika (dry and wet eczema) were selected from the OPD of SVS) hospital attached to the IPGER. To all the cases Tuvaraka Taila in the form of capsules was given once daily in a dose of 500 mg for 10 days followed by 500 mg twice daily for 10 days.

Duration of illness ranged from 3 months to 3 years.

Diagnosis was based on the following features:

1. Kandu (pruritus)
2. Pidaka (inflammatory lesions of eruptions)
3. Syavrna (pale discolouration)
4. Vahusrava (exudative discharge).
5. Vali (furring of the skin).
6. Ruksha tvacha (roughness of the skin i.e., scally deformity of skin).

Besides above features, one patient has complaint of breathing difficulty as similar to Tamaka Swasa and one patient had complaint of symptoms similar to Grahani. After treatment of 20 days, following results were observed.

Table 1.4: *Showing Percentage of Clinical Improvement*

Symptoms	*No. of Pts. Complaints B.Treat.*	*No. of Pts. Relieved After 20 Days Treatment*	*Percentage of Cure After Treatment*
1. Kandu	11	11	100%
2. Pidaka	11	11	100%
3. Syaba	9	7	77.77%
4. Vahusrava	10	8	80%
5. Vali	5	3	60%
6. RukshaTvacha	11	9	81.80%

The symptoms like swasa (breathing difficulty) and Grahani (Stetorrhea) were managed conservatively. Routine laboratory investigations done before and after treatment showed no significant abnormalities. However fungus cultures were not done due to nonavailability of culture media, instruments etc.

The observations showed that Tuvaraka has a definite role on Vicarcika. Further study can give us a new avenue to treatment approach.

Andharia M.J., Kasavan M., Mistry I.U., Shastry M.S.: *The Aetiopathological Study of Vicarcika and Its Management with Special Reference to Nimbadi Quath, Auy. Sam.,* 14:10:1992.

18 patients of Vicarcika were treated with Nimbadi Quath in a dose of two tolas twice a day for 30 days. For the purpose of the study, the recipes from Sahasra yoga was selected. The ingredients of Nimbadi Quath were as follows: Nimba twak, Haridra, Guduchi, Vasa, Hareetaki, Amalaki, Vibheetaki, Patol, Nidigdhika, Shunti and Vishata. According to Ayurvedic classics, Nimbadi Quath has got the predominance of Tikta rasa and acts as a kapha and pittahara. It has got laghu and ruksha guna; therefore, it must be acting on vitiated kapha. Due to its properties of ushna veerya, it acts as kapha and vatahara. Due to predominance of katu vipaka, it has got subsiding capacity for kapha. Thus it is evident that Nimbadi Quath is Tridoshahara.

During the course of treatment, patients were given only salt free diet which included chapatis and milk or chapatis or salt free dal and vegetables.

Observations

1. The drug is effective for all doshas but more effective on kapha and pitta.
2. It acts on kandu (kapha) and daha (pitta); also effective on the symptoms of ruksha, tvak vaivarnya which are related to vata.
3. 100 per cent relief was obtained in the symptoms like srava, kandu, and daha.
4. More than 60 per cent improvement was obtained in the symptoms like Kharasparsha and Parusha.

Table 1.5: *Effect of Nimbadi Quath on Vicarcika (n=18)*

Results	*No. of Pts.*	*Percentage*
1. Cured	8	50%
2. Marked improvement	5	27.1%
3. Moderate improvement	3	16.1%
4. Poor improvement	1	5.5%
5. Unchanged	Nil	Nil

Note: For Samprapti, Sushruta mentioned the Vicarcika as Pitta predominant; while Charaka says it is Kapha predominant. Vagbhata, Bhavaprakasha, Sarangadhara completely follow the opinion of Charaka in the consideration of Dosha predominance.
Separate nidana have not been mentioned for Vicarcika in classics; therefore, the general nidana for Kustha vyadhi may be considered.

Gandhi D.B., Chhaya M.K., Yeriswamy H., Sharma H.S.: *Efficacy of Rasa Karpura in Kshudra Kushta with Special Reference to Vicarcika, Auy. Samachar,* 15:2:1992.

Rasakarpura comprises of two words—Rasa means Parad (mercury) and Karpura is a substance with white colour and particular smell. Rasakarpura is a pharmaceutical product in which rasa is the main ingredient and the end product is white in colour.

Rasakārpura is in use since twelfth century A.D., but under the name of mercuric preparation. From the fourteenth century onwards it was named as Rasakarpura. Total of 40 references are available on Rasakarpura in various classical texts. In the preparation of Rasakarpura, three types of drugs are used—from mineral, animal and vegetable origin.

Study

15 cases of Vicarcika were selected irrespective of the age, sex, occupation, duration of illness etc. from O.P. and I.P. Depts of IPGT&R Hospital, Jamnagar.

Following classical features were noted in diagnosis:

Pidika—Syava pidika, Raga pidika, Syava lihita pidika, Parisuska pidika.

Srava—Bahu, Lasika, Praklinna.

Paka—Ati Rajyah, Visarpanah

Some signs which are not explainable in texts but are considered as common signs and symptoms of kustha are found in several cases. Totally, 11 features have been considered for the diagnosis among which kandu, pidika, vedana and srava were present in more than 60 per cent of the patients. Kandu and pidika were present in all the 15 cases (100 per cent). Srava is found in 10 patients (75 per cent) and Vedana is found in 9 cases (60 per cent).

Drug

Rasakarpura was prepared according to the reference of Rasatarangini and clinically used.

Mode of Administration of the Drug

Rasakarpura and Dalcini (Cinnamomum zeylanicum Blume) were powdered, mixed well in ratio of 1:40 and capsulated. Each capsule contains 3.126 mg of Rasakarpura and 121.875 mg of Dalcini. These capsules were administered only internally.

Dosage

Dosage was fixed on the basis of duration of illness and the severity of the disease as follows:

(a) Below 1 year duration of illness—1 X twice daily.

(b) Above 1 year duration of illness—1 X thrice daily.

(c) In children below 5 years of age—1 X twice daily.

Capsules administered with water.

Duration of Treatment

Fixed to 21 days only.

Diet

Though there are so many dietetic restriction recommended in the texts, patients were advised to wear clean cotton dress and to use medicated soap.

Prakriti

9 patients out of 15 are of Pitta-Kapha prakriti which supports the doshic involvement as per the classics.

Site of Lesion

More prominent on legs in 11 patients (73.32 per cent) and on hands in 8 patients (53.44 per cent).

Duration of Illness

Less than 1 year in 7 patients (60 per cent) and 1-6 years in 6 patients (40 per cent).

Symptomatic relief was prominent in Kandu, Srava, Pidika, Vedana, Paka, Daha, Tvak Vidaran and Tvak sotha. The symptomatic relief in Kandu is 86.66 per cent, in Pidika 46.66 per cent, in Srava 100 per cent, Vedana 77.71 per cent, Paka 50 per cent, in Daha, Tvak vidarana and Tvak sodha 100 per cent. The relief obtained is significant at the level of 2 per cent probability, statistically.

Table 1.6: *Results of Treatment in 15 Patients of Vicarcika.*

Result	*No. of Pts.*	*Percentage*
1. Cured	7	46.66
2. Marked improvement	6	40.00
3. Improvement (Mild)	2	13.33
4. No improvement	0	00.00

The commencement of relief was noticed in the second and third week in most number of patients. No side effects or poisonous effects had been found during this period and follow up for a period of six months after the clinical study was undertaken. Only 2 patients have complained the relapse of clinical features after 10 days and 42 days respectively after the completion of the treatment.

Toxicity of Rasakarpura

Regarding the toxic effects of Rasakarpura the authors of Rasasastra have not mentioned much; but while we go through proper way, it causes Kustha, Sandhivata and it increases Kapha dosha. Management of toxic effects of Parada and Rasakarpura:

1. Rasakarpura should be discontinued and the symptomatic treatment should be followed.

2. Drinking Mahisha Mala Jala (Buffalo dung water).
3. Sarkara (sugar) mixed with the Dhanyaka jala (Coriandrum sativum).
4. Oral administration of Dugdha (milk) and Taila (oil) extracted from the Varti prepared by Suddha Gandhaka (purified sulphur) and Ghrita (ghee).
5. Gargling with the kwath (decoction) of Babbula (Acacia arabica) or Badara (Zizypus jujuba) Twak alongwith Kanksi (alum) and Tuttha (copper sulphate).
6. Oral administration of Kusumanda rasa (Aloevera), Kadali svarasa (extraction of banana plant).

Vyas P.P., Mistry I.U., Desai K.R.: *A Clinical Study on the Role of Vaman and Virechan in the Management of Ksudra Kustha, Ayu. Samac.* 15:1:1992.

Skin diseases are narrated in Ayurveda Samhitas under the heading of Kustha. These skin disorders manifest in variety of forms and innumerable types of presentation are observed. They can be identified and be named according to involvement of Dosha, Dushya Sthan etc. on Auyrvedic lines.

In Ayurveda, all types of Kustha are considered as Tridoshaja. They have been included in Rakta Pradoshaja and Raktaja disorders. There is no clear-cut demarcation for the Ksudra and Mahakustha in classical texts. But when the pathogenesis of Kustha manifests in milder form due to less involvement of Samprapti Ghatakas, then these skin diseases are observed under Ksudra Kustha and if greater involvement of Samprapti Ghatakas is there, then it calls as Mahakustha—as stated by Chakrapani.

Panchakarma Chikitsa a well reputed speciality of Ayurveda is known not only for uprooting the disease, but provides immunity against diseases also. Thus it has both therapeutic as well as prophylactic value. It is specially recommended in classics for Bahudosha vyadhi like Kustha.

Out of five therapeutic measures used, Shodhan Basti is contraindicated in kustha. Nasya is advised for Urdhwa Jatrugata

Kustha and Kilas. Sushruta mentions Udhyato shodhan i.e. vaman and virechan even in purvarupa stage of kustha. Charak empasises on vaman, virechan and Rakta Mokshan in Kustha according to doshic vitiation. Vaman is the best for kapha dusti. Virechan is indicated not only for pitta, but also in Rakta dusti. Snehan is indicated for Vataja Kustha; so these measures were selected for the present study.

Method and Materials

Irrespective of age, sex and religion, 14 patients were selected at random under study from Indoor Hospital of IPGT&R, Jamnagar.

Diagnosis was made principally on the basis of clinical feature of disease and specially observed the doshik stage of the disease. Detailed and routine investigations were done for assessment. Male and female ratio was 6:8 respectively. Occupation—Study (8), Service (3), Housewife (2), and Retired (1). Age Group—10-20 years (3), 20-30 years (4), 30-40 years (4), 50-60 years (20), and 60-70 years (1) case. Duration of illness—1-6 months (4), 6-12 months (4), 12-24 months (1), and more than 24 months (5) cases.

In this study, two groups were made. First group Shodhan was performed by vamana and virechan having 6 patients. In second group directly virechan was given to the patients for shodhan having 8 patients; prior to shodhan, snehan and swedan were conducted as purva karma.

For snehan, Panchatikta Ghrita was used in increasing dose from 30 gm to 210 gm in seven days. Ghrita was given in the morning with warm water orally. After completion of snehan, Mridu Abhyanga and virechan was carried out for sufficient period.

After samyak snehan and swedana, sanshodhan was administered. On the prior evening of the vamana day, kaphotklesh diet was given to patients.

For shodhana therapy vamana was administered. To induce vamana, Madanaphaladi yoga was used. It contains Madanaphal, pippli powder 10 gm, vacha 5 gm, Saindhava 3 gm. It was well mixed with honey and given with decoction of Yastimadhu.

For virechan karma, Aragvadhadi kwath with castor oil was used. It contains Aragvadha 15 gm, Draksha 15 gm, and Haritaki 15 gm. Decoction of these drugs was prepared and in the decoction 30 ml castor oil and 4 gm of Katuki powder was mixed before administration.

Sansarjana karma was done by Peya, Vilepi, Akrit, and Krit Yusha. This diet had given 3 times to patients.

Criteria of assessment was based on clinical signs and symptoms. Results were tabulated.

Table 1.7: *Scored and Percentage Relief in Symptoms of 6 Patients of Ksudra Kustha Treated with Ubhayto Shodhana*

Symptoms	*Symptom Score*		*Percentage Relief*
	B.T.	*A.T.*	
Shveta varna	8	0	100%
Rakta varna	4	0	100%
Kanduta	12	2	83.33%
Pidaka	6	1	83.33%
Utsedha	6	0	100%
Srava	8	0	100%
Shitya	6	0	100%
Sneha	6	0	100%
Paka	2	0	100%
Raktasrava	2	0	100%
Putigandha	6	0	100%
Daha	2	0	100%

Table 1.8: *Percentage Relief in Each Symptom Scored of 8 Patients of Ksudra Kustha Treated with Virechana*

Symptoms	*Symptoms Scored*		*Percentage Relief*
	B.T.	*A.T.*	
Daha	16	0	100%
Rakta varna	14	2	85.71%
Syava varna	4	0	100%
Aruna varna	8	1	87.5%
Kandu	6	0	100%
Pidika	14	2	85.71%
Shula	4	0	100%
Srava	8	0	100%
Paka	12	0	100%
Putigandha	8	0	100%
Vibhanda	10	0	100%

Table 1.9: *Total Effect of Therapy on 14 Patients of Kushdra Kushta*

Result	*Group I*		*Group II*	
	No. of Pts.	*%*	*No. of Pts.*	*%*
Cured	4	66.66%	6	75%
Marked improvement	2	33.34%	2	25%

Conclusion

On the basis of these observations, it can be concluded that shodhana has a beneficial effect in patients of Kshudra Kustha. A classification which was based on dominance of dosha was useful for the treatment and it was provided significant relief to the patients.

INFECTIOUS DISEASES (SKIN)

Clinical Reports

Preliminary In Vitro Study on Asvatha and Udumbara in Certain Skin Pathogenic Microorganisms: T.M. Unnikrishnan and J.M. Sharma, *Ayurved Samachar:* 13:12:1991.

Asvatha (Ficus religiosa) and Udumbara (Ficus glomerata) are the two widely used Ayurvedic drugs in the external management of skin diseases. It is reported in the wealth of India that an aqueous extract of the bark of Asvatha shows antibacterial activity against staphylococcus aureus and E.Coli. In the present study using standard microbiological techniques of growth of bacteria and their culture and antibiotic sensitivity tests (using Gentamycin and Nystatin for control sensitivity), in the in vitro study of the bark of these two drugs, it is found that they haven't got any action against common skin pathogenic bacteria and fungus i.e. Staphylococcus pyogenes, Streptococcus pyogenes, Pseudomonas pyocyanea (concentration of drug used 16 mg/ml, 30 mg/ml, 40 mg/ml) and Fungus: Candida albicans (Concentration 20 mg/ml, 40 mg/ml, 80 mg/ml). All have shown resistance except the two control antibiotics, Gentamycin and Nystatin.

Therapeutic Effect of Coconut Shell Extract in Dermatophytosis: P.K.S. Nair, N.G.K. Pillai, P.B. Kurup, and C.P.R. Nair: *JRAS*: VIII: 1-2:1987.

The effect of alcoholic extract of coconut shell, 2 per cent ointment with petroleum jelly as an external medication on 31 cases of Dermatophytosis is observed in this study. The decrease of symptoms, itching, burning sensation, erythema, vesicles, oozing and hyperpigmentation are observed in second week, fourth week, and sixth week and compared with the initial stage, the drug showed significant antifungal activity.

Coconut shell is very cheap and easily available in Kerala. The oily liquid obtained from the coconut shell on pyrolysis at temperature 160-240° was found to be highly active against six types of fungal organisms viz. Aspergillus niger, Penicillium chrysogenum, Candida albicans, Trycophyton mentagrophytes, Rhizoctonia solani and R. bataticola (Anonymous, 1976).

Coconut shells on analysis gave moisture 8.0, ash 6.0, solvent extractives 4.2, lilignin 29.4, pentosans 27.7, uronic anhydrides 3.5; cellulose 26.6; methoxyl content 5.6, and nitrogen 0.11 per cent. The pentosans of the shells are largely xylosans and good yields of xylose can be obtained by hydrolysis with 4 per cent sulphuric acid. The oily exudation from the shells obtained by heating is used as an application for wounds. Destructive distillation of shells obtained charcoal 35 per cent, pyroligeneous acid 38.2 per cent, settled tar 5.6 per cent and gas. The tar obtained by distillation upto 280 contains 25 per cent pitch. Phenols constitute over 30 per cent of the total settled tar, and of this a large proportion is ordinary phenol. In this study alcoholic extract of coconut shell (2 per cent ointment with petroleum jelly on external application) was taken up to evaluate the effect on dermatophytosis.

31 cases of Tinea cruris and Tinea corporis belonging to either sex and various age groups were selected. The following features were taken into consideration: Kandu (Itching), Vaivarnya (Hyperpigmentation), Ulsheda (Raised patch), Mandalakrithy (Circular shape), Pidakas (Pustules/Vesicles). Clinical and microbiological assessment was also done.

The drug was given to the patients in the form of ointment and they were advised to apply it over the lesions three times daily, after washing with tepid water, and leave it, therefore, atleast three hours each time. Patients were advised not to use any soap or any other antiseptic for washing and also advised to take necessary precautions to avoid any chance of reinfection.

Observations and Results

Out of the 31 patients selected for study 14 were males and 17 were females and their mean age was 24.8 years. Among the selected cases 13 had tinea corporis and 4 had tinea cruris. Both the complaints were present in the remaining 14 cases. Majority of cases (n=19) did not have any treatment before. Of the remaining 17 cases, 5 cases were tried with modern treatment and 7 with Ayurvedic drugs. The duration of the disease ranged from one week to 2 months. Both literate and illiterate had the disease. Most of the patients (n=28) had annular lesions, while 3 cases showed polycyclic lesions. The degree of inflammation of the lesions was assessed as minimal, significant, highly inflammatory and granulomatous. The cases taken up for study come under the group of minimal (16 cases) and significant (15 cases).

Even though 31 patients were entered in this study, 4 patients were forced to discontinue the treatment due to the flare-up of lesions during the second week. All other patients completed the period of study (6 weeks). In terms of scoring of symptoms, there was significant decrease in itching, burning sensation, erythema, vesicles, oozing and hyperpigmentation. The response to each symptoms (in second, fourth and sixth week) is compared with that of the initial stage. In the cases that responded 11 cases showed no fungal mycelium on microscopic examination in the first week of treatment. In 14 cases smear became negative in the second week and in 2 cases in the fourth week. All the cases that showed response to treatment were followed up for a period of 3 months. Only 4 cases had relapse of the complaints during this period.

Conclusion

The evaluation of anti-fungal activity of coconut shell extract is undertaken in this study. It shows significant anti-fungal activity in the patients undergone the treatment. Out of the 31 cases of dermatophytosis taken up for study, 23 cases got complete cure without relapse of the complaints. In 4 cases that did not respond developed flare-up of symptoms during the second week of treatment. All other patients tolerated the external application, without any side effects. Detailed studies with various extracts of coconut shell in comparison with standard drugs are being undertaken.

Effect of Resottamadilepa, a Herbomineral Formulation in the treatment of Dermatophytosis: P.K.S. Nair, S.S. Nair, K.C.B. Amma, D.R.N. Nair, N.G.K. Pillai, B.K.R. Pillai, P.B. Kurup, and C.P.R. Nair: *JRAS*: X:1-2:1989.

Twenty-three cases of dermatophytosis belonging to both the sexes and various age groups were treated with a herbomineral preparation Resottamadilepa. The drug was applied externally over the lesions. 11 cases got complete relief, 7 cases showed marked improvement, 2 cases did not respond. 3 cases discontinued the treatment.

The Ayurvedic line of treatment mainly depends upon the dosha-dusyadusti in the disease (Charaka Samhita). The lakshanas of each dosha predominant condition in Kustha-roga are mentioned (Charaka Samhita). The dermatophytosis appears to be vata-kapha predominant condition with tvak and lasika as dushyas.

A herbomineral preparation named Resottamadilepa is extensively used in kaphadika diseases of skin in Kerala. Its origin can be traced to an unpublished manuscript in a family of traditional physicians. One of whom was the Principal of the Government Ayurvedic College, Trivandrum and who introduced this Yoga in the Government Pharmacopoeia (Anonymous, 1962). It contains 8 ingredients:

1. Paradam (Mercury);
2. Gandhaka (Sulphur);
3. Manasila (Arsenic rubrum);
4. Girisindura (Red oxide of mercury);
5. Bakuchi (Psoralia corylifolia);
6. Marica (Piper nigrum);
7. Haridra (Curcuma longa);
8. Daruharidra (Berberis aristata).

The ingredients are taken in equal parts and powdered. It is sprinkled on to a hot mixture of melted wax and coconut oil. The ratio of the powder, wax and coconut oil is 1:10:40. All the ingredients have ushna veerya, kaphavataharatva and kriminasakatva properties.

After the clinical and microscopical examination, all the patients were given Resottamadilepa for external application over the lesions at least for three hours every time. No dietary restrictions were imposed. Patients were advised not to use any soap or antiseptic for washing, to change the clothes which were in contact with the lesion, and to wash it with hot water before the next use.

Criteria for Assessment

The clinical criteria for assessing the response was based on subjective symptoms like itching sensation (Kandu), burning (daha), and objective observations like erythema (raga), vesicles (acca pidika), oozing (laseka srava), hyperpigmentation (syava varna) etc. Assessment of the effect of the drug was done once in every 7 days for individual symptoms. Microscopical examination of smear (Potassium Hydroxide) from dermal lesions was also conducted every week.

Results and Discussion

There were 14 males and 9 females among the 23 cases studied. The majority of them in the age group of 16-30. It was observed that 5 patients had tinea cruris and 11 cases had tinea corporis while the remaining 7 patients had both types of lesions. The duration of the disease varied from one month to one year.

Even though 23 cases were taken for study, only 20 cases completed the full course of treatment. Out of these 20 cases, 11 got complete cure, 2 did not respond, and the remaining 7 cases showed marked improvement of their symptoms. On microscopical examination (using KOH), 11 cases showed no fungal mycelium during the third week. However, 2 cases showed positive formycelia even after fourth week. All the treated cases were followed up for a period of one month.

Conclusion

The compound drug Resottamadilepa, has a significant antifungal effect. Out of 20 cases treated, 2 cases did not show any response. Out of the treated cases, 55 per cent of them completely recovered within the specific period, the remaining cases showed 55 per cent to 100 per cent relief for individual symptoms. All the patients tolerated the external application and no side effects were noted.

Action of Patolakaturohinyadi Kvatham and Gopatmajadi Keram on Skin Diseases: A Clinical Trial (A. Geetha, K.G.S. Pillai, P.B. Kurup, C.P.R. Nair: *JRAS*: 1-2:1980).—Short Research Communication.

Patolakaturohinyadi Kvatham is a well-known yoga described in the Sodhanadiganasamgrahadhyaya of Astangahridayam (Sutra Sthanam). The phalasruthy in the stanza shows its importance in the treatment of skin diseases and Kaphapittadhika rogas. Tiktarasa is a common property of the six drugs mentioned in the stanza (i.e. Patolam—Trichosanthes cucumerina, Kadurohini—Picrorrhiza kurroa, Chandanam-Santalum album, Madhusravam—Chonemorpha macrophylla, Guduci—Tinospora cordifolia, Pata—Cyclea peltata). It is having the property of kaphaharatvam. Moreover, Patola is a common ingredient in most of the yogas enlisted by Charaka, Sushruta, and Vagbhata, for the treatment of Kustha and Visarpa. Patolakaturohinyadi kvatham was given internally to 30 selected cases of kaphadhika, vatakaphadhika, and kaphapittadhika rogas.

The external application used was Gopatmajadi keram under this trial (Sahasrayoga). This is a popular yoga of Kerala mentioned in Sahasrayoga. Even though there are so many other yogas which can be used as external application in diseases of skin, this particular yoga was selected since the ingredients of Gopatmajadi keram (i.e. Durva—Cynodon dactylon, Sariba—Hemidesmus indicus, Chandanam—Santalum album, Usiram—Vetiveria zizaniodes, Madhuyasti—

Glycyrrhiza glabra, Asvattha—Ficus religiosa, Nyagrodham—Ficus bengalensis, Udumbaram—Ficus glomerata, Plaksam-Ficus retusa, Bisam—Nelumbo nucifera (stalk), Ulpalam—Minochoria hastaefolia) have the common properties of Sitavirya, Tiktarasa, Kaphapittasamanatvam and Vranaropanatvam which match with those of the ingredients of the internal medicine—Patolakaturohini kvatham.

The study was aimed to watch the effectiveness in diseases of skin and to compare the results with those of the single drug treatments carried out by the authors.

2 oz. of Patolakaturohinyadi kvatham was given thrice daily internally to 30 patients. Though not very palatable, the decoction had a mild laxative effect in the majority of patients and it increased the appetite. 5 patients had regular loose motions. Initial nausea in 3 was not found after the third day of therapy. 8 cases with severe pyoderma received wet dressing with Thespesia populanea decoction before starting the external application of Gopatmajadi keram. Table 1-10 shows the types of cases treated, their numbers and average number of days taken for ropana—control of exudation and formation of crusts, subsidence of bahyalakshanas—morphological cure and relief of kandu—pruritus.

Criteria for ropana are: 1. Drying of pakvapidikas—pustules, 2. Control of lasikasravam and pooya sravam—exudation, 3. Ragam—erythema, 4. Tapam—burning sensation, 5. Sotham—oedema, 6. Ruk—pain, and 7. Formation of cipitika—crusts.

The response to the treatment was much faster in these cases, compared to cases treated with preparation of Aragwada—Cassia fistula and Nimba—Azadirachta indica. The difference was very well marked in Pithadika cases. 10 cases of Pundarikam (Allergic eczematous dermatitis 8 cases and Bacterial eczema 2 cases) were cured in two weeks time. This result was not achieved with either Aragvadha or Nimba. The response was not so good in the cases of Pama-infected scabies and Dadru—Psoriasis. Kidibham—non-exudating allergic eczema also responded better than the single drug treatment.

Table 1.10: *Shows the Clinical and Treatment Aspects of the Diseases Treated*

Disease	*No. of Cases Treated*	*Modern Medical Diagnosis*	*Average No. of Days Taken for Ropana*	*Average No. of Days Taken for Subsidence of Bahya-lakshanas*	*Average No. of Days Taken for Relief of Kandu*
Kidibham (Vatakaphaja)	7	Endogenous and atopic eczema	5	8	11
Vicarica (Kaphaja)	4	Chronic follicular eczema, Dariers disease subcorneal pustular dermatoses of Sneddon and Wilkinsons and sycosis barbae	9	13	15
Pundarikam (Kaphapittaja)	10	Bacterial eczema, stasis, dermatitis, nummular eczema, contact dermatitis, dermatitis medicamentosa.	8	13	15

Pama (Kaphapitaja)	1	Infected scabies	13	22	32
Dadru (Kaphapitaja)	2	Discoid psoriasis, pustular psoriasis and Lichen planus	20	32	34
Sidhmam (Vatakaphaja)	3	Seborrhoeic dermatitis	8	19	23
Gajacarma (Vatakaphaja)	3	Disseminated neurodermatitis circumscripta and Dermatomycosis	7	13	14

FILARIASIS (SLEEPADA)

Essential Features

1. Recurrent attacks of appearance at irregular intervals of lymphangitis, lymphadenitis, fever, orchitis.
2. Hydrocele, chyluria, elephantiasis of legs, arms, genitalia, or breasts.
3. Characteristic microfilariae in the blood.
4. Eosinophilia; positive skin or complement fixation tests.
5. Filariasis is caused by infection with one or two filarial nematodes, Wucheraria bancrofti and Brugia malayi.
6. *Differential Diagnosis:* Diagnosis of the early febrile and inflammatory episodes may be difficult, particularly when the patient has moved from an endemic area, because clinical features are transitory and microfilariae may be rare in the blood. Filarial funiculitis, orchitis, and epididymitis may suggest gonococcal infection, but there is no urethral discharge in the uncomplicated case. Among the late manifestations, elephantiasis may be confused with hernia, Milroy's disease, multiple lipomatosis, severe congestive heart failure, venous thrombosis, and obstructive lesions of the lymphatics, which may produce nonfilarial elephantiasis of the extremities. The last three named diseases can be distinguished readily from filariasis. Multiple lipomas may produce a massive soft lumpy swelling of the proximal part of a limb. In contrast, the filarial lesion starts distally and becomes hard as it enlarges. Milroy's congenital elephantiasis usually involves both legs below the knees. The skin is smooth, there is esnophilia, and the patient often has never visited the tropics.
7. *Prognosis:* In early and mild cases, the prognosis is good with treatment and if the patient avoids reinfection. Drug treatment will not significantly influence the course of advanced filariasis.

Ayurvedic Concept

A disease entity known as Sleepada described in Ayurveda more or less resembles filariasis. Sushruta has firstly enumerated environmental conditions like water stagnated areas (varidosha), cold weather in whole year wherein the incidence of this disease is more high. The term 'Sleepada' is used since the swelling is hard as stone. The concept of disease is modified at each stage of the development of pathology in keeping with the level of knowledge. Ayurvedic concept of holding the host as responsible in the pathogenesis of diseases including infectious diseases is quite logical. (Sushruta Samhita-Sutrasthana).

As per the current concept of maintenance of homeostasis (internal and external) of the body, the ancients too, as in the case of other diseases, recognised only the doshas—vata, pitta and kapha (structural and functional factors) of the body in the causation of this disease. Particularly, kapha is the main dosha causing the disease, as gurutwa and mahatwa (heaviness and enlargement) are qualities of kapha (Madhavakara: Madhava Nidana). They have recognised this endemic disease, a disease commonly occurring in anupadesha.

Sushruta describes six kriyakalas in the evolution of disease. (Sushruta Samhita-Sutrasthana). The deranged doshas, checked and subdued in the samchaya stage (stage of accumulation of dosha) fail to exhibit any further development, but if left untreated, they gain strength and intensity in the course of their further development. If the samchaya stage is the microfilarial, the sthana samsraya to bheda stages are represented by elephantiasis or sleepada.

The objective of Ayurveda is not only the cure of disease but also prevention of the same before its actual onset (Charaka Samhita-Sutra Sthana). Though improvement in environmental sanitation will prevent the incidence of this disease to some extent, still, the treatment of the disease in (microfilaria) samchaya stage with suitable Ayurvedic medicines should have anti-microfilarial effect.

Prevention of microfilaria with Ayurvedic drugs can be planned as per Ayurvedic principles on doshic lines. Since sleepada is a kapha (Madhavakara) dominant disease prevalent in anupadesha, microfilaria, which is nothing but its sanchaya phase can be treated with kaphahara drugs with advantage. Ayurveda prescribes Sudarshana choornam not only as an effective anti-pyretic drug in conditions caused by Varidosha (water pollution) particularly in endemic area. The other drugs which can be used with advantage are: Kiratatiktaka (Swertia chirata) is well-known for its antipyretic property, which form 50 per cent of Sudarshan churna known as antipyretic compound. Saptachada (Alstoniascholaris) described as digestive and good in healing of ulcers is used as one of the ingredients in a number of kashayas prescribed in fever. Katuki (Picrorrhiza-kurroa) is described as having digestive, antipyretic and anthelmintic effect with particular place in Arogyavardhini vati (Bhavamishra: Bhavaprakash Nighantu-Guduchyadi Varga-Hareetakyaivivara), a well-known compound used in hepatic and splenic disorders, containing Katuki amounting to 50 per cent. Lathakaranja (Vaghbhata: Rasaratna Sauchya-Kushtadhikara) or Kuberakshibeeja (Caesalpinia bonducella) is described as an anthelmintic. However, in tradition it is used in filaria and malaria as antipyretic. All the above four are of mainly katu and tikta rasa, used singly or in combination in fevers, particularly vishama jwara, exhibiting periodicity of rise in temperature and rigor. They are more kaphahara than Sudharshan Churna. This is one of the reasons for the better action of Ayush-64-CCRAS when compared to Sudarshana churna.

As said earlier, the prognosis of this disease is unfavourable if elephantiasis sets in. The Ayurvedic literature also indicates that the disease of more than one year standing and those with large swelling are incurable (Madhava). Nothing is said to be helpful in this stage of the disease.

Clinical Reports

Therapeutic Assessment of Shakhotaka Ghana Vati on Sleepada (Filariasis)—P.N. Pandey and U.K. Das) *JRAS*:XI:1-2:1990.

The incidence of Sleepada-Filariasis is high in the coastal areas. As such large number of patients of Sleepada are seen in the Puri Town. The study has been conducted during the period from January 1985 to March 1986, 40 patients of either sex were selected for the present study. An effort has been made to study the effect of Sakhotakaghana vati in 25 patients and Diethyl carbamazine in 15 patients. Sakhotakaghana vati has been found to be effective in the manifested disease as well as on microfilaria.

Efforts to study its role in the treatment of filariasis (Sleepada) have been taken up earlier (Singhal 1963) and has been referred to as the drug of choice for Sleepada in the Ayurveda text as well (Sarangadhara).

The patients have been studied in two groups:

Trial Group A: Sakhotaka ghana vati—Powder 500 mg in capsular form thrice daily with water for three months. (Total No. 25 patients).

Trial Group B: (15 patients) Diethyl carbamazine tab 100 mg thrice daily with water for three weeks.

The patients were advised to take their routine diet but to avoid late night meals, excess rice, jaggery and constipative foods and also to avoid excess walking, cycling, standing duties etc. The assessment of the result was made on the basis of the clinical improvement and laboratory investigations.

The disease has been more prevalent in the persons accustomed to Kaphaja Ahar (75 per cent), Vataja Ahar (17.5 per cent) and Pittaja Ahar (7.5 per cent) and in the non-vegetarians (80 per cent) followed by vegetarian (20 per cent). However, extremities of either side were mostly affected (57 per cent) than the upper extremities. Swelling was present in all the cases, regional lymphadenopathy, pain, burning sensation over the affected part was frequently observed.

Microfilaria was positive in 8 cases (6 in group A and 2 in group B) which became negative after the treatment in both groups.The eosionophil count was raised in almost all the cases ranging from 5-25 per cent with a mean value of 9.04 per cent before treatment in Group A which came down to mean value of 3.8 per cent after treatment with a difference mean value of 5.32 per cent; similarly in Group B the mean value of eosinophil count was 11.13 per cent which came down to 3.33 per cent with a difference mean value of 7.8 per cent. Hookworm was positive in 8 cases, Round worm in 15 cases and E. histolytica cyst in 3 cases. An appreciable (84 per cent) reduction in swelling in Gr A and 50 per cent in Gr B has been observed. Complete relief (100 per cent) achieved in the constipation, 80 per cent relief in pain, 30 per cent in lymphadenopathy with trial drug whereas 60per cent relief in swelling and pain, 80 per cent in tenderness and 63 per cent in lymphadenopathy with the control drug was seen.

The overall results of the treatment as classified according to criteria mentioned earlier showed marked improvement in 6 (24 per cent) fair improvement in 15 (60 per cent) in Gr A; whereas it was 3 (20 per cent) and 6 (40 per cent) respectively in Gr B.

Discussions

The incidence is more frequent in the persons accustomed to kaphaja ahara (75 per cent) and in the non-vegetarian 32 (80 per cent). The reason behind this may be due to the fact that Puri town and surroundings fall under Anupadesa and the non-vegetarians taking fish (Udaka Mansh) and the diet predominantly for kapha vruddhi may be the important factor for the disease. It is evident that the cardinal features like swelling, fever, pain, tenderness, and lymphadenopathy responded better to the trial drug than the control. The trial drug also relieved constipation in almost all the cases. The possible mechanism of action of the drug may be attributed to its Katutikta ras, antipyretic, antiinflammatory and antifilarial activities (Sarangadhar). Both the trial and control drug reduced the eosinophil count but it was more rapid with the control drug than the trial. Shakotaka vati has also been effective on microfilaria as the microfilaria in all the six positive cases became negative after the treatment. Hence Shakhotaka (Streblus asper Lour) an easily available nontoxic single herbal drug can be safely employed for microfilaria as well as on manifested disease in the rural health programme.

Prevention of Sleepada (Elephantiasis) with Ayurvedic Compounds—S. Venkataraghavan, N. Gowri, R. Sitaraman, K. Srinivasan, K. Janaki—*JRAS*:1:1:1980.

Two Ayurvedic compounds Kiratadi and Sudarshana choorna were studied using modern standard drug, Diethylcarbamazine as control in 61 cases having microfilaria in the blood for their effect in prevention of sleepada.

The description of sleepada described in the classical Ayurvedic literature compares well with the description in modern medicine. The term sleepada is used since the swelling is hard as stone. Particularly kapha is the main dosha causing the disease, as gurutwa and mahatwa (heaviness and enlargement) are qualities of kapha (Madhavakara-Madhavanidanam). They have recognised this endemic disease, a disease commonly occurring in anupadesa.

If the samchaya (stage of accumulation of dosha) stage is the microfilaria, the sthana samaraya to bheda stages are represented by the elephantiasis or sleepada. Though improvement in environmental sanitation will prevent the incidence of this disease to some extent, still, the treatment of the disease (microfilaria) in samchaya stage with suitable Ayurvedic medicines would have anti-microfilarial effect.

Prevention of micro-filaria with Ayurvedic drugs can be planned as per Ayurvedic principles on doshic lines. Since sleepada is a kapha dominant disease prevalent in anupadesa microfilaria which is nothing but it is samchaya phase can be treated with kaphahara drugs with advantage.

Ayurveda prescribes Sudarshana choornam not only as an effective anti-pyretic drug, but also as an effective drug in conditions caused by Varidosha (water pollution) particularly in endemic area. Since Kiratatikta forms 50 per cent of Sudarshan choorna, a compound (Ayush-64) with Kiratatikta, Saptachada, Katuka, and Latakaranja is also considered to be effective in the prevention of this disease where it is endemic. Modern medicine prescribes Diethyl carbamazine for 12 days in the treatment of microfilaria.

In the study, Diethylcarbamazine (Hetrazan), Sudarshana choorna, prepared as per Sarangadhar Samhita was used. Kiratadi compound (Ayush-64) containing the ghanasatva (dried aqueous extract prepared by using standard Ayurvedic procedure) of Kirata (Swertia chirata), Saptachada (Alstonia schoiaris) and Katuka (Picrorrhiza kurroa) and powders of Kubherakshibeeja (Caesalpinia bonducella) was prepared and used.

Diethylcarbamazine (50 mg drug + 450 mg starch), Kiratadi compound (125 mg + 375 mg starch), Sudarshana choorna (500 mg drug) were encapsulated and administered to patients in a dose of two capsules thrice daily for 12 days. Follow-up night blood smears of the patients were taken on the 15th and 60th day after the completion of the treatment period, at about the same time of taking the initial blood smear. The cases who could not be contacted in their given addresses for takIng the confirmatory blood smear were excluded from the final analysis. Thus, total of 61 cases, 15 in Kiratadi (Ayush-64) group, 22 in Sudarshana choorna group, and 24 in Diethylcarbamazine group of treatment were considered as active participants in the present trial. Complete absence of microfilaria (Microfilaria bancrofti) in the confirmatory night blood smear was fixed as the criterion of response for the assessment of the drug effect. The results were statistically analysed. In the study, side effects like joint pain and fever, were noted in 4 cases in Diethylcarbamazine group and abdominal pain was noted in one patient who received Kiratadi compound treatment and no side effects were noted in Sudarshana choorna treatment group.

Discussion

From the results, it is seen that the effects of Kiratadi and Diethylcarbamazine at the end of 15 days are not alike but at the end of 60 days showed results identical to that of Kiratadi and at the end of 60 days results equivalent to the effect of Diethylcarbamazine than at 15 days. This may be due to the probability of the drug causing the desired action at a later stage. When Sudarshana is compared with Kiratadi, it is found that the effects of the two treatments are alike. However, when the response, based on the complete disappearance of microfilaria is considered, the percentage of response in Sudarshana group is bound to decrease at the end of 60 days follow-up when compared with the 15 days follow-up. This may be due to the inadequate dosage of Sudarshana choorna. Since this is the first controlled study with these drugs, the dose was fixed arbitrarily on the basis of experience of use. Kiratatikta (Swertia chirata) is well known for its antipyretic property, which forms 50 per cent of Sudarshana choorna, known antipyretic compound. Saptachada (Alstonia scholaris) described as digestive and good in healing of ulcers is used as one of the ingradients in a number of kashayas prescribed in fever. Katuki (Picrorrhiza kurroa) is described as having digestive, antipyretic and anthelmintic effect with particular place in Arogyavardhini vati (Bhavamishra-Bhavaprakasha Nighantu), a well-known compound used in hepatic and splenic disorders, contains Katuki amounting to 50 per cent. Lathakaranja or Kubeerakshibeeja (Caesalpinia bonducella) is described as anthelmintic (Vagbhata—Rasaratna Samuchhya-Kushtadhi-kara). However, in tradition, it is used in filaria and malaria as antipyretic. All the above four are of mainly katu and tikta rasa, used singly or in combination in fevers particularly Vishama jwara, exhibiting periodicity of rise in temperature and rigour. They are more Kapha hara than Sudarshana choorna. This is one of the reasons for the better action of Kiratadi when compared to Sudarshana choorna.

Since the tolerance of the patients of present dose with exhibition of no side effect, is known, the efficacy of the two Ayurvedic compounds can be improved with higher dose in further studies. Once this is achieved the Ayurvedic formulations will prove useful in microfilarial infection as also as an antipyretic agent, which will be effective not only in subclinical but in clinical phase also.

Table 1.11: *Response Distribution Among Three Different Groups*

	Ayush-64	*Diethyl-carbamazine*	*Sudarshana choornam*
I Follow-pup (15 Days)			
Responded	60.6% (9)	95.9% (25)	81.8% (18)
Not Responded	39.4% (6)	4.1% (1)	18.2% (4)
II Follow up (60 Days)			
Responded	73.3% (11)	95.9% (23)	68.2% (15)
Not Responded	26.7% (4)	4.1% (1)	31.8% (7)

Note: Figures in parentheses represent the number of cases. Response means that there is absence of microfilaria in the blood with the treatment.

Clinical Trial of Ayush-64 in Sleepada (T. Seshagiri Rao, P.V. Rao, K. Kusuma Kumari, B. Netaji, K. Nisteswar, and C.R.R. Sharma: *JRAS*:1-2:1982).

Clinically diagnosed cases of Sleepada were treated with Ayush-64, a known antimalarial drug which was incidentally found to be effective in cases of Microfilariasis. Results of the treatment have been encouraging and point out the need for a planned study in large number of cases.

A disease entity known as Sleepada described in Ayurveda more or less resembles filariasis. Sushruta has firstly enumerated environmental conditions like water stagnated areas, cold weather in whole year wherein the incidence of this disease is more high.

A few clinical studies carried out so far with single as well as compound indigenous drugs have not shown satisfactory results. Recently, research workers pointed out to the beneficial effect of Sudarshana choornam and Ayush-64 in cases of Microfilariasis. Venkataraghavan et al (1980, IRAS). In the present study an attempt has been made to assess the effect of Ayush-64 with Sarshapa lepa in clinically confirmed cases of Sleepada.

Twenty cases of Sleepada belonging to both sexes and of different age groups (10-70 years) have been selected with the following criteria.

1. Chronic painless residual swelling appearing on various parts of the body especially the lower limbs, upper limbs, genitals etc.
2. History of attacks of swelling in Vankshana (groin) generally associated with jwara and then spreading to other parts of the body.
3. Increase in size of swelling during periodical attacks with or without pyrexia.

Treatment consists of both internal and external medication. Ayush-64 was administered internally at the dose of 1.5 gm per day for a period of 100 days along with Sarshapa lepa with gomutra externally. Affected part along with duration of illness of the included mostly of lower limbs and duration of illness of 2 months—10 years.

Assessment of size of the swelling has been made by taking measurements at various points of the affected part as follows: Below knee-middle of calf; below calf-middle of ankle; middle of foot-metatarsals.

These measurements have been assessed initially and finally. Results have been statistically analysed by applying paired 8 X 8 test.

Results and Discussion

The drug Ayush-64 at the dose of 1.5 gm a day for 100 days with Sarshapa lepa has reduced significantly the swelling of the affected limb (less than 0.01). The symptoms like jwara, vankshana shotha which were present in a few cases have disappeared after drug administration. Ayush-64 consisting of katu and tikta rasa drugs might have acted as kaphahara and medohara. Side effects like burning sensation have been complained with Sarshapa lepa where as atisara and chardi of mild form have been observed in a few cases with Ayush-64. Course of treatment was not affected by the above side effects as these are of short duration and disappeared with/without treatment. Microfilaria in blood was absent in all the cases.

It is hoped that by increasing the dosage and cutting down the duration better results may be obtained.

Clinical Evaluation of Certain Herbal Preparations in the Treatment of Chronic Sleepada—Elephantiasis. (Prem Kishore and M.K.Chaturvedi: *JRAS*: VII: 1-2:1986).

An attempt has been made to assess the efficacy of certain Ayurvedic herbal preparations—Sudarshana Choorna/ Sudharshana Ghanavati and Punarnavadyarishta in the treatment of chronic patients of Sleepada which have been considered so far incurable. The observation indicates that the disease may effect individual of any age group irrespective of sex and it usually runs a chronic course, though many patients have been observed with recent history (1-3 years). The effect of the treatment has been quite significant since most of the patients who completed the full course had shown definite effect of the treatment.The effect of Sudarshana Ghana Vati appears to be more pronounced than that of Sudarshana Choorna. The relationship of chronicity and age with the effect of treatment is also significant.

The Ayurvedic literature indicates that the disease of more than one year standing and those with large swelling are incurable (Madhava). Nothing could be helpful in this stage of the disease. So far no trial has been reported specifically for this form of disease. Though the observations on Nityananda Rasa (Mishra et al 1979), Ayush-64 and Maha Sudarshana Choorna (Venkataraghavan et al 1980) have been published on other stages of disease. The studies on few patients of chronic sleepada with the Sudarshana Choorna and Punarnavarishta have shown encouraging response (Kishore et al 1981). As such a trial has been planned on a series of patients to assess the efficacy of this regimen of treatment.

The trial had been conducted on forty patients. Sudarshana Choorna was provided to 21 patients and 19 patients were treated with Sudarshana Ghanavati, while Punarnavadyarishta had been prescribed to all patients. The patients were provided 30 days course to treatment with:

1. Sudarshana Churna, 3 gm, thrice daily with warm water or Sudarshana Ghanavati 2 tabs (Bhaisajya Ratnavali: Jwara Chikitsa)
2. Punarnavadyarishta, 20 ml twice daily after meals with water (Bhaisajya Ratnavali: Soth Chikitsa).

The patients have been provided normal hospital diet consisting of rice, chapati, dal, vegetable, upama and milk.

The disease affected the individuals in all the age groups above the age of 11 years. The disease affects the males relatively more than females. The duration of illness varied from one year to thirty years though majority suffered from one to three years.

The selection of the drug was based on the preliminary experience on a few patients (Kishore et al 1981) and the potential of Sudarshana Choorna in providing relief of jwara and its potent of kaphahara effect and the sothhara potential of Punarnavadyarishta. The criteria for the selection of patients and the methodology for the trial adopted was largely based on clinical objective parameters. Nevertheless, these were also in consonance with Ayurvedic fundamentals. The general characteristics of the patients taken up for trials show that the disease may affect the individual in any age and sex. The involvement of the parts i.e. lower limb in most of the patients is also in conformity of the observation made earlier (Dey and Dey 1970). The absence of microfilaria in most of the patients is also according to the textual description. The complete relief of the disease has been relatively better in the patients who have been given Sudarshana Ghanavati than Sudarshana Choorna. Relatively more efficacy (complete relief) of the treatment in the younger age group of patients and those with short history of the disease i.e. upto 5 years are also quite significant. The effect of the treatment on ESR and microfilaria though not consistent has been significant. The reduction of the swelling was obvious in a few days though substantial reduction would take a week or so. The observation of increase in pain after reduction of swelling may be attributed to sudden decompression of the affected tissue.

It is possible that the reduction in the swelling may be due to the parasiticidal (Pandey et al 1980) and kaphahara (Sharma 1975) effect of Kiratatikta (the main ingredient of the Sudarshana Choorna). The sothhara i.e. anti-inflammatory and also diuretic effect of Punarnavadyarishta would also help in reduction of swelling. The observations, first of this kind i.e. specifically in the chronic cases of Sleepada-Filariasis, definitely provide important conclusive evidences of the efficacy of this approach.

Clinical Assessment of the Effect of Ayush-64 in the Acute Cases of Sleepada-(Filariasis): Prem Kishore and M.K. Chaturvedi (*JRAS*:VII:3-4: 1986).

Attempt was made to evolve the treatment of acute filarial lymphangitis. Ayush-64, the formulation developed primarily for the treatment of Malaria was taken up for trial on the basis of its properties and actions. The preliminary observations on beneficial effect on 20 patients at O.P.D. level (Kishore 1980) and its effect in eliminating microfilaria (Venkataraghavan 1980) were guiding factors for further trials. The cases (total

No. 31) selected for the studies were of less than one year duration which is considered as Sadhya in Ayurveda (Madhava). It was observed that most of the patients suffering from the acute stage of the disease taken up for trial were of 11 to 30 years of age and the males were predominantly affected. About 2/3 of the patients were suffering for less than 3 months. The involvement of lower limbs was more frequent. The cardinal manifestations of the disease i.e. pain and swelling was invariably observed in all patients except those suffering from Chyluria. It was observed that the patients were quickly relieved to a great extent within few days and complete relief could be observed within 2-4 weeks of the treatment. The reduction in measurements of the affected parts was also confirmed these observations. It is interesting to note that the effect was more obvious in the patients in the younger age group i.e. 11 to 30 years of age. It was noted that the drug did not have any effect on microfilaria in the blood of the patients which it was found to be present. It may be conclusively stated that the formulation Ayush-64 is best suited for the treatment of acute attacks of filarial lymphangitis. The possible mechanism of the action of the drug may be attributed to the Visama Jvaraghna and Krimighna properties of the ingredients of this formulation (Sharma 1975). The parasiticidal effect of the Kiratatikta demonstrated experimentally (Pandey et al 1980) may also contribute to its efficacy.

Evaluation of the Effect of Ayurvedic Drug (Internal and External) in the Treatment of Sleepada (Filariasis)—A Pilot Study: T. Seshagiri Rao, C.R.R. Sharma, K.K. Kumari and T. Bikshapati: JRAS:VII: 3-4:1986).

A study of 30 clinically confirmed cases of Sleepada (Filariasis) occurring in one of the lower limbs was conducted with an Ayurvedic drug (internal and external) evolved by the centre. In Ayurvedic texts, Sleepada is classified into three varieties according to symptoms as Vatika, Paittika and Saishmika. In this pilot study, 11 Vatika Sleepada cases and 19 Salishmika Sleepada cases were studied and treated for 40 days in In-patient Department.

A trial drug consisting of vata and sleshmahara drugs in the form of capsules was administered internally 1 gm tds. along with external application (vide caption drug) for a period of 40 days. The results of the treatment was mainly based on the objective assessment of reduction in swelling.

Drug

Internal: Fine powder of drugs given below are mixed and soaked in gomutra and dried. The powdered medicine is filled in capsules.

Vata Sleepada Capsules: 1. Amruta–1 part; 2. Guggulu–1part; 3.Sunti–1 part; 4. Punarnava–1part; 5. Shakotra twak–1 part; 6. Rasna–1 part.

Slaishmika Sleepada Capsules: Amrutha–1 part; 2. Guggulu–1 part; 3. Sunti–1part; 4. Punarnava–1 part; 5. Shakotra twak–1 part; 6. Haritaki–1part.

External: Sarshapa 1 part, Haridra 1 part were mixed together and made paste with water. This paste was applied on the affected part once a day.

Conclusion and Discussion

Out of 30 cases (leaving 3 drop-outs, 2 cases with no relief and one case with aggravation) 24 cases have shown relief in varying degrees. This study suggests that age, sex, and duration of illness have no influence over the disease and results of the treatment. Results are encouraging in spite of the classical statement that Sleepada of more than one year duration is Asadhya (Sushruta). This pilot study has prompted the authors to conduct further study.

Epidemiological Studies and Therapeutic Trials on Sleepada (Filariasis) in the Village Malipada (Puri District of Orissa): M.M. Padhi and Prem Kishore: *JRAS*:IX:3-4: 1988.

An attempt has been made to present the observations on epidemiological studies and the therapeutic trials in different stages of the disease Sleepada—Filariasis in a village located near Bhubaneswar. The disease was found to be highly prevalent in the selected population (28.3 per cent). The microfilaraemia was almost equally prevalent as the manifest disease. The individuals in the age range below 30 years were more frequently affected with microfilaraemia while those of age range above 30 years were mostly affected with chronic dormant stage of the disease. The high incidence may be due to the unhealthy living habits of the people. Peripheral blood smear became negative in 7 out of 23 cases who completed two weeks of treatment with Nityananda Rasa. This was administered to microfilaraemia patients with dose of 2 tabs. (500 mg) thrice daily with water for 2 weeks. Complete relief was observed in 4 patients and partial relief in 10 patients of manifest disease out of 15 patients completing four weeks of treatment with Sudarshana Ghanavati (2 tabs. 700 mg) thrice daily with water for 4 weeks.

The effect of 14 days of course of Nityananda Rasa in microfilaraemia is reasonably good considering the short course of the treatment, since the parasite could be eliminated in about 60 per cent of the cases after 3 months of treatment reported in earlier studies (Mishra et al 1979).

The effect of Sudarshana Ghanavati on the various stages of the manifest disease taken for trial also appears to be consistent with earlier observations. All the cases in acute stage of the disease in which complete course of the treatment was taken were completely relieved. The patients in chronic dormant stage of the disease also invariably relieved to a great extent although complete relief was possible in one patient.

LEPROSY (KUSTHA)

Essential Features

1. Pale, anaesthetic macular or nodular and erythematous-skin lesions.
2. Superficial nerve thickening with associated sensory changes.
3. History of residence in endemic area in childhood.
4. Acid-fast bacilli in skin lesions or nasal scrapings, or characteristic histologic nerve changes.
5. Leprosy is a chronic infectious disease caused by the acid-fast rod Mycobacterium leprae. The mode of transmission is unknown but probably involves prolonged exposure in childhood. Only rarely, have adults become infected (e.g. by tattoing).
6. *Differential Diagnosis*: The skin lesions of leprosy often resembles those of lupus erythematosus, sarcoidosis, syphilis, erythema nodosum, erythema multiforme, and vitiligo. Nerve involvement, sensory dissociation, and resulting deformity may require differentiation from syringomyelia and scleroderma.
7. *Complications*: Intercurrent pulmonary tuberculosis is common in the lepromatous type, probably because of deficient cellular immunity. Amyloidosis may occur with longstanding disease.
8. *Prevention*: At present prevention through vaccines or drugs is not yet possible. Social hygiene is only the best answer.
9. *Prognosis*: Untreated lepromatous leprosy is progressive and fatal in 10-20 years. In the tuberculoid type, spontaneous arrest usually occurs in 1-3 years; it may however, produce crippling deformities. With treatment, the lepromatous type regresses slowly (over a period of 3-8 years). Recovery from the tuberculoid type is more rapid. Recrudescences are always possible; and it may be safe to assume that the bacilli are never eradicated. Deformities

persist after complete recovery and may markedly interfere with function and appearance.

AYURVEDIC TREATMENT

Clinical Reports

S. Chaudhury, S.K. Hajra, B. Saha, V. Mazumder: *New Multidrug Regimen with Indigenous Drugs and Dapsone in Treatment of Lepromatous Leprosy: Ayurved Samachar:* 15:2:1992.

Treatment of leprosy by Multidrug Regimen (MDR) is not the final answer. Need for development of new drug and new drug regimen is an urgent necessity. Present communication is a report of therapeutic assessment of a combination of active principles of two indigenous drugs from Chaulmoogra oil (Hydnocarpus oil) and Centella asiatica and plus Dapsone. Preliminary report indicating that the new drug regimen is comparable to MDR, clinically and bacteriologically and reactional episodes are negligible in comparison to MDR.

Among the many indications, drugs used from the time of Charaka and Sushruta for leprosy, the most important of this was Chaulmoogra oil (Hydnocarpus oil) which was the only medicine for Leprosy from 600 B.C. to 1950. The other being Centella Asiatica till widely used in Sri Lanka and coastal region of India.

Hydnocarpoic acid from Hydnocarpus oil has been recently proved to be bacteriostatic to M. leprae in mice foot pad model. Chaulmoogric acid has also been shown to be incorporated into cell wall lipids of Mycobacteriathan might explain its chemotherapeutic activity. As regards Centella asiatica, known antileprotic, the recently isolated glycoside asiaticoside claimed to dissolve the covering of M. leprae; the bacilli become fragile and be easily be destroyed by tissue and by drugs. It has also been reported that asiaticoside has inhibitory effect on biosynthesis of acid mucopolysaccharide which is one of the important nutrient for Mleprae. Chaudury et al have reported its both clinical and bacteriological importance in lepromatous leprosy cases and have demonstrated that serum mucopolysaccharide level depends on activity and type of the disease, its concentration falls as the disease regresses and when treated with asiaticoside, there is rapid fall in mucosaccharide concentration.

As regards Dapsone it is the most trusted drug till date and a major dependent of all the available multidrug regimens.

Material and Method

Hydnocarpus oil was procured from the source which having the specifications of Indian Pharmacopoea (1966). Hydnocarpic acid was isolated by process of alkaline hydrolysis followed by crystallisation and LD 50 was estimated in mice—it was 325 mg/kg.

Asiaticoside was isolated from the whole plant by alcoholic extract and by counter current principle of extraction with Aquous ethanolis Chloroform and LD 50 of Asiaticoside was estimated in mice and found to be 150 mg/kg.

This was followed by combined acute and chronic toxicity studies in mice by using double the human dose taking standard 50 mg a daily dose for Dapsone i.e. Dapsone 100 mg. Hydnocarpic acid 100 mg and Asiaticoside 100 mg daily. It was found to be absolutely nontoxic to mice.

Subsequently the combined drugs using proposed human dose (Dapsone 50 mg, Hydnocarpic acid 50 mg and Asiaticoside 50 mg) were fed to mice after foot pad innoculation of M. leprae though result has not been completed yet up to date. Information being 3 mice from control group showed plenty of AFB from the foot pad harvest, whereas among six test group mice AFB could not be detected in four; in other two mice there were only few faintly stained AFB detected. Being encouraged it with this observation of toxicity study and preliminary finding of mouse foot pad results, this drug was put on human trial as experimental chemotherapy in 25 highly bacilliform lepromatous leprosy cases.

Up till now 25 active untreated highly bacilliferous lepromatous leprosy cases selected from O.P. Department of

Leprology, School of Tropical Medicine, Calcutta were taken. Their initial clinical, bacteriological, histopathological, immunological findings were recorded in internal case records. Initial liver function test, urine examination, haematological examination done and repeated at intervals. They were given Dapsone 50 mg, Hydnocarpic oil 50 mg, and Asiaticoside 50 mg. in their separate capsules daily.

Similarly 25 active untreated lepromatous cases was taken as control and findings were recorded as in experimental group and they were given Rifampicin 600 mg daily for 14 days. Clofazamine 100 mg daily for 30 days; and Dapsone 100 mg daily for 30 days; then on the first of next month they were given Rifampicin 600 mg and Clofazamine 300 mg and Dapsone 100 mg; later only Clofazamine 100 mg alternate day and Dapsone 100 mg and the course repeated on the first day of the month dose.

Results

In the test group, all the patients accepted the drug very well. Out of 25 patients 7 patients completed 18 months, 3 completed 12 months, rest completed 6 months treatment. Clinical improvement was noteworthy in all the cases. Bacteriologically there was steady fall in BI in all the cases. In one case BI became negative; in another BI fall from 4 to 0.75 and in 3 cases, BI fall from 4 to 1.26; and in the rest 3 cases from 4 to 2. Morphological index became 0 in all the cases. In two cases, there was mild ENL type of reaction and in none there was any neurological complication. Initially histopathology was a typical picture of Leproma and with plenty of AFB. Repeat histopathology after 12 months of therapy showed appreciable reduction in the quantum of granuloma and bacilli. There was no change in the immunological status as regards Lepromin test is concerned. There was no significant alteration of the liver function test and haematological findings. In the control group clinical and bacteriological improvement was at par with test group. Out of 25 cases, in 10 cases there was ENL type of reaction. In 4 cases within 3 months of therapy and in 2 cases, it was very severe along with multiple joint pain and constitutional symptoms. Steroids were given in all the 4 cases in heavy doses and later antileprosy drug except Clofazamine had to be withdrawn in two cases and to prevent deformity, perineural injection of steroid had to be introduced in one case. Out of 25 cases, 18 cases are still on Multidrug regimen (MDR) as per Government of India regimen but none became bacteriologically negative yet.

Lepromin test remained negative as before. Histological picture was comparable with test group, and there was also no change in the liver function test and in the haemogram.

Discussion

This is a preliminary report on a comparative study between a new multidrug regimen and modern multidrug regimen in highly bacilliform cases of Lepromatous leprosy.

Preliminary report showed that the combination of Dapsone, Hydnocarpic acid and Asiaticoside is well tolerated as well as accepted by the patients and complications like ENL reaction and neuritis are uncommon in comparison to MDR. The bacteriological findings are comparable to modern multidrug regimen.

Long term study in large number of cases are essential for drawing any conclusion.

Traditional Treatment of Leprosy and Leucoderma by the Tribals of Bundelkhand in Uttar Pradesh: A.P. Saxena and K.M. Vyas: *JRAS*: II:2:1981.

The Chitrakut-Dham, a sacred place and important in natural vegetation in Bundelkhand region (24° 0'-26° 30'N and 78° 10'-81° 30'E) was surveyed in 1980 with the purpose of collection of folklore records on medicines and treatments of the tribals (Gujars and Lodhs). They treated their ailments with local medicinal plants. Several folklore claims and practices on various diseases were recorded. Interestingly, the treatment of leprosy and leucoderma appeared to be most promising for the successful eradication of these diseases.

Leprosy: The medicine is a powdered mixture of air dried seeds of Psoralia corylifolia Linn. (Sanskrit Bakuchi); roots of Plumbago zeylanica Linn.(Sanskrit Chitrak) and plants of Alectra parasitica A. Rich Var. chitrakutensis Rau (Sanskrit Nirgund). All the three taken in equal amounts are mixed together with the expressed juice of some fresh leaves of Eclipta alba Hassk (local name Ghamra) so as to make it into a paste. This paste is then applied externally on the diseased part of the body of the patient. About three grams of the powdered mixture of air dried seeds of Psoralia corylifolia and plant of Alectra parasitica is recommended for oral administration twice a day along with 50 cc of cow's urine.

Leucoderma: The air dried plants of Alectra parasitica and seeds of Psoralia corylifolia are taken in equal quantity and powdered. The powder is then mixed with a small amount of cow's urine and the paste is applied externally in the form of poultice on the white patches. About three grams of the powdered mixture is given orally twice a day with about 50 cc of cow's urine.

Note: Alectra parasitica is now being collected from nearby localities of Banda and Kalinger areas of Bundelkhand region. Its vegetation is rare in almost all the states. Therefore, its preservation is urgently called for by the authors of this paper).

ACNE VULGARIS (TARUNYA PEETIKA)

Essential Features

1. Pimples (papules or pustules) over the face, back, and shoulders occurring at puberty.
2. Open and closed comedones.
3. Cyst formation, slow resolution, scarring.
4. The most common of all skin conditions.
5. Acne vulgaris is a common inflammatory disease of unknown cause that is apparently activated by androgens who are genetically predisposed. Eunuchs are spared. Similar involvement may occur in identical twins. Contrary to popular belief, they may last even upto sixth decade of life.

6. *Differential Diagnosis*: Distinguish from acneiform lesions, caused by bromides, iodide, and contact with chlorinated naphthalenes and diphenyles.
7. *Complications*: Cyst formation, severe scarring, and psychic trauma.
8. *Prognosis*: Untreated acne vulgaris often remits spontaneously, but the condition may persist throughout adulthood and may lead to severe scarring. The disease is chronic and tends to recur in spite of treatment. Remissions following systemic treatment with Isotretinoin tend to be lasting, though the drug has risk of teratogenicity.

Ayurvedic Treatment

Charaka Samhita describes Acne Vulgaris as 'Tarunya Peetika' meaning a disease of adolescence. A variety of drugs have been used in Ayurveda to treat this condition. These agents are Sookshma Triphala, Mahamanjishthadi Quath etc. and are claimed to be safe and effective (Sharangadhar Samhita) but their effectiveness has not been tested in controlled clinical trials.

Clinical Report

Prakash Paranjpe: *Clinical Evaluation of Mahamanjishthadi Quath and Sookshma Triphala in the Management of Acne Vulgaris—A Single Blind Study. NIMA*:XXXVII:10:1995.

Forty patients with Acne vulgaris were randomised into four groups. Three different Ayurvedic treatment schedules were given orally for 8 weeks; while one group received Placebo. Gr A—consisted of Sookshma Triphala + Mahamanjishthadi Quath; Gr. B—Mahamanjishthadi Quath; Gr. C—Sookshma Triphala; and Gr. D—Placebo (Charcosal).—Manufactured by Ayurved Rasashala, Pune. Sookshma Tiphala contains (250 mg tablet): Harida (Terminalia chebula—66.66 mg), Beheda (Terminalia bellerica 66.66 mg, Amalaki (Embelica officianalis 66.66 mg); Parad (Mercury pure 5.0 mg), Gandhak 5.0 mg), Placebo (250 mg tablet) contains: Amalaki mashi—Embelica officinalis (ash), Takan lahi (Borax pure), Sajjikshar (salt), Hing (Asafoetida)—150 mg., 33 mg., 33 mg., and 16 mg. respectively. Mahamanjishthadi Quath is a known compound.

Physical and clinical investigations were carried out at every two week intervals. A significant reduction in lesion count was observed in patients receiving combination of two drugs (Group A) when compared with Placebo and other two Ayurvedic formulations, which failed to produce any significant difference from the pretreatment condition. The drugs were well tolerated. Treatment in Group A showed a significant improvement in the severity of both inflammatory and non-inflammatory lesions. However, treatment in groups failed to show any significant improvement in the severity of acne. The response to treatment in Group A is comparable to the results reported from other well controlled trials using antibiotics and other agents. The exact mechanism of action of this novel Ayurvedic combination (Group A) has not yet been worked out.

ALOPECIA AREATA (KHALITYA)

Essential Features

1. Characterized by sudden loss of hair either in patches (Alopecia areata), all over scalp (Alopecia totalis) or throughout the body (Alopecia universalis).
2. Patches are bald and the skin surface is smooth with few (exclamatory mark) stumps at the edges of the patches.
3. The cause is not exactly known.
4. *Differential Diagnosis*: Alopecia areata should be differentiated from: Tinea capitis—surface of the affected skin is scaly, not smooth; woodlamp shows fluorescence and potassium hydroxide preparation shows fungus. In black dot ring worm, diagnosis depend upon finding fungus microscopically.

   Syphilitic alopecia—The patches are smaller, are not completely bald, have indefinite margins and no exclamation mark hairs. Hairs appear moth eaten. Other stigmata of syphilis are present. Lesions causing scar on the scalp especially cicatrial alopecia—Presence of scarring and empty hair follicles, and a few exclamation mark hairs.

5. *Prognosis*: Prognosis is good if the condition begins before puberty. The shorter the duration, the better the prognosis. Multiple patches or rapid extension are bad prognostic signs and the chances of complete recovery diminish with each succeeding mark. Exclamation mark hairs signifies recovery; firmly implanted hair present at the periphery means that the alopecia has become stationary while loose hair at the periphery implies that the disease is still active. After the condition has reached the state of alopecia totalis, recovery is rare and no chances of curability in alopecia universalis.

Ayurvedic Concept

Etiology

There is no specific reference of etiological factors of Khalitya in Ayurvedic literature. Referring to the etiological factors scatterily described in various ancient Ayurvedic classics, the following are the causes thought to be involved in the pathogenesis of Khalitya.

1. Excessive use of Kshera and salt (Charaka Vimana 1/17, 18).
2. Vata and Pitta Prakopaka ahara and vihara.
3. Excessive exercise (Madhava Nidana).
4. Srtovarodha 55/28, 29.
5. Disturbance of menstrual cycle (related Vimansh to females only).
6. Non-application of hair oil (Charaka Samhita, Sutra 5/82,83).

According to Videha (Madhava Nidana 55/Vimarsha), the ladies are not affected by this disease as they don't do excessive exercise and further due to menses they are not having srotoavarodha; hence, don't suffer from Khalitya. Earlier studies also show that males were more affected than female and in females marked increase in incidence of disorder about the age of fifty. As this is the age of menopause, the sexual involution in the females has definite etiological significance. But the recent studies show equal distribution in both sexes.

Classification

In Ayurvedic texts, the Khalitya is classified on the basis of site of the disease in view and doshik involvement. There is a quoting in Madhava Nidana that Kartikeya has classified this disease keeping in mind the site involved. He has used the term Indralupta, Khalitya and Ruhya. Indralupta refers to loss of hair from beard and moustach, while Khalitya and Ruhya stands for loss of hair from scalp and whole body respectively. In Ashtangha Sangraha, four types of Khalitya are described basing on doshik involvement e.g. Vataja, Pittaja, Kaphaja and Sannipataja.

Clinical Features

Charaka has mentioned that falling of hair is only sign of the disease. Sushruta has narrated two signs i.e. falling of hair and cessation of regrowth of the hair (Sushrutha Nidana 13/32, 33). According to Ashtanga Sangraha, in Indralupta there is an abrupt fall of hair where as a gradual loss of hair is a sign of Khalitya. Further, there is a mention of clinical features based on doshik involvement in Ashtanga Sangraha (28/20).

Pathogenesis

Regarding samprapti, Charaka opines that the provoked teja (Pitta) alongwith vata etc., after burning the kesha-bhumi (hair-follicles), abruptly produces the disorder Khalitya (Charaka Chikitsa 26/132). In Sushruta Samhita it is mentioned that pitta along with vata goes into Romakupa, the hair follicles and sheds the hair. Later, kapha mixed with rakta closes the hair follicles, which inhibits the regrowth of the hair (Sushruta Nidana 13/32, 33).

Prognosis

The disesase Khalitya having colours of nails and/or burns, with complete loss of hairs or which is caused due to burn is incurable. Further, the disease which is caused due to initiation of all the three doshas is also incurable (Ashtanga Hridaya 23/28).

Treatment

It is mentioned in Charaka Samhita that for treatment of Khalitya, first of all samshodhana measures like vamana and virechana are to be applied, followed by the use of nasya, oil massage on the head, pralepa on the face etc. (Charaka Chikitsa 26/262-265); while Sushruta has emphasized more on the measures like Siravedha (Venisection) and Raktamokshana (blood letting). According to him, after performing the above measures, the lepas are to be applied on the part (Su. Chi. 20/24-26). Scholars of later period have also agreed to the above principles. Ashtanga Sangraha opines that vamana and virechana procedures are to be used in proportion to the predominance of doshas (kapha and pitta). According to Vangasena, it is necessary to rub the lesion of indralupta with rough leaves and then only the topical applications are to be used (Vangasena, 694/134-151). For successful treatment it is necessary to rub the lesion repeatedly.

Ayurvedic formulations as indicated for the treatment of Khalitya in different texts are given below:

1. Charaka Samhita—Chikitsa Sthana:
   - (i) Sanjanana-Yoga consist of ash made of skin hair, horn and bone of the body of quadruped (25/118).
   - (ii) Vidari gandhadiataila for nasya (26/262).
   - (iii) Anutaila for nasya (26/263).
2. Bhaishajya Ratnavali–Kshudra–Roga Chikitsa:
   - (i) Lepa made up of kalkas of Maricha, Mainshila, Kasees and Tutiya.
   - (ii) Lepa of Ghunghachi Kalka.
   - (iii) Lepa made up of antar dhooma dagdha hasti danta and rasaunta.

(iv) Yasthimadhukadya Taila
(v) Adityapaka Guduchi Taila
(vii) Chandanadya Taila.

3. Yoga Ratnakar–Kshudra Roga Chikitsa
(i) Lepa of Gunja-phala
(ii) Lepa of Hilava svarsa
(iii) Lepa consist of ash of white horse khusra along with butter
(iv) Lepa of Katupatola patra
(v) Lepa made of gokshuru, Tila flower
(vi) Snuhyadi Khalityahar Taila
(vii) Jatyadi Taila
(viii) Bhringaraja Taila

4. Vangasena has mentioned following single drugs:
(i) Svarsa of Katu patola patra
(ii) Jatiphala
(iii) Barikateri moola
(iv) Chautali moola—Vangasea 694/134-151.

(*Article*: Pawan Kumar and D. Ojha: Critical appraisal of Khalitya vis-a-vis Alopecia Areata; *Ayurved Samachar*. 16:2:1993).

Clinical Report

A Simple Siddha Remedy for Puzhuvettu (Alopecia areata)—A Pilot Study—G. Ponniachamy, S. Rajalakshmi, P.R. Saroja, M. Sundaram, and G. Veluchamy; *JRAS*:X:1-2:1989.

To evaluate the effect of Keedari Thailam, a Siddha preparation, as external application on Puzhuvettu (Alopecia), a pilot study was conducted at the Outpatient Department of Central Research Institute for Siddha, Arumbakkam, Madras on 20 cases of Puzhuvettu. The response was 100 per cent within the range of 3 weeks to 8 weeks of treatment.

In Siddha literature forty-six types of diseases confined to scalp are explained in which Puzhuvettu or otherwise called Uroma Kirumivettu or Kabalapura Kiruminoi is one among them. In Kabalapura Kiruminoi, scar like bald patches appear due to continuous falling of hair. Pruritus is present as that is caused by lice. Mild scaling as that of ashes is also present (Siddhar Aruvai Maruthuvamp, 115).

Keedari Thailam is a simple preparation given in Therayar Thaila Varga Churukkam specially for the treatment of dandruff.

Materials and Methods

The cases were selected based on the following criteria:

1. Single or multiple bald patches in the scalp brow or beard.
2. Glossy appearance of the surface of the skin in the affected area.
3. Pruritus.

Detailed history and examination were done to exclude—congenital alopecia, ehrpes zoster, and fungal infection, burns, scalds, injury, chemical injury, history of cancer treatment etc. were ruled out. Apart from routine blood investigation VDRL, was done to rule out STD. Skin scrappings for fungus, AFB for tubercular skin and Hansen were done. Mantoux test was also done.

Mode of Preparation of the Drug Tested

Keedari Thailam—Juice extracted from the leaf of Poduthalai (Lippia nodiflora), onion and lime fruit, one part each was mixed with one part of gingely oil and quarter part of pepper. The whole mixture was exposed to sun till the water content was evaporated.

Method of Treatment

Keedari Thailam was applied to the affected part daily for three days and the fourth day affected area was thoroughly washed. This type of treatment was continued till hair growing over the bald patches.

Criteria for Assessment

Regrowth of hair over the lesions and disappearance of pruritus were considered the main criteria for assessment of prognosis. The cases were clinically assessed once in a week and clinical photos were taken periodically. The patients who were not attending O.P. Department regularly for following up were dropped from the study.

Results and Discussion

20 cases of Puzhuvettu in the age range of 9 years to 40 years are included in the study. Age and sex incidence—the disease is more in males than in females.

The duration of the treatment for complete recovery varies from 3 weeks to 8 weeks. 10 per cent of the cases recovered completely in 3 weeks, 40 per cent in 4 weeks, 20 per cent in 5 weeks, 10 per cent in 7 weeks and 20 per cent of the cases in 8 weeks of treatment. Even though all the cases responded to treatment, the variation in response may be due to the chronicity of the disease and the individuals care in applying the oil regularly.

It is clinically observed that there is no adverse side effects during the course of treatment.

VITILIGO (SHVITRA)

The term shvitram is derived from the Sanskrit dhatu' shvitra i.e. to become white. The word vitiligo comes from the Latin word 'vital lus' which means veal, that is pale, pink and flesh.

The disease is world wide in distribution. 4 per cent to 6 per cent of Indian population is suffering from vitiligo. It means nearly 40 million (4 crores) of Indians are facing the problem. It is vividly described in Vedas even. Vitiligo otherwise known as leucoderma is a much despised disease, mainly because of failure of pigmentation resulting in patches in the body. The patient is not accepted socially due to the ugly sight. Its social stigma is aggravated because of the age old belief that it is a kind of lepromatous disease and is named Swedakuttam or Venkuttam in Tamil. Actually this disease has nothing to do with lepromatous group, which in fact is a bacterial infection. About 1 per cent of the world population is affected with this condition.

Charaka has described the disease in detail for the first time with its three synonyms viz. Darunam, Charunam, and Shvitram. Vagbhata also described it is an undischarging (Aparishravi) nature of disease which is a main characteristic. Kilasm is another term used. But later the synonym shivtra became popular term. It gives the literal meaning to become white.

Site

Regarding the site of the disease Charaka opines that third layer of skin is the seat of disease. Vagbhata also follows Charaka but Sushruta says that fourth layer is the seat of the disease. The idea of Sushruta is verified by Sharangadhara. Shvitra involves rakta (blood), mamsa (muscular tissue) and meda (adipose tissue).

Aetiology

(i) Vitiation of asthi, mamsa and meda is the causative factor.

(ii) Lessening of pitta is the causative factor of whiteness of skin.

(iii) Shvitra is caused due to pathological changes in blood.

(iv) Incompatible cereals.

(v) Telling lies, indebtness. Practising abuse to divine soul, disobedience to teachers, sinful acts of previous life contributed to shvitra.

(vi) Excessive use of kaphakara eatables.

(vii) All the other aetiological factors responsible for kustha.

(viii) Shvitra is a garbhaj disease. The disease of this group are caused due to faulty dietary habits of the pregnant women. The disease are of two types: annarasajanya and due to nonfulfilment of the desire of pregnant women. Shvitra is one of the diseases of this group.

Pathogenesis

Sushruta says that the aetiological factors vitiates all the three doshas of an individual and this vitiation in blood makes the skin white or pale. Thus, it is tridoshaja vyadhi (vata, pitta, and kapha); yet is predominantly manifested due to the disturbance of kapha and pitta. It is not a contagious disease. According to Ayurveda, normal function of Bhrajaka pitta is responsible for colour pigmentation of the skin (Vagbhata) and its functional defect results in svitra. Brajaka Agni is one of the five subvarieties of Pachaka Agni having its site as skin (Twak). In svitra, the tissues affected are: Twak (skin), Rakta (blood), Mamsa (muscular tissue), and Medas (fatty tissue), and the metabolism of Brajakagni is vitiated by Tridoshas (Charaka Samhita; Ashtanga Hridaya).

Classification

According to Charaka, the disease is of three types: 1. Darunam; 2. Charunam; 3. Shvitram.

According to colour of lesions, it is of 3 types:

1. Raktavarna shvitra—When the vata dosha involves the rakta, the lesions have red colour.
2. Tamravarna shvitra—When the pitta dosha involves mamsa, the lesions have coppery colour.
3. Shvetavarna shvitra—When the kapha dosha involves the meda, the lesions have white colour.

According to Sushruta, kilasa is of 3 types, according to involvement of doshas.

1. Vataja kilasa—Reddish white colour lesions with horripilation of hairs of the lesions.
2. Pittaja kilasa—lesions are similar to lotus leaves and with burning sensation.
3. Kaphaja kilasa—The lesions are white, smooth and thick with itching.

According to involvement of dhatus, there are three types:

1. Rakta involved shvitram—lesions are reddish white in colour.
2. Mamsa involved shvitram—lesions are coppery white in colour.
3. Meda involved shvitram—lesions are absolutely white in colour.

Clinical Features

It is superficial and involves only skin of the body and it has no discharge. According to Vagbhata, the lesions of vataja Shvitra are dry, red and seat of shvitra is rakta. The lesions of pittaja shvitra are coppery, similar to lotus leaves with burning sensation, and also cause horripilation of the hairs of the lesions. The seat of shvitra is in mamsa. Kaphaja shvitra is absolutely white, dense, thick with itching and the seat of shivtra is in meda.

Leucoderma or secondary depigmentation may complicate atopic dermatitis, lichen planus, psoriasis, alopecia areata, lichen simplex chronicus, and such systemic conditions as myxedema, thyrotoxicosis, syphilis, and toxaemias. It may follow local skin trauma, or various sorts, or may complicate dermatitis due to exposure to gold or arsenic. Antioxidants in rubber goods, such as monobenzyl ether of hydroquinone, cause leucoderma from the wearing of gauntlet gloves, rubber pads in brassieres, etc. This is most likely to occur in blacks.

Differential Diagnosis

One must distinguish true lack of pigment from pseudoachromia, such as occurs in tinea versicolour, pityriasis versicolour, pityriasis simplex, and seborrheic dermatitis. It may be difficult to differentiate true vertigo from leucoderma and even from partial albinism.

Complications

Solar keratoses and epitheliomas are more likely to develop in persons with vitiligo and albinism. Vitiligo tends to cause pruritus in anogenital folds. There may be severe emotional trauma in extensive vitiligo and other types of hypopigmentation, particularly when they occur in naturally dark-skinned persons.

Prognosis

There is no increase of pigment in partial or total albinism; return of pigment is rare in vitiligo; in leucoderma, repigmentation may occur spontaneously. Therapy of vitiligo is long and tedious.

According to Ayurveda—Shvitra situated in meda dhatu is relatively most difficult to treat than in mamsa and rakta. Shvitra in which the lesions are collapsed, extensive, the hair have become red in colour and are of long duration is incurable. If the lesions have not turned grey, the lesions are few and reddish in colour and are of not long duration, then in such cases, shvitra is curable.

Thus shvitra is incurable when the lesions have collapsed, the sites of involvement are the lips, plantar surface of feet, palmar surface of the hands, the genital area and the hairs of the lesions have turned grey and the lesions similar to burn.

According to Vagbhata shvitra is worse than kushta, because it attains incurability in a very short time period. Hence it is necessary to start the treatment very soon in the same way as people run immediately to pacify the fire of a burning home.

It is worth mentioning as the Ayurvedists described as early as first century B.C. that the recent patches which were not continuous and extensive and not caused by burns were curable and the rest had to be avoided (Ashtangahridaya).

Treatment

Samsodhana—Vaman, Virechan (Kakodumbar and guda especially for virechana).

The luke warm water prepared out of the powder udumbara is to be used in shvitra, and also used in the lesions; vesicles are formed and they are perforated for draining. Afterwards, the ash obtained after burning of Sugandhabala along with Vibhitak oil may be applied locally as an ointment. In the texts there are so many lepas described which can be used locally (e.g. Tuthadi, Tilvakadi, Haritakyadi, Bhallatakadi etc.)

Ghrita—Neela Ghrita, Mahaneela Ghrita.

Taila—The topical application of Kushthadi followed by exposure of the lesions to sun rays cures recent vitiligeneous lesions within a month (other taila used are Vibhitaka, Bhallataka etc.)

Anjana—Mustadya Netranjana Varti.

Dhooma—Shvetadi Seerso Virechan Dhooma.

Surgical measures—Lekhana.

Oral Medicaments

Single drugs—Guggulu, Rasona, Chitraka, Bavachea, drugs of Asanadigana.

Choorna—Mustadi, Hapushadi, Khadiradi.

Kashaya—Patolmuladi, Kakodumbarikadi

Asava-arishta—Lodhrasava, Madhvasava, Kanakabindurishtam, Abhayarishta, Madhukasava, Punarnavadyarishta.

Ghrita—Neela, Mahaneela, Avartaki, Tiktaka, Mahavajraka.

Gudika—Kshara.

Yoga—Chitrakadi, Bramyadi

Guda—Manibhadra, Vidangadi, Pathyadi, Chandrasakaladi

Rasayana—Chitraka, Bakushee

Topical-Lepa—Bojapatragranthyadi, Araghvadhadi, Farinjakadi, Manhasiladi, Baksheebijadi, Mulakbeejadi, Neelotpaladi etc.

Here, two combination of drugs which are highly effective and selected after extensive trials in SS Hospital, IMS, Banaras Hindu University, Varanasi are being given which will be helpful in treating the patient suffering from shvitra (R.K. Mamgain, Mrs. Pratibha Mamgain, and D. Ojha, *Shvitra (Vitiligo) and Its Ayurvedic Management (Ayurved Samachar,* 15:1:1992).

Compound Drug A: It contains:

Drug	*Latin Name*	*Parts Used*	*Qty in 12 gms*
1. Khadira	Acacia catechu	Khadira sara	1 gm
2. Haridra	Circuma longa	Rhizome	1 gm
3. Chakramarda	Cassia tora	Seeds	1 gm
4. Chakshushya	Cassia absus	Seeds	1 gm

5. Rajodumbara	Ficus carica	Fruit	3 gms
6. Bakuchea	Psoralia corylifolia	Seeds	5 gms

Compound Drug B: It contains:

1. Bakuchea	Psoralia corylifolia	Seeds	2 gms
2. Khadira	Acacia catechu	Khadirasara	2 gms
3. Nimba	Azadirachta indica	Panchang churna	2 gms
4. Haridra	Circuma longa	Rhizome	2 gms

Both the two drugs are used orally as well as locally. Prepared compound drug is poured in one cup of water at night. Early in the morning the water was decanted from the cup. With this filtrate, 6 gms of powder taken orally after breakfast and the remaining residue in the cup is mixed thoroughly and applied as a thin paste over shvitra patch, after one and half hour of oral intake of drug. It is allowed to dry for half an hour. Now, it is exposed to sunlight for 5 minutes only. Morning single dose treatment was given. The results with this treatment are excellent.

Clinical Reports

A Clinical Study of Vitiligo with Ayush–57. T. Seshagiri Rao, K. Kuppurajan, V. Rajagopalan, and K.K. Janaki: *JRAS*:1:4:1980).

Vitiligo is one of the incurable diseases described in ancient Ayurvedic literature. Ayurveda describes majority of the chronic skin disorders under the title 'Kushta' (wrongly equated as leprosy) and this has been attributed to have similar etio-pathogenesis as Kushta (Ashtanga Hridaya). According to Ayurveda, the pigmentation of the skin is due to the metabolism of 'Bhrajaka Agni,' one of the five sub-varieties of 'Pachaka Agni' having its site as skin (twak). In Shvitra (Vitiligo), the tissues affected are twak (skin), rakta (blood), mamsa (muscular tissue), and medas (fatty tissue), and the metabolism of Brajaka agni is vitiated by Tridoshas (Charaka Samhita; Ashtanga

Hridaya). It is worth mentioning that the Ayurvedists described as early as first century B.C. that the recent patches which were not continuous and extensive and not caused by burns were curable and the rest had to be avoided (Ashtanga Hridaya).

It is a common observation that many claims are made about some recipes having highly beneficial effect in Shvitra. Ayush-57 which among others has Sulphur, Rakta chitraka (Plumbago rosea Linn.), Hirakash, Hartal, Triphala (Haritaki—Terminalia bellerica, Vibhitaki—Terminalia chebula Roxb., and Amalataki-Emblica officinalis Gaertn) and Yavatikta (Andrographis panniculata Nees) is one such recipe being investigated at various centres under the aegis of CCRAS for its efficacy. This paper presents the preliminary observations made and also the analysed results of 50 cases who had completed 12 weeks of treatment conducted at Dr. A. Lakshmipathy Unit for Research in Indian Medicine (CCRAS).

To assess the results of the treatment scientifically, one or two prominent, isolated well demarcated medium patches were selected and graphs were drawn and area was measured in sq. cms. initially and periodically. Drug was issued to the volunteers with the following instructions:

1. The selected patch is to be cleaned well.
2. The stick is to be rubbed on a stone slab with little water and made into a paste.
3. Paste is to be applied on the selected patch, twice a day.
4. While applying the paste, gentle massage for about 15 minutes is to be done.
5. Exposure to sun for 15 minutes is recommended after the massage.

   Diet and conduct to be avoided.
6. Incompatible foods like (a) fish with milk, (b) channa with milk, (c) channa and common grams like green gram, Bengal gram with milk, curd etc.
7. Intake of food before the previous food is digested.
8. Exercise and excessive sexual indulgence.
9. Cold water bath, after taking food.

10. Intake of food articles like potatoes which are difficult to digest.

General

1. Soapnut powder or green gram powder is to be used for cleaning the part.
2. Soap is any form should not be used.
3. The patient has to report for following-up every 4th week periodically for 3 months without fail.
4. Any complication such as itching, blister formation etc. should be reported to the unit immediately for advice.

Observations

Of the 90 cases screened and included in the trial, 49 were males and 41 were females; Age range: 3 months and 78 years; Age of onset of diseases—less than 16 years; duration of disease—less than 10 years. Site of first appearance of the disease was face, chest, limbs, genitals, waist, and back. In this sample, the disease had made its first apperance on limbs and face in majority of cases. Majority of patients have taken allopathic treatment with Psoralin compounds with/without multivitamins.

Assessment of Prakriti in the study group brings to light the equal dominance of pith and kapha in males and the preponderance of kapha in females. It is also noted that the dominance of vata was least among both the cases.

Observations on Drug Application

Blister formation on application of the paste prepared out of Ayush-57 was reported in one case only. Pruritus was complained occasionally on exposure to sun which however, disappeared on discontinuation of the same. Appearance of a few spots of natural pigments over the untreated patches which might probably be due to activation of Brajaka pitta. Though no definite causative factor could be established for the disease, the effects of the disease are far reaching. Patients had inferiority and introverted tendencies.

Results and Discussion

Out of 90 cases screened and admitted into the trial, 50 cases had completed the stipulated treatment period of 12 weeks, which was arbitrarily fixed to indicate the response to treatment. To assess the effect of the drug, the change in the area (measured in sq. cms.) of the selected patches between the initial and final graphs was considered. Reduction of at least 1 sq. cm. of area between initial and final graphs was considered as improvement; increase of reduction of the area by less than 1 sq. cm. as neither improvement nor aggravation of the disease; increase in the area by 1 sq. cm. and above as aggravation of the disease.

According to the criteria mentioned above, 20 cases of vitiligo were registered as having improvement (40 per cent), 19 maintained status quo (38 per cent), and 11 showed aggravation (22 per cent) out of 50 completed cases (100 per cent) taken for analysis.

The possible association between sex and improvement; age and improvement; duration of disease and improvement were tested by means of 't' test and 'X2' test. It was found that improvement was not significantly different within the groups (less than 0.05). The results demonstrate that the chances of total cure in the cases of vitiligo are remote and the improvement shown was also not spectacular. However, the slight improvement noted in the above small sample is encouraging. Appearance of spots of natural pigmentation in certain untreated vitiligo patches suggests that the stimulation of the pigment metabolism and not the tanning effect. In the improved cases, small spots of natural pigmentation appeared which expanded and converted together to form islands of natural skin colour within the treated patches. Similar pattern of skin pigmentation was noted in patients who were treated with Mepacrine internally by A.K. Banerjee et al, 1965.

The stimulation of pigmentation in this study justifies the continuance of the drug for longer periods on bigger samples to declare the utility of the drug. Internal medication with laxatives and svitrahara drugs may enhance the therapeutic effect of the drug which is in agreement with the Samhitas.

Clinical Evaluation of Ayurvedic Preparations in Vitiligo—P.R. Nair, M.N.S. Namboodiri, P. Madhavikutty, and V.A. Prabhakaran; *JRAS*:VIII:1-2:1987.

Two sets of medicinal preparations were evaluated for their efficacy in Shvitra (Vitiligo). 60 vitiligo patients were grouped into two sets based on random number generation. To first group Nimbapanchanga (Azadirachta indica) powder 4 gm. thrice daily was administered internally and a paste of Gunja (Abrus precatorius) and Chitraka (Plumbago zeylanica) was applied externally. Group II received powder of Amalaki phala (Phyllanthus embelica), Khadira sara (Acacia catechu) and Avalgujabeeja (seeds of Psoralia corylifolia) 4 g thrice daily. A paste of Avalgujabeeja (1 part) and Harathala (1/4 part Arsenic Tersulphurecticum) was applied on the affected area. The patches were exposed to sunlight for 10 minutes duration after the external application of the paste. Encouraging improvement was noted in both the groups after the treatment. The result obtained with the second set was better than that of the first one.

A research study conducted with Ayush-57 (a coded drug) for external application in Shvitra revealed that the external application of the preparation alone is not sufficient to initiate repigmentation of the lesions. Hence it was decided to conduct clinical trials with medicines given internally (oral) along with the external application of medicines on white patches in Shvitra.

Out of 60 patients, 15 at random were included in Group I and 45 in Group II. 12 gm of Nimbapanchanga Churna (Shastri 1969) (Powder of root, and stem bark, leaves, flowers, and fruits of Neem tree—Azadirachta indica Meliaceae) was given orally in 3 divided doses of 4 gm each one hour before the meals with hot water in Group I. Gunjachitrakavarthi (Shastri 1969) paste (Gunja—Abrus precatorius Linn. Leguminoseae and Chitraka—Plumbago zeylanica Linn. Plumbaginaceae) was applied on the lesions. In Group II,

Dhathryadi Churnam (Shastri 1969) (Powder of Dhatriphala fruits of Phyllanthus embelica Linn Euphorbiaceae), Khadira sara (stem of Acacia catechu Leguminosae) and Avalgujabeeja (seeds of Psoraea corylifilia Linn. Leguminosae) were given orally in a dose of 12 gm per day in 3 divided doses of 4 gm each one hour before meals with hot water. Avalgujabeejadi Varthi (Shastri 1969) (paste of Avalgujabeeja 4 parts and Haratala 1 part—Arsenic tersul-phurecticum) was applied on the lesions. The patches were exposed to sunlight for 10 minutes after application of the paste in all the cases (both the groups). The paste was retained on the patches as long as patients tolerated the application and were advised to apply the medicine twice a day (morning and evening). The minimum duration of treatment was fixed as 90 days in all the cases to assess the improvement. Maximum duration of treatment was not fixed as a slow and steady improvement was noticed in majority of the cases and the treatment was continued till the patches completely disappeared or till the patients discontinued the treatment. Results of the patients who have not completed 90 days treatment was not taken into consideration while assessing the efficacy of the therapy. No changes were made in the patients usual diet.

On analysis of the results, it is observed that the duration of the disease has not influenced the results in Group I. Chronic cases respond well to the treatment where as no improvement was obtained in some short duration cases in this group. Improvement was better in fresh cases in Group II. It has been found that complete relief (complete repigmentation of the patches) could have been obtained in majority of the cases, if the treatment were continued for longer period.

Side Effects

No side effects has been observed in patients in Group I. In Group II in 11 cases vesication was noticed after the application of Avalgujabeejadi Varthi. Three of these patients discontinued the treatment. The condition became severe in two patients due to infection of the lesions. However, the blisters disappeared after withdrawal of the medication and the infection was controlled by applying pure coconut oil. The repigmentation of the white patches was quicker in the above stated cases. Four cases from this group (out of 11) showed complete relief, two cases showed moderate relief. In two cases, white patches reappeared on withdrawal of medicines but on reapplication of the same group of medicine, improvement was again noted.

Conclusion

Two sets of medicines i.e. 1. Nimbapanchanga Churna and Gunjachitraka Varthi and 2. Dhathrayadi Churna and Avalgujabeejadi Varthi are proved to be effective in Shvitra. Effect was better in Dhatrayadi Churna Group (II) in comparison with Group I. Hence Dhathrayadi Churna internally and Avalgujabeejadi Varthi externally can be effectively employed in the treatment of Shvitra and a minimum period of 18-24 months treatment is required for a complete relief from Shvitra. (Ambikadatta Shastri:1969: Bhaishajyaratnavali, Vidyotini Commentary; Chowkamba Sanskrit Series Office, Varanasi).

PSORIASIS

Essential Features

1. Psoriasis is a common benign, acute or chronic inflammatory skin disease that apparently is based on genetic predisposition.
2. Silvery scales on bright red plaques, usually on the knees, elbows and scalp.
3. Stippled nails.
4. Itching is mild unless psoriasis is eruptive or occurs in body folds.
5. Psoriatic arthritis may be present.
6. Histopathologic features are specific.
7. Differential diagnosis: Differentiate in the scalp from

seborrheic dermatitis; in body folds from intertrigo and candidiasis; and in the nails from onychomycosis.

8. Prognosis: The course tends to be chronic and unpredictable, and the disease may be refractory to treatment.

Ayurvedic Concept of Psoriasis

There is no particular single kushtam (Skin disease) which can be compared to the Psoriasis in Ayurveda. So, based on symptomatology of Psoriasis, this can be compared to the following kushtas mentioned in Ayurvedic texts.

And by observing the following chart, we can also know that only the Dadru Kushtam shows the maximum similarities to the Psoriasis. When we observe the Sadhya-Sadhyata of the disease Dadru, Charaka and Vagbhata mentioned as Kasta Sadhya Vyadhi. Sushruta quoted it as the Asadhyavyadhi. Bhela says that it becomes asadhya only when it enters the dhatus like resho-majja and asthi.

General Line of Treatment of Kushtas

In all types of kushtas Snehapan is recommended at the early stages. And they have also mentioned that the treatment is to be done on the basis of their dosha predominance.

InVata Predominance—Medicated ghee to be administered, e.g., Dasamoola, Amruta etc.

Pitta Predominance—Medicated ghee like Thikthaka ghrita.

Kapha Predominance—Medicated ghee preparation like Nimba, Chitraka and Maricha etc.

In Ashtanga Hridaya, Tuvaraka Tailam and Sarsapa Tailam are indicated in all types of Kushtas.

According to Charaka

In Vata Pradhanam—Snehapana

In Pitta Pradhanam—Blood letting after giving virechana to patient.

In Kapaha Pradhanam—Vamana

Table 1.12: *Comparative Study of Kshudra Kushtas to Psoriasis*

Symptoms of Psoriasis	*Ayu. Terminology*	*Diseases Mentioned in Ayu. having the Same Symptoms*				
		Dadru	*Kitibha*	*Eka*	*Sitma*	*Charmadala*
Itching absent	Kandu	+	+	–	–	+
Raised non-indurates	Utsannamadaka	+	–	–	–	–
Erythematous						
Dry	Rooksha	–	+	–	+	–
Silvery scaling	Twak Vigalana (Mestyasakala Sannibha)	–	–	+	+	–
Candle greeze sign	Sweta utsanna					
	Mandala	+	–	–	–	–
Pin point bleeding (Auspitz sign)	Raga pitika	+	–	–	–	–
History of previous attacks	Anushangini	+	+	–	–	–

In Ashtanga Hridaya and Sushruta Chikitsasthan, the schedule for Sodhana therapy of kushta is as follows: The patient has to undergo:

Vamana	–	once in 15 days
Virechana	–	once in a month
Nasya karma	–	once in 3 days
Raktamokshana	–	once in 6 months.

Clinical Reports

Based on the above statement given by Acharyas, they have conducted a clinical trial on 20 patients of Dadru kushta. (A. Sankar Babu et al. *Kshudra Kustha-Clinical Research with Special Reference to Psoriasis: Ayurved Samachar:* 14:12:1992).

Poorva karma	Snehapana
	Sweda: Anagneya sweda
	Vamana
	Virechana

In some cases which had reccurrences, thakra dhara was conducted additionally.

20 cases of psoriasis were selected as per the criteria given below for the clinical trial from the O.P. Department of Government Ayurvedic Hospital, Trivandrum.

Criteria for Selection

Age between 15 to 60 years; Duration of the disease not more than 15 years; sex—either sex.

Presence of Cardinal Signs and Symptoms of the Disease

1. Rounded elevated erythematous plaque; 2. Silvery scaling; 3. Pinpoint bleeding; 4. Itching.

Administration of Medicine

The patients taken for research study were kept on Placebo therapy for three days. All the routine investigations and examinations were carried out during the period.

After enquiring the appetite and digestive power, from 4th day onwards 'Snehapana' was commenced. The snehadravya was administered in all the patients in the form of 'accha snehapana.' 'Vajraka' mentioned in Ashtanga Hridaya Chikitsa Prakarana was used for snehapana.

The administration of medicine (ghrita) was started with an initial dose of 50 ml. at 6 a.m. on the first day. The patient eyes were covered with a piece of cloth and nostrils were closed, with perfumed cotton, in order to prevent the aversion towards the sight and smell of sneha.

Soon after snehapana, a little quantity of warm water was given in order to cleanse the mouth and for proper digestion of sneha. Patients were advised not to sleep during day time and when he feels thirst the warm shunthi water was given for drinking. After getting good appetite only, patients were permitted to take peyadi karma. Next day onwards, the quantity of ghee was increased depending the agni bala and pachana shakti of patients. Snehapana is continued till samyak snigdha lakshanas were manifested.

We found samyak snigdha lakshanas within 7 days in most of the cases. The maximum quantity consumed on the last day was 350 ml. Out of 20 cases 14 cases consumed the maximum dose.

In cases, where samyak snigdha lakshanas was not seen with in 7 days, were given sadhya snehas till they obtain prescribed lakshanas.

'Kanji' was given to the patients in moderate quantity and asked to continue the same through the snehapana period. Patients were instructed to take hot water bath for two consecutive days after samyak snigdha lakshanas to get a mrudusweda, since in all the kushthas, sweda is contraindicated.

Vamana Karma

7 days after samyak snigdha lakshanas patients were subjected to undergo vamana karma. A day previous to vamana karma, the patients were instructed to take masha and milk

diet which have the quality of kaphatklesha. After examining the pulse, respiration and blood pressure etc., on the day of vamana karma during kaphakala (i.e. morning period) the patients were subjected to local abhyanga with shuddha doorvedi karma (Doorvo+coconut oil) and mridu bhaspa sweda to chest and back before starting the process.

Patients were asked to take boiled milk as much as they can be consumed. After that vamana drug was given as a single dose, which contains Madanaphala Churna 3 gm, Vacha Churna 5 gm, Saindhava 5 gm and honey 25 ml. All were mixed well by grinding and this paste was mixed with 50 ml milk and administered.

In most of cases spontaneous vomiting was started within fifteen minutes. The proper vamana symptoms were noted by observing the vomitus. The factors such as Antyaki (order of dosha expelled), Vaigiki (number of Vegas), Laingiki (signs and symptoms) were observed.

Soon after Vamana, Dhoomapana was conducted with Haridra Churnavarthi. Then patients were instructed to follow the samsarjana karma i.e. Peyadi karma in order to obtain a normal appetite.

After samsarjana karma, again sneha dravya was given in the form of Vicharna sneha for 5 days in the dose of 25 grs twice daily to patients. Instead of sweda, hot water bath was advised for two days after attaining proper sneha symptoms. During the process shuddha doorvedi karma was also used for external application.

Virechana karma was performed on the next day morning by giving 20 grs. of Avipathi Churnam with honey in order to eliminate the extrinsic dosha (i.e. doshas persist after vamana) and observe to samyak virechana lakshanas.

Samsarjana karma was again followed to regain the normal appetite. Investigations repeated and results were noted. Once again the patients were undergone samsarjana karma and vicharna sneha.

Afterwards nasya oordha shodhana was conducted for 7 days in uttama matra with Anutailam.

Then the patients were discharged. Vajraka Ghrita was given as samana for a period of one month. Advise to report the Hospital O.P. Department in every month for the follow up study for 6 months. After second follow up, it is seen that out of 20 patients, only 6 were shown significant response to the treatment. Hence it is advised to conduct a second course of shodhana therapy to the remaining 14 patients and conducted.

Observations and Results

20 patients were admitted in Ayurvedic Hospital, Trivandrum, out of which 14 were males and 6 were females.

Most of the patients were lower socio-economic group having incompatible food habits and also having the habits of Viruddhasana, Adhyosana and Madhyasevana etc.

Among the 20 patients, 12 had attacks of the disease for more than once i.e. 4 of them have second attack, 6 has third attack and 2 had fourth attack. 8 patients approached the hospital with the first attack. Out of 20, only 2 showed family history of the same disease. Seasonal variation also noticed in some patients. Some of the patients complain that itching aggravated during cold and subsides during summer; others complain vice versa. Maximum persons were having the duration of the illness between 3-4 years.

The size of lesion were varied from 5 mm to 15 cm approximately. All the plaques were dry in nature. The common affected areas observed in most of the patients were scalp, elbow, knees, sacral regions, forearm, legs and trunk. Most of the patients complains that the lesions was initially started in scalp. The Auspitz's sign was observed in all patients. This was noted by scratching the scales. Total area affected by the plaques were estimated on the basis of burning's scoring formula i.e. Rule of nine.

Table 1.13: *Shows Decreasing Percentage of Psoriatic Lesions Before and After Treatment.*

Sl. No. Area	*No. of Patients*	*Before Treatment* % of Psoriatic Lesions Over Body	*After Treatment* % of Psoriatic Lesions Over Body
1. Scalp	4	60%	20%
2. Back	4	40%	0%
3. Elbows	5	80%	40%
4. Knees	5	80%	20%
5. Whole body	2	60%	10%

Regarding the mental state in 8 patients, stress and strain was observed markedly. This was because of their isolated feeling in society, about their marriage, association, and future of their life. (The age of the patients: 11-30 (7); 31-50 years (12); 51-60 years (1) .)

Investigations showed Haemoglobin percentage was slightly below the normal in many patients. Other investigations did not show any notable abnormality before treatment.

Changes Observed in Clinical Features

Itching: Before treatment it was present in all patients with different severity. After snehapana all of them showed remarkable relief from itching. And after shodhana therapy in all patients itching has subsided totally.

Scaling: After snehapana in 10 patients, the scaling were reduced remarkably. Others also showed reduction even though it is not significant. In 4 patients, it was completely absent. 14 patients showed highly significant reduction in scaling after first course of shodhana procedure. In one patient, scaling was increased mildly after shodhana. But the case which was not responded initially has shown significant response after the second course of shodhana procedure.

Erythema: It was present in all patients with different grades. After snehapana, no notable changes were observed in any patient. But, after shodhana, 14 patients showed gradual reduction of erythema and it was almost completely absent after the second course of shodhana karma.

Auspitz's sign was not observed after second course of shodhana therapy; the dryness of the lesion subsided markedly in 12 patients out of 20 patients after the first course of shodhana itself. It was also absent after the second course of shodhana therapy.

Thus, after first course of shodhana therapy, 6 patients (out of 20) showed significant response; and after second course of therapy 10 patients (out of 12) showed significant response.

The mental state of the patients were improved during the trial period and all the patients were quite happy with this mode of treatment even though, the shodhana procedure and dietic restrictions are difficult to follow. No significant changes was observed in haematological and biochemical values after the treatment since the values before and after the trial were within normal range.

Table 1.14: *Degree of Relief Obtained with Therapy*

Degree of Relief	*No. of Patients*
Complete	5
Moderate	4
Mild	3
Nil	8
Total	20

Charaka and Vagbhata considered it as Kashtasadhya and Sushruta as Asadhya vyadhi. Acharyas give prime importance to the vitiated doshas for the management. So, they gave maximum importance to eliminate the vitiated doshas from the body through shodhana therapy especially by vamana, virechana and nasya.

From the above results, it may be concluded that the treatment adopted for the trial with Pancha Karma Therapy is necessary and to conduct further research work in large number of patients for the final and fruitful results.

(A. Sankar Babu; Jayaram Jinde; P. Sankaran Kutty: *Kshudra Kusta-Clinical Research with Special Reference to Psoriasis: Ayurveda Samachar:* 14:12:1992).

Clinical Study of Vetpalai (Wrightia tinctoria Linn) Oil in the Treatment of Kalanjaga Padai (Psoriasis)—J.R. Krishnamurthy, S. Kalaimani, G. Valuchamy: *JRAS*:II:1:1981.

Amongst Siddha Practitioners, "Kalanjaga Padai" is adopted as a term representing Psoriasis; although it does not find a place in the Ancient Siddha Literatures. The leaves of Vetpalai (Wrightia tinctoria) with coconuts and gingely oil is very widely used in cases of skin disorders by the people living around Kunrathur, Chengalpattu District, Tamil Nadu with remarkable results. To confirm it on scientific lines, a study of this drug in cases of Kalanjaga Padai was planned. For the purpose, 14 cases of Kalanjaga Padai were selected from the Out Patient Department of Central Research Institute (Siddha), Arambakkam and admitted there in the In-Patient Department. To all these 14 cases, Vetpalai oil was administered orally in 5 ml. dose thrice a day along with milk and the same oil was applied externally for local application on the affected areas. The duration of treatment was for five weeks to 15 weeks. 50 per cent of cases responded well to the treatment. Four cases were followed up for six months without any recurrence. Vetpalai oil has been found to be safe and without any toxic or other side effects.

Plant (Wrightia tinctoria) (Vetpalai) Description

It is an apocyanaceae tree growing throughout India. Its flowers are white and fragrant. The leaves are the source of blue dye called Mysore Pala Indigo.

An analysis of the leaves from Tamil Nadu showed that the leaves possess proteolytic properties and contain indigo-yielding glucosides. There are no known Siddha textual references regarding the therapeutic and pharmacological action of the leaves of Vetpalai for Kalanjaga padai and similar skin diseases. Hence, the leaves of Vetpalai are taken up for clinical trial, and microbiological and pharmacological studies at CRIS and CSMDRI, Arumbakkam.

The drug was found to be microbiologically active on Gram positive Staphlococcus aureus, Staphylococcus albus and Staphylococcus citreus at a concentration of 0.2 per cent and 6.0 per cent. It is resistant against gram negative bacteria and fungi.

In the clinical trial, a majority of the cases showed improvement within ten days. Total response to treatment was 50 per cent which was very encouraging. The oil of Vetpalai clears ugly condition of the skin in a matter of ten days and gives a psychological boost to the patient who has been subjected to cuticular disfigurement and consequent mental depression for a number of years. Recurrence of the episode in 28.57per cent of cases after observation for over a period of six months is low. Vetpalai has been found to be safe and without any toxic or other side effects.

REFERENCES AND NOTES

1. Rajasekharan S., Pillai, N.G.K.P., Kurup P.B., Pillai. K.G.B., Nair C.P.R; Effect of Nimbidin in Psoriasis—A Case Report: *JRAS*:1:1:1980.
2. Venkataraghavan S., Gowri N., Sitaraman R., Kanchana Srinivasan, Janaki K.: Preventionof Sleepada (Elephantiasis) with Ayurvedic Compounds; *JRAS*:1:1:1980.
3. Geetha A., Pillai K.G.S., Kurup P.B., Nair C.P.R.: Action of Patolakaturohinyadi Kwatham and Gopatmajadikeram on Skin Diseases—A Clinical Trial: *JRAS*:1:2:1980.
4. Seshagiri Rao T., Kuppurajan K., Rajagopalan V., Kanaki K.: A Clinical Study of Vitiligo with Ayush-57: *JRAS*:1:4:1980.

5. Krishnamurthy J.R., Kalaimani S., Valuchamy G.: Clinical Study of Vetpalai (Wrightia tinctoria R.Br.) Oil in the Treatment of Kalanjaga Padai (Psoriasis): II:1:1981 (*JRAS*).
6. Saxena A.P., Vyas K.M., Traditional Treatment of Leprosy and Leucoderma by the Tribals of Bundelkhand in Uttar Pradesh: *JRAS*: II:2:1981.
7. Masilamani G., Showkath Ali, Subbalaxmi V.: Study on Karappan (Eczema): *JRAS*:II:2:1981.
8. Seshagiri Rao T., Vishwanatha Rao P., Kusumakumari K., Netaji B., Nisteswar K., R.R. Sharma C.: Clinical Trial of Ayush-64 in Sleepada: *JRAS*:III:1&2:1982.
9. P. Kishore and Chaturvedi M.K.: Clinical Evaluation of Certain Herbal Preparations in the Treatment of Chronic Slipada—Elephantiasis: *JRAS*: VII:1&2:1986.
10. P. Kishore and Chaturvedi M.K.: Clinical Assessment of the Effect of Ayush-64 in the Acute Cases of Slipada (Filariasis): *JRAS*:VII:3&4:1986.
11. Seshagiri Rao, R.R., Sharma C., Kusuma Kumari K., Bikshapathi T.: Evaluation of the Effect of Ayurvedic Drug (Internal and External) in the Treatment of Slipada (Filariasis)—A Pilot Study: *JRAS*: VII: 3 and 4: 1986.
12. Ramachandran M.N.S., Namboodiri P., Madhavi Kutty and V.A. Prabhakaran: Clinical Evaluation of Ayurvedic Preparation in Vitiligo: *JRAS*:VIII:1&2:1987.
13. Rajeshwari R.H., Hiremath G.G.: Kitibha (Psoriasis) and Its Management with Special References to Jalaukavacharana: *JRAS*:VIII:1&2:1987.
14. Sudarshana Nair P.K., Pillai N.G.K., Kurup P.B., and Nair C.P.R.: Therapeutic Effect of Coconut Shell Extract in Dermatophytosis: *JRAS*: VIII:1&2:1987.
15. K.R. Kalavati, Chellamal R., Sivanandan G., Krishnamurthy J.R., Veluchamy G.: Associated Medical Problems in Psoriatics (A Statistical Analysis Based on Laboratory and Clinical Parameters): *JRAS*: VIII: 3&4:1987.
16. Nair R.B., Nair P.K.S., Pillai N.G.K., Kurup P.B., Nair C.P.R.: Psoriasis—A Review—Short Research Communication: *JRAS*:IX:1-2:1988.
17. Padhi M.M., and P. Kishore: Epidemiological Studies and Therapeutic Trials on Slipada (Filariasis) in the Village Malipada (Puri District of Orissa).: *JRAS*:IX:3-4:1988.
18. Rao K.K., Krishnamurthi J.R., Shetty B.M.V., Pandiyarajan., Veluchamy G.: Herbal Treatment (Siddha) for Psoriasis: *JRAS*: IX: 3-4:1988.

19. Nair P.K.S., Nair S.S., Amma K.C.B., Nair D.R.N., Pillai N.G.K., Pillai B.K.R., Kurup P.B., Nair C.P.R.: Effect of Resottamadilepa, a Herbomineral Formulation in the Treatment of Dermatophytosis; *JRAS*:X:1-2:1989.

20. Ponniachamy G., Rajalakshmi S., Saroja P.R., Sundram M., Veluchamy G.: A Simple Siddha Remedy for Puzhuvettu (Alopecia areata—A Pilot Study: *JRAS*:X:1-2:1989.

21. K. Kalavathy, Shetty B.M.V., Ramachandran J.R., Krishna Murthy and Veluchamy G.: Effect of 777 Oil on Nonspecific Dermatitis (777 Oil—A Siddha Herbal Coded Preparation): *JRAS*:X:3-4:1989.

22. P. Kishore and Pandey P.N.: Effect of Ayush-64 and Saptaparnaghana Vati on Microfilaraemia; *JRAS*:XII:3-4:1991.

23. P.R.C. Nair., Menon T.V., Vijayan N.P., Prabhakaran V.A.: A Comparative Study of Patolatriphaladi and Panchatiktaka Kwatha Yogas in the Treatment of Pama.: *JRAS*:XII:3-4:1991.

24. Ananadan, Sivanandam G., Suresh, Veluchamy G.: Clinical Trials of Certain Siddha Drugs in Padarthamarai (Dermatophycosis): *JRAS*:XII:3-4:1991.

25. Sivaprakasam K., Kalavathy K. Rao, Yashoda R., Veluchamy G.: Effect of Kandankathiri in the Management of Venkuttam (Vitiligo): *JRAS*: XII: 3-4:1991.

26. Das U.K., Pandey P.N.: Therapeutic Assessment of Shakhotaka Ghanavati on Slipada (Filariasis) *JRAS*:XI:1-4:1990.

27. Sharma P.C., Mehandale V.V., Yelne M.B.,: Kocha (Lepidagathes cristata Willd.) A Traditional Drug for Measles: *JRAS*:XI:1-4:1990.

28. Sivaprakasam K., Yashoda R., Anandan T., Kalavathy K. Rao, Veluchamy G.: *JRAS*:XI:1-4:1990. Screeing of Certain Siddha Drugs in Venkuttam (Vitiligo).

29. J. Sangeeta, Mahajana R., Sharma J.M.: A Study of Amragandhi Haridra in Kandu: *Ayu. Samachar*:13:12:1991.

30. Mishra P.K.: Dermin Pulv-A Herbal Preparation Useful in Kushtha (Skin Diseases), *Ibid.*

31. Unnikrishnan, Sharma J.M.: Preliminary In Vitro Study on Asavatha and Udumbara in Certain Skin Pathogenic Microorganisms: *Ibid.*

32. Sharma B.P., Ojha D.: Indigenous Drugs Compound in the Management of Vitiligo (Shvitra): *Ibid.*

33. Das B., Joshi D.: Pathogenesis and Management of Kushta with Special Reference to Rasousadhi: *Ibid.*

34. Swain M., Mistry I.: Management of Ksudra Kushta (Pama, Dadru, Vicarika) with Related to Female Genital Organ: *Ayu. Samachar*:14:2:1991.

35. Mirani K.J., Vaidya A.R., Mistry I.U., Shastry M.S.: A Study of Anti Sidhmakushta Actions of Nimba in Accordance with Pathogenesis of Kushtha: *Ayu. Samachar.*14:4:1991.
36. Biswas T.K.: A Clinical Evaluation of the effect of Tuvaraka (Hydnocarpus castanea) Triil in Vicharchika: *Ayu. Samachar: Ibid.*
37. Bhatt K., Anadkat H.: Study of Ksudra Kushta with Its Management by Rasamanikya: *Ayu. Samachar:* 14:9:1992.
38. Andharia M.J., Kasavan M., Mistry I.U., Shastry M.S.: The Aetiopathological Study of Vicharchika and its Management with Special Reference to Nimbadi Quatha: *Ayu. Samachar.* 14:10:1992.
39. Babu A.S., Jinde J., Sankarankutty: Kshudra Kusta-Clinical Research with Special Reference to Psoriasis: *Ayu. Samachar.* 14:12:1992.
40. Mamgain R.K., Mamgain P. (Mrs)., Ojha D.: Shvitra (Vitiligo) and Its Ayurvedic Management: *Ayu. Samachar.* 15:1:1992.
41. Medh K.G., Dahiya J., Baghel M.S., Singh G.: Management of Shvitra with Certain Ayurvedic Compounds: *Ayu. Samachar. Ibid.*
42. Sharma P., Sharma N.P.: A Short Discourse of the Body Colours: *Ibid.*
43. Vyas P.P., Mistry I.U., Desai K.R.: A Clinical Study on the Role of Vaman and Virechan in the Management of Ksudra Kushtha: *Ibid.*
44. Sharma P., Sharma N.P.: A Brief Discussion on Savarikarana Drugs-Varnya Dravyas: *Ibid.*
45. Chaudhury S., Hajra S.K., Saha B., Mazumder V.: New Multidrug Regimen with Indigenous Drugs and Dapsone in Treatment of Lepromatous Leprosy: *Ayu. Samachar.* 15:2:1992.
46. Gandhi D.B., Chhaya M.K., Yeriswamy H., Sharma H.S.: Efficacy of Rasa Karpura in Kshudra Kustha with Special Reference to Vicarcika: *Ibid.*
47. Sharma P., Sharma N., Mukherjee P., Ghosh S.: Herbs for Hair Care Pharmacognosy and Phytochemistry of Amalaki and Henna: *Ayu. Samachar.* 15:3:1992.
48. Kumar P., Ojha D.: Critical Appraisal of Khalitya vis-a-vis Alopecia areata: *Ayu. Samachar.* 16:2:1993.
49. Paranjpe P., Kulkarani P.H.: Treatment of Acne Vulgaris—A Randomised Clinical Evaluation with Combinations: *NIMA*: XXXV: 11: 1993.
50. Paranjpe P.: Clinical Evaluation of Mahamanjishtadi Quath and Sookshma Triphala in the Management of Acne Vulgaris: *NIMA*: XXXVII: 10:1995.

2

NEUROLOGY AND RHEUMATOLOGY

CONNECTIVE TISSUE (COLLAGEN) DISEASES

The connective tissue disorders are a protean group of acquired diseases in which genetic factors appear to play a role. They have in common widespread immunologic and inflammatory alterations of connective tissue. A variety of other names have been given to the groups (e.g., collagen diseases, collagenoses, diffuse vascular diseases, collagen vascular diseases, visceral angitides), but no completely satisfactory term has been found. This group of acquired diseases must be distinguished from rare heritable disorders of connective tissue.

The acquired connective tissue diseases generally include the following clinical entities: rheumatoid arthritis, systemic lupus erythematosus, polymyositis, scleroderma, necrotizing vasculitis, rheumatic fever, mixed connective tissue disease, relapsing polychondritis, and Sjogren's syndrome.

These entities have certain features in common, and differentiation among them is often difficult because of overlapping features. Common findings include synovitis, pleuritis, myocarditis, endocarditis, pericarditis, peritonitis, vasculits, myositis, changes in skin, alterations of connective tissues, and, in some cases, nephritis. Laboratory tests may reveal Coombs-positive hemolytic anaemia, thrombocytopenia, leukopenia, B and T cell alterations, immunoglobulin excesses or deficiencies, impaired or accentuated delayed hypersensitivity, antinuclear antibodies, antibodies to DNA and ENA (extractable nuclear antigen), rheumatoid factors, cryoglobulins, false-positive serologic tests for syphilis, elevated muscle enzymes, antithyroid antibodies, alterations in serum complement, and changes in acute phase reactants.

Although the connective disorders are regarded as acquired diseases, the underlying causes cannot be determined in most instances, and it is unlikely that the established clinical entities have similar causes. Heredity, infection or other environmental antigen, immunoglobulin deficiency or inappropriated control (T cells), drug allergy, antigen-antibody-complement immune complexes, anaphylaxis, cytolysis, or some combination of all of these factors appear to play varying undefined roles. Investigations into the etiologic role of viruses appear promising.

Some of the laboratory alterations that occur in this group of disease (e.g. false-positive serologic tests for syphilis) may also occur in asymptomatic individuals and may suggest the possibility of the presence of or future development of one of the connective tissue diseases. It is interesting to note also that these alterations in laboratory values may be demonstrated in certain asymptomatic relatives of patients with connective tissue diseases, in older persons in association with certain drugs and infections, and in patients with abnormalities of the immune system.

RHEUMATIC DISEASES

Introduction

Rheumatic diseases have affected mankind since antiquity. Even the Dinosaurs who inhabited earth 100 million years ago their fossils have shown the evidence of arthritis. The Neanderthal man is considered to be the initial human being suffered from osteo-arthritis. Egyptian mummies estimated to be of 8,000 years old have also shown the evidence of arthritis. Obviously for such an age-old disease various remedies and cures must have been tried over the ages world over.

I believe the very initial, authentic, systemic and clearcut description of arthritis alongwith its logical management finds mention in Charaka Samhita which is estimated to be 600 years. B.C. Bhrugh has also described the synovial fluid and changes in arthritis. The major break through occurred in its understanding when Madhava in Madhava-Nidana described a separate entity Amavata. Later on Chakradatta first time illustrated the principle line of treatment for 'Amavata'. Later on Chkradatta first (Table 2.1) gives brief account of historical milestones in understanding of and treatment of Amavata.

If one searches for rheumatic diseases mentioned in Ayurvedic literature on the basis of clinical descriptions given in the ancient texts some of the names come forward which are given in (Table 2.2). In this table alongwith the Ayurvedic names of which share certain similarities. It would be unwise to find for the exact description of the diseases in ancient Ayurvedic literature which we understand today, since basic approach in understanding the disease is different. So also the nature of the disease gets modified over the period of years; however the hallmark of clinical presentations would remain same in whatever may one tries to understand a disease.

Etiopathogenesis

The rheumatic diseases are conditions in which pain and stiffness of some part of musculo skeletal system are prominent. These diseases can be grouped as inflammatory, metabolic and degenerative, on the bases of connective tissue pathology.

Inflammatory diseases of connective tissues are Rheumatoid arthritis and infective arthritis, spondyloarthritis, diffuse connective tissue diseases with multi-system organ pathology, systemic disturbance and immune disregulation diseases like systemic lupus erythematosus (S.L.E.), Progressive systemic sclerosis, polymyositis, dermato-myostis etc.

Metabolic disorders include crystal deposition diseases like Gout, Chondro-calcinosis etc.

Degenerative disorders are osteo-arthosis, spondylosis and a number of painful soft tissue syndromes etc.

Most of the conditions or diseases mentioned above, can be included under 'Amavata' according to Ayurveda. It is necessary to explain the meaning and application of both the terms i.e. Ama and Vata.

Vata: The proof of life are (1) movement, (2) Heat and metabolism and (3) Protoplasm or matter. These three are represented by the term Vata, Pitta and Kapha i.e. three doshas or Tridoshas. From multicellular animal like an elephant and in any cell, tissues, organs, system to a combination of many systems i.e. in the human body, these three (i.e. movement, heat or metabolism and protoplasm or matter or in other words Vata, Pitta and Kapha) are present. These three work in coordination and cooperation. If any of these three are disturbed, the matter, functionally and structurally will be disturbed, resulting into disease, decay, degeneration or death. In the disease Amavata, Vata is predominantly disturbed.

Tridoshas have certain special sthanas (areas or organs or parts) where their special function is more marked. Thus there are Vata-sthanas, Pitta-sthanas and Kapha-sthanas.

These three are further divided according to their special functions e.g. in G.I. Tract, Vata will produce peristaltic and swaying movement. This vata is called 'Saman Vayu.' In excretory organs i.e. rectum, urinary system, uterus, vagina their special function is excretion i.e. to expel out. This is called Apan Vayu. In Heart, the special function is contraction and expansion, producing circulation of Rasa (Plasma) and blood (R.B.C., W.B.C., Platelets) and O_2. This is performed by Vyana Vayu. The air exchange in the respiratory tract and production of sound specially alphabets etc. are due to udana vayu and the ultimate control of all these vayus lies with the brain. This vayu is called 'Prana Vayu.' The movement of joints etc. are also due to Vayu. This movement is disturbed due to the obstruction, decay or degeneration; it is called vata vyadhi which is a type of Rheumatic disorder.

Due to the length of the subject, other doshas are not described. This is enough to understand rheumatic disorders.

Ama: The concept of Ama is the most important and fundamental principle in understanding the physio-pathology of most of the diseases and specially Amavata.

'Ama' is an accumulation of unutilized, unmetabolized, undigested material or some foreign material which can neither be digested, utilized nor metabolized. The body has a capacity to aclimatize even the changes in weather. But when these two i.e. digestion and metabolism is poor or aclimatization cannot properly take place, some foreign material is accumulated. This accumulation is called Ama.

There are mainly 3 types of Ama viz. (1) Ama annarasa (untransformed food material) at the gastro-intestinal level, (2) Mala-Sanchaya (accumulation of metabolic waste) and (3) Prathama dosha-dusti (sudden vitiation of dosha due to extrinsic factors).

Properties of Ama—Ama is avipakwa (undigested,), Asanyukta (not well formed) i.e. it may be unformed or very sticky and greasy or mucoid in nature, durgandhi having some types of unpleasant odour; when such thing collects in the body it produces looseness of body.

Thus even hypercholesterolemia, hypergycemia, hyperuria, hypertriglyceridemia and all the biochemical values when in the excess and cannot be utilized for the body functions are called Ama.

The product of digestion and metabolism is generally utilized or excreted out. But if this type of foreign body cannot be utilized or excreted, they remain in the body and vitiate the body tissue mechanism. The tissues lose their structural or functional integrity. The immune mechanism become disturbed, resulting in any type of connective tissue disorders like RA, S.L.E. or systemic sclerosis.

The present day understanding of rheumatic disorders is altered immune response and persistent Antigenic stimulation. In the same way S.L.E. is a multisystem tissue disease characterised by the presence of numerous autoantibodies, circulating immune complexes and widespread immunologically determined tissue damage.

Progressive systemic sclerosis is characterized by fibrosis and degenerative changes in the skin (scleroderma) and many internal organs. It is believed to be one end of the spectrum of connective tissue diseases where immunologically determined inflammation is followed by thickening of small blood vessels and excessive production and cross-lining of collagen.

From the above pathology process, it will be clear that Sanchaya (accumulation) of immune bodies leads to various types of connective tissue disorders. The body requires a certain quantity of immune antibodies. The excess should be excreted out or utilized; but if they cannot be excreted or utilized, they are deposited in tissues resulting in destruction of tissues and replacement by immune bodies.

Ayurveda says

The tridoshas when they are normal in quantity, quality and function serve as Dhatu i.e. they support the body; when slightly vitiated, they serve as Doshas (Vitiators) and when they excessively vitiate they are termed as 'Malas.' The immune bodies, when normal in quantity, quality and function support the body, but when in excess or less they produce disease.

Thus the immune complexes serve as Ama. That is the reason why majority of diseases of connective tissue are to be treated like 'Ama-Vata.'

In metabolic disorders like gout, chondrocalcinosis and such other disorders, crystal deposition takes place. In gout mono-sodium urate monohydrate derived from hyperuricaemic body fluids give rise to inflammatory arthritis, tenosinovitis, bursitis, cellulitis, urolithiasis and renal diseases. Diminished renal excretion of uric acid is a major problem. It may be genetic predisposition or aquired due to faulty diet and exercise. Specific enzyme defects resulting in an increase in purine synthesis should be suspected.

In these diseases also, the pitta (enzyme) required for utilization of uric acid, produced by faulty diet and sedentary habits, is either diminished or not up to the standard required to utilize or excrete uric acid, resulting in deposition.

This type of mala sanchaya i.e. accumulation of excessive uric acid is called 'Ama' i.e. undigested, untransformed material. The cause is 'Agnimandya' i.e. weakness of digestive and metabolic enzymes.

Mala: The body elements are briefly of two kinds (Prasada Bhutha) (useful to the body or beneficial) and Mool Bhutha (impure). They are malaboota which are harmful to the body. The uric acid, in normal quantity is useful to the body. Thus normal value of uric acid is Prasada bhoota or beneficial, and excess is harmful. These mala boota materials are excretas issuing outwards from the orifices of the body in various forms; purescent body elements (Dhatvas) 'vitiated Vata, Pita and Kapha and also such other materials or properties (Bhav) which tend to injure (upadhaya) the body.' The excess of uric acid in hyperurecaemia or gout, or C.P.P.D (Calcium pyrophosphate deposition) in chondrocalcinosis, or copper deposition, all these fall under the group of Malasanchaya or Amadhosh.

It can from the above discussion, be inferred that:

1. Ama is undigested and unmetabolized product produced by the weakness of digestive and metabolic enzymes (Agnimandh)
2. Ama is also called waste matter which should be removed from the body.
3. If Ama mala remains continuously in the body, it is likely to hurt (Aabadhkar) the body.
4. Ama is stickly (pichil) in nature.
5. The excess of collagen materials, immune bodies or crystals like uric acid, are to be considered as Ama.
6. Ama when mixes or reacts with Vata, produces stiffness of joint, Atheroscelerosis, deposition and dryness in the body tissue e.g. Sl E or Scleroderma or Sclerosis.
7. The external manifestation for which patient consults a doctor is stiffness and pain in the body specially joint pain and swelling and muscular pain etc.

Madhava has comprehensively described the etiopathogenesis of 'Amavata.' He says 'A person having inherent suboptimal digestive capacity when exposed to contradict ory diet and physical activities "Ama" is produced.' The Ama gets

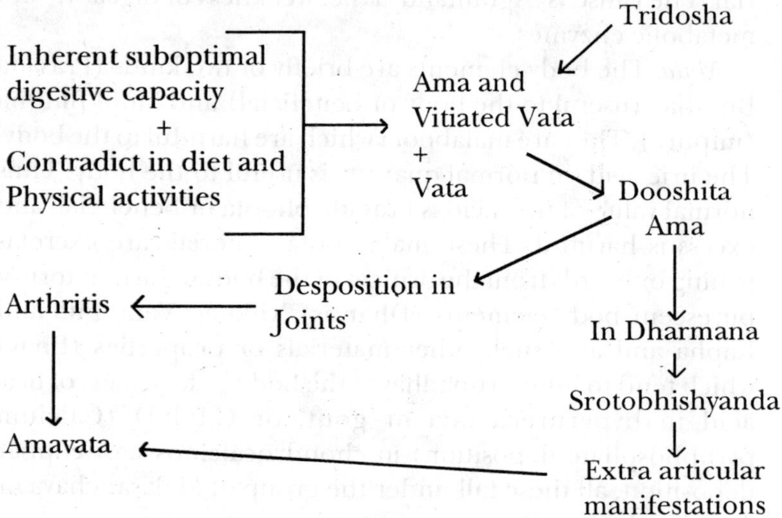

Fig. 2.1. Pathogenesis of Amavata

further vitiated by 'tridoshas' and leads to the formation of 'dooshita Ama'; this vitiated 'Ama and Vata' simultaneously get deposited in joint spaces and produce 'Amavata.' Dooshita Ama in Dhamani due to 'Srotobhishyanda' also leads to extra articular manifestations of the disease (Figure 2.1). It is obvious from the above description that in 'Ama' Srotobhishyanda Virechana (Purgation), Snehapana (oleation) and Basti (medicated enemas) are employed to alleviate and control the vitiated vata.

Besides above therapy 'Rasayana therapy' is recommended for complete remission of disease and prevention of relapse.

Table 2.1: *Milestones in Understanding and Treatment of Amavata*

Text	*Chapter*	*Period*
Charaka Samhita	Chikitsasthana Vatavyadhi	600 B.C.
Madhava Nidana	Amavatanidana Adhyaya	700 A.D.
Chakradatta	Amavata Chikitsa Adhyaya	Eleventh Century
Rasaratna Samucchaya	Vatavyadhi Chikista	Thirteenth Century
Bhavaprakash	Uttaratantra	Sixteenth Century
Bhaijshajya Ratnavali	Amavata Chikitsa	Seventeenth Century
Yogaratnakar	Amavata Chikitsa	Eighteenth Century

Table 2.2: *Rheumatic Disorders in Ayurvedic Literature*

Sandhigat Vaata Niram	Osteoarthritis degenerative
Sandhigat Vaata Miraam Saam	Osteoarthritis inflammatory
Vaatrakt Vuthaan	SLE? Scleroderma, MCTD
Vaatrakt Gambhir	Crystal induced arthritis
Amavaat	Rheumatid disease
Avabhajuk	Frozen shoulder
Krosh Kasheersh	Infective Arthritis
Sandhigat Jwar	Rheumatic fever
Grudhsi	Sciatic neuralgia
Vishwasichi	Brachial neuralgia
Snugthvaath	Ebtgesioaty
Mamsgathvaath	Fibromyalgia

Management

Line of treatment in most of the cases of connective tissue disorders are:

In first stage removal of Ama. Ama can be removed in the following way according to Ayurveda.

The drugs having Tikta, Katu rasa, (i.e. bitter and pungent taste) and deepaniya property (enhancing digestive ability) will get rid of 'Ama.' Langhana (Fasting) and swedana (sudation) (digestive ability) Virechana (Purgation), Snehapana (oleation) and Basti (medicated enemas) are employed to alleviate and control the 'vitiated vata.'

Besides above therapy 'Rasayana therapy' is recommended for complete remission of disease and prevention or relapse.

Langhana

Ten types of langhana are described in the text. Here the types of langhana undertaken for therapeutic purpose is 'Upavasa-Kshudha Nivrutti.' It has been amply demonstrated by number of short term studies that fasting is beneficial in arthritis and it does reduce subjective as well as objective indices of disease activity. In many patients with rheumatoid arthritis, ironically it is usually observed that following withdrawal of fasting, continuation of response is not maintained. At this junction, application of Ayurvedic concepts of 'Sansarjana Karma' and 'Pathyaapathya' may help to overcome the problem. In this strategy following fasting, regular diet is reintroduced gradually from liquid to solid viz. Yusha, Manda, Peya, Vilepi, Yvagu and Odana. This reintroduction is further fine tuned by incorporating certain dietary articles which have therapeutic potential and may have possible insulating role (Apathya). We have noted in our study survey that community has a strong belief and experiences that certain diet articles play a role in the management of arthritis. Case studies have been reported in the literature where food articles have been demonstrated as the main culprit in the induction of arthritis.

It means that langhana is the treatment of choice. Langhana means either absolute fasting or light diet. It may be clear in the minds of both, Ayurvedic and modern physicians that both sciences believe in digestion and nutrition. The modern medical science lays more emphasis on nutrition than digestion. While Ayurvedic science lays more emphasis on digestion than nutrition. The body has got the innate capacity to the best use of all materials including waster matter. It is the duty of the physician to help the body in its such beneficial work. Langhana (fasting) or less quantity of food (Laghu aahar) tries to utilize the excess of biochemical substances like uric acid, sugar urea etc. and also the excess of collagen substances, immunological substances and other substances.

The plan of langhana may be as under but can be changed according to Desha and Kala (Patient and Season).

For the first five days a very small quantity of double boiled rice and Thin mung (green grams) soup.

Next five days 1 roti morning and evening can be added.

Then every five days a small quantity of food can be added.

Throughout these days no unctous material like ghee, oil, mutton should be given.

The above course can last for about a month or so. This increases the digestive and metabolic power: also this can utilise the excess or accumulated Ama. The body may become (Nirama) devoid of Ama.

Swedana

The process by which sweating is induced is called swedana. It relieves stiffness, heaviness and antagonises all sheeta properties.

Dry swedana is indicated in inflammatory joint diseases while in noninflammatory degenerative joint diseases other swedana procedures which include decoctions, poultice, oils shall be used. In non-articular diseases upanaha sweda or patra sweda is employed while in polyarticular diseases dhara sweda, parisheka sweda or avagah sweda is used. There are published reports about hydrotherapy and magneto otherapy which indicate objective improvement in some rheumatoid arthritis patients following this therapy. When medically processed water is used for such hydrotherapy (avagah sweda) it would have an added advantage.

Virechana Snehapanam

Eranda Sneha (Castor oil) avails a special reference in Ayurvedic text. It is said that 'An elephant like disease activity of Amavata can be controlled only with lion like castor oil.' There are many encouraging clinical studies on or role of castor oil in rheumatoid arthritis. The major drawback of this drug is its unpatability but with advancement in pharmaceutical techniques we should be able to overcome it.

Basti

Basti means medicated enemas. Basti chikitsa has been elaborately described in Ayurvedic literature. It is considered as an important therapeutic modality particularly for 'Vata diseases.' There are various types of bastis depending on the retention time. Types of fluid used and duration of retention is an important pathogenetic factor. To alleviate this vitiated vata and get complete control over vata dosha basti chikitsa is very much beneficial.

For excretion purpose a small quantity (10 to 15 ml) of castor oil with ginger juice or decoction of dry ginger should be given early morning on empty stomach daily. Throughout, bitter digestive substances like cheratta can be given. This is the treatment in Ama stage.

By this treatment, there is likelihood of some weight loss but there is no need of worry. The body becomes light, the digestion improves. The body channels (srotham) open with the nutrious material (ras) and the malas (metabolic by-products) etc. are properly exchanged. The nutrients are well utilized. And overall the accumulation of Ama doshas (collagen excess immune bodies and certain excess biochemical substances are reduced utilized or excreted. The stiffness and pain are reduced to a great extent.

After about a month treatment, ghee, better medicated, may be started. The advantage of ghee is certain fat soluble substances are dissolved and they are properly excreted.

Side by side Basti (enemata) be started. There are two types of bastis (1) Anuvasana or Basti with oil and (2) Asthapana (with decoction). The maximum period of Basti is 1 month. There are 3 types of Bastis according to the number of Bastis (1) Kala (2) Yoga and (3) Karama. It is better to treat with Basti for a month i.e. 30 in number.

After a period of break, the same above treatment should be started. Thus the treatment last for about two years.

Once the acute inflammatory condition, has subsided exercise should be started. In the beginning passive movement and afterwards active movement should be started to minimise or avert permanent joint and muscular changes. For the active movement two methods are suggested (1) Oil massage and sweda (fomentation) both together and (2) Yoga-asanas. Both the treatment are necessary. The patient should be trained by a proper Yoga teacher. I always teach the patients some type of light yoga exercises e.g. 'Uttana-ada-asana' (lifting the legs straight). Then Pavana-muktaasana (folding of feet from position) and Shalabhaasana. Then Padmasana (Lotus position), Matsyaasana. Then Bhujangaasana (snake position) and Shalabhaasana. Then Padma sana (Lotus position) and last 'Shavasana' (lying down with loose body like dead man). By these asanas (Yogic positions), permanent deformities can be averted or minimised to a very great extent.

Tikta Deepana Katu

The drugs having tikta-katu rasa, deepaniya-guna and amavataghna karma are indicated to be useful in 'Amavata.'

In our preliminary survey of Ayurvedic literature it was found that various types of preparations are recommended for rheumatic disorders. These are on various types like powders, decoctions, pills, medicated confectionaries, medicated ghee, oils, etc. Most of them are for internal use and few are for external use. It is apparent that many of these formulations are composed of multiple ingredients. It seems that these are composed with the aim of having the site of action at all levels of pathogenetic mechanisms having the actions of amapachana, vatashamana, srotoshaodahana and rasayana. To quote a few commonly used formulations—Yogaraja- gugullu, Rasnadi kwath, Ajmodadi choorna, Amritbhallatak, Vatavidhvansa rasa etc. for internal use while Vishagarbaha taila, Lepa guti, Nirugundi taila, etc. are recommended for external use.

In our study of Yogaraj guggulu in rheumatoid arthritis diseases activity was controlled in more than 50 per cent of cases with Yogaraj guggulu alone. In one of the major study at Banaras Hindu University of 'Àmritbhallatak' has shown very encouraging results in diseases like rheumatoid arthritis, osteoarthritis and sciatica).

Drugs

1. Guggulu is a drug of choice. Yogarajaguggulu, Mahayogaraja guggulu with gold are drugs of choice. If there is urinary trouble Gokshuradi guggulu and Chandraprabhavati are the drugs of choice. In lymphadenopathy, Kanchanar guggulu can be prescribed. If associated with heart disease Pushkarmoolaguggulu should be prescribed. All these drugs are from ancient Ayurveda literature. Certain proprietory preparation are also available in the market.
2. Agni-Tundic vati is another drug of choice.
3. Ashwagandha, chopachini, rasna, lashuma, methi, pippalimoola, yastimadhu can be given single or in mixture form.

Rasa Preparations: Certain Rasa preparations are also prescribed. They are Mahavatvidhavansa rasa, Vatagajankush rasa, Vatakulantaka rasa, Brihadvatachintamani rasa. These drugs contain Mercury, Sulphur and certain metals. Parad (mercury) is considered as Yoga-vahi i.e. activator of the properties.

There are two types of mercurial preparations viz. (1) Nirghandha (not containing sulphur) and (2) Sagandha (containing sulphur). The sagandha preparations are not at all harmful. Not only this, it activates the other drug preparations. So they can freely be used in proper dose and at proper time. The criticism for Rasa preparations is not based on copying the modern and for proving one's own superiority without understanding.

In conclusion, it may be said that many Rheumatoid arthritis patients are treated by Ayurvedic method successfully by the Ayurvedic physicians. Even S.L.E. and Systemic Sclerosis cases have also been relieved by Ayurvedic treatment. The necessity for the Ayurvedic physician is to keep proper records, follow up etc. according to both the sciences i.e. Ayurvedic and modern and proper canvassing of Ayurvedic. Of course proper understanding is highly necessary.

The idea is to relieve the patient from ailing may be by any method. The unscientific criticism should be totally condemned.

(Abstracts from: Shukla C.P.: A*mavata (Rheumatic Disorders and Diseases of Connective Tissues;* Raut A.A.: *Management of Rheumatic Diseases-Ayurvedic Concepts: NIMA*:XXXVIII:1:1996).

RHEUMATOID ARTHRITIS (AMAVATA)

Essential Features

1. A systemic disease.
2. *Aetiology*: Not defined.
3. *Ayurveda*: Causative factor—Ama; Predisposing factor—Viruddha ahara, viruddha chesta, mandagni, nischesta, snigdha bhojana with vyayama.
4. *Pathogenesis*: A chronic systemic inflammatory disease, chiefly affecting synovial membranes of multiple joints with involvement of connective tissues (collagen tissue) locally and systemically. Ayurveda: Production of Ama,

Srotobhishyanda and vitiated vata are main factors of pathogenesis.

5. *Prodromal symptoms*: Malaise, fever, weight loss, and morning stiffness.
6. *Onset*: Usually insiduous and in small joints; progression is centripetal and symmetric; deformities common.
7. *X-ray findings*: Juxta-articular osteoporosis, joint erosions, and narrowing of the joints spaces.
8. Rheumatoid factor test usually positive.
9. *Extra-articular manifestations*: Vasculitis, atrophy of muscle, subcutaneous and systemic nodules (granulomae), pleurisy, pericarditis, pulmonary fibrosis, lymphadenopathy, splenomegaly, and leukopenia.
10. *Differential diagnosis*: Difficult often. Clinically can be differentiated from—Rheumatic fever, Systemic lupus erythematosus, Degenerative joint disease (osteoarthritis), Gouty arthrits, Pyogenic arthritis.
11. *Management*: Often unsatisfactory; prolonged therapy with variable results.
12. *Prognosis*: Totally unpredictable, although spontaneous remissions and relapses are common early in the disease. Although the disease is commonly progressive and some degree of permanent deformity may result—it must be emphasized that after 10 years, half of the patients are still capable of self-care and fully employable.

Management

Management depends upon the pathogenesis (Samprapti) of the disease. The aim of Ayurvedic treatment is not only the radical removal of those causative factors, but also the restoration of the doshic homeostasis. Various measures to treat the disease Amavata have been described in all the available Ayurvedic literature. The measures applied for the management of Amavata may be summarised as follows:

1. Measures to stop the formation of Ama.
2. Measures to digest or excrete already formed Ama.
3. Measures to clean the srotas and to improve digestion.

4. Measures to pacify vata dosha, and
5. Measures to prevent the disease.

According to the concept of etiopathogenesis in Ayurveda, the disease is caused by hypofunctioning of the gastro-intestinal system (Madhava, 1960). The treatment of this disease in Ayurveda is based largely on the improvement of the functioning of gastro-intestinal system (Yogaratnakara, 1955). In recent years, a number of clinical and experimental studies have demonstrated efficacy of the Ayurvedic treatment (Desai, 1964, Kishore et al, 1980, Kishore and Tripathi, 1966; Tripathi and Kishore, 1967.) The observations also demonstrated the hypo-functioning of gastro-intestinal system by way of diminished gastric acid secretion, deranged liver functioning and impaired intestinal absorption (Tripathi and Kishore, 1966; Shatin, 1967). The treatment with drugs having gastro-intestinal stimulant effect has also showed an improvement (Kishore and Tripathi, 1966; Kishore 1980). The modern treatment of this disease is only non-specific due to the lack of precise knowledge of the process of the disease and its etiology. The available treatment is attended with many side effects.

Considering the efficacy of the Ayurvedic treatment of this disease, and the absence of any specific modern medical treatment, the Ayurvedic system of treatment offers immense potential. However, these treatments need standardisation through clinical trials. Evolution of certain new treatments is also necessary.

Clinical Reports

Role of Sunthi-Guduci in the Treatment of Amavata-Rheumatoid Arthritis (Prem Kishore, P.N. Pandey, S.D. Ruhil, *J.R.A.S.* 1: 3: 1980).

Considering the powerful gastro-intestinal stimulant action and its extensive mention for the treatment of Amavata in various forms, Sunthi (Latin. Zingiber officinale) has been taken up for trial. The other drug Guduci (Lat. Tinospora cordifolia) has also been recommended for the treatment of joint diseases. Roth these drugs have been recommended in the form of decoction for the treatment of Amavata (Yoga Ratnakara). In order to have a comparative assessment of its efficacy another group of patients have been treated with a combination of Yograja-guggulu, Vata-Gajankusha Rasa and Maharasnadi Kvatha, commonly prescribed by Ayurvedic physicians. It may also provide an opportunity to assess the relative efficacy of treatment primarily based on correction of gastro-intestinal function and other approach.

A total number of 77 patients have been taken up in two groups for trial on the basis of following signs and symptoms: 1. Morning stiffness; 2. Pain on motion; 3. Painful swelling of atleast one joint; 4. Tenderness; 5. Painful swelling of more than one joint; 6. Symmetrical joint involvement.

All the patients have been subjected to thorough clinical investigation including routine pathological examination, blood, stool and urine. The gradation of function and stage of disease has also been taken up. The patients suffering from other joint diseases have been excluded from the study.

Drug Administration

The following drugs have been administered daily to both the groups for a period of 6-8 weeks.

Group A (40 patients)

Yogaraja Guggulu—1 gm. thrice
Vatagajankusha Rasa—250 mg thrice
Maharasanadi Kvatha—50 ml thrice

Group B (37 patients)

Sunthi Guduchi Kvatha—50 ml thrice

In both the groups Baluk Sweda, Doshagna or Dasanga lepa, Virechana with Ichhabhedi Rasa, Snehana with Ghrita and Matravasti with Eranda Taila and Dasamula Kvatha is given according to Amavastha and Niraamavastha. Apart from routine course of treatment, certain symptomatic treatment was also given according to the needs.

Diet

All the patients in both groups have been prescribed diet as per schedule given below:

Breakfast: Suji 55 gm; Onion 5 gm.; Oil 6 ml.;
Lunch: Rice 250 gm.; Dal 45 gm.; Vegetable 200 gm.;
Evening: Milk 150 ml.; Sugar 15 gm.;
Dinner: Atta 250 gm.; Dal 25 gm.; Vegetable 250 gm.

Classification of Results

On the basis of clinical features, ESR and functional tests, the results have been classified under following categories.

Complete relief—No pain or sign of joint inflammation. No remaining impairment of joint immobility other than that associated with irreversible change.

Partial relief—Major signs of inflammation resolved; movement of the joint improved but not fully.

No improvement—The patients did not respond for the treatment at all.

Drop out—The patient left the treatment during the course of study.

The patients were followed up for a period of one year periodically.

Results

The reduction in pain and swelling of joints have been noted in 1-2 weeks which gradually subsided in 5-6 weeks of treatment and in the patients who have been completely relieved. The functional capacity of the patients also improved gradually and became normal except those due to irreversible changes. With the beginning of Niramavastha the patients have been prescribed Sodhan chikitsa consisting of Snehana, Virechana and Vasti. The ESR was reduced to normal range where it was increased. The patients who have shown partial relief did not fully recover though substantial reduction of pain and swelling has been noted.

The treatment of both the groups showed clinical efficacy. However, the treatment of Group B Sunthi-Guduchi Kvatha has shown better effect than treatment of Group A Yogaraja Guggulu, Vata Gajankusha Rasa and Maha Rasnadi Quath.

Though the percentage of complete relief has been equal in both groups, but relatively more percentage of patients have been classified as partially relieved with Group B treatment. The percentage of 'no relief' has also been comparatively less in the patients of Group B.

Though all patients did not report for follow up, yet many of them who reported did not show any reoccurrence for over 2 years.

Discussion

The observations shows that the disease affects males more frequently than females and is more common in the age range of 21-30 years. The type of cases included confirm to previous observations and are more or less evenly distributed in either groups.

The results show relatively better efficacy of Sunthi Guduchi Quath. The action of Sunthi Guduchi Quath may be due to potent Deepano-Paachana and Vata Shamaka effects of these drugs. Sunthi has been specifically recommended for Amapachana and treatment of Amavata. It is also used for the treatment of Agni-Dosa, Grahani Dosa, the root cause of the disease. Its clinical efficacy has been demonstrated in the patients of Grahani Roga. Guduchi has also been considered as a best Dipana and Vibandha Prasamana drugs, in addition to its possessing Vatahara and Vatasamaka effects (Charaka). This drug has also demonstrated anti-inflammatory, antipyretic and analgesic effects. Recent clinical trials of the drug in rheumatoid arthritis has also shown significant effect.

The other set of treatment Yogaraja Guggulu, Vata Gajankusha Rasa and Maharasnadi Kvatha has been mentioned in Ayurvedic treatment and has been evolved on the basis of long experience. Relatively better efficacy was observed with Sunthi Guduchi which may perhaps be attributable to their potent effect on the impaired gastro-intestinal function, which is the root causes of the disease.

These observations give definite lead to the evolution and practice of such simple prescriptions which have been discussed in classics. The futility of poly-therapy involving many compound formulations is also demonstrated. Such prescriptions may also be helpful in providing primary medicare by way of self-medication since these drugs are commonly available everywhere.

Clinical Studies on the Treatment of Amavata-Rheumatoid Arthritis with Sunthi-Guggulu: Prem Kishore, K.V. Devi Das and S. Banerjee (*JRAS*: III: 3&4: 1982).

Efforts have been made to assess the clinical efficacy of Sunthi-Guggulu in the treatment of this disease in relation to the prevalent set of medicines consisting of Yogaraja Guggulu, Vata Gajankusha Rasa, Amavatari Rasa and Maharasnadi Kvatha. The observations on 63 patients indicate that the disease is more prevalent in the age group of eleven to forty years; and males suffer from it more than females. The results indicate better effects of Sunthi-Guggulu as compared to the other set of medicines taken up for trial.

Drug Administration

The patients were given two sets of treatment for six weeks as per details given below:

Group A (36 patients):

Sunthi—Rhizome (Zingiber officinalis)—1 gm
Guggulu—Purified resin of Commiphora
Mukul—1 gm
} 1 × 3

Group B (27 Patients):

Yogaraja Guggulu—1 gm
Amavata Rasa or Vatagajankusha Rasa—0.5 gm
Maharasnadi Kvatha—25 ml
} 1 × 3

The drug has been given in powder form. External application of Doshagna lepa and Baluka Sweda has also been made on the affected parts. Apart from the routine course of treatment, the symptomatic treatment was also given according to the needs.

Diet

See under Section I above (P. Kishore et al).

Further Clinical Evaluation of Sunthi-Guggulu in the Treatment of Amavata-Rheumatoid Arthritis: P.Kishore and M.M. Padhi. (*JRAS*:IX:3-4:1988).

Sunthi-Guggulu combination has already demonstrated its efficacy in the treatment of Amavata in early studies (see above). Therefore, further studies have been undertaken on more specific and quantifiable parameters for diagnosis and assessment of the effect. A score system with the maximum 100 points have been evolved on the basis of various objective and subjective findings. The observations on 50 patients demonstrated cardinal clinical features of the disease—pain, swelling, tenderness, muscle weakness, restriction of joint movement and morning stiffness in all the patients. A substantial number of patients were also having manifestations of gastro-intestinal dysfunctions. The ankle, knee, wrist, elbow and the smaller joints of the hands and feet were most frequently affected. Most of the patients were suffering with moderate severity (50-74 per cent) while remaining were suffering from very severity of the disease.

The effect of the treatment assessed separately on each of the cardinal clinical manifestations of the disease shows significant effect on them since about 80 per cent of these patients who completed the full course of treatment got relief. The associated gastro-intestinal symptoms were also relieved to a great extent. The functional ability of the patients have also shown significant improvement. The overall effect of treatment is very obvious since about 80 per cent of the patients who completed full course of treatment showed either marked relief or complete relief. These observations further confirmed the efficacy of the drug and its possible effect on dissolution of the Pathogenesis.

Treatment

1. *Drug, dose, vehicle and duration of treatment:* Sunthi-Guggulu (fine powder of Zingiber officinale dry mixed well with purified resin of Commiphora mukul in equal proportion) in the doses of 4 gm. thrice daily was prescribed with warm water for a period of 6 weeks. The patients were also prescribed Baluka sweda during the course of treatment.

2. *Diet:* Mixed diet consisting of Upma/loaf and milk in breakfast; rice, dal, vegetable curry in lunch and roti, dal vegetable and milk in the dinner was prescribed throughout the course of treatment.

Results of the Treatment

The treatment showed gradual effect within 1-2 weeks of treatment and substantial relief in most of the patients who completed the full course of treatment. The effect of the treatment on each of the cardinal features has been tested. The effect of the treatment as per overall score of the severity of disease has been found to be statistically significant. There has been a reduction of ESR in those patients who showed an increase in levels in the beginning. The effect of treatment in relation to chronicity and age of the patient did not show any uniform relationship.

No side or toxic effect was observed in any of the cases.

It may be seen that the present study has been able to conclusively demonstrate the efficacy of the combination Sunthi-Guggulu in the treatment of Amavata—rheumatoid arthritis, on quantifiable parameters. The study also provides therapeutic evidence to the Ayurvedic concept of its etiopathogenesis. The mechanism of action of the preparation may possibly be attributed to the Guna and Rasa of the drugs of the combination which are opposite to the properties of the Dosa and Dushya of the disease.

Clinical Evaluation of Rasonadi Kvatha in the treatment of Amavata-Rheumatoid Arthritis: P. Kishore, and S.N. Banerjee (*JRAS*: IX: 1-2: 1988).

The observations on the effect of Rasonadi Kvatha—a combination of Rasona, Sunthi and Nirgundi in the patients of Amavata—Rheumatoid Arthritis (n=50) have been tested. The preparation has been selected on the basis of effect of its ingredients on Samprapti of Amavata. The ingredients have been individually recommended for treatment of rheumatic disease in general and Amavata—rheumatoid arthritis in particular. All these three drugs—Sunthi (dry ginger), Rasona (garlic), and Nirgundi (five leaved fomentory) are Kaphavata Samaka and Ama Pachana and their Sarira Gunas are appropriate to the Dosa and Dusya involved in the pathogenesis of this disease.

Treatment

The Rasonadi Kvatha has been administered in the dose of 25 ml three times a day for 6 weeks. The daily dosage of Kvatha represents 25 gms of each of the ingredients, the patients have also been prescribed external application of Dasanga or Doshagna lepa and Baluka sweda during acute inflammatory stage. The diet consisting of rice, chapati, dal, vegetable upama and milk has been provided to the patients during the six weeks trial period.

During acute exacerbation of pain, Pippalimoola Churna or Visatundika vati was administered for relief of pain. This was an open trial without control.

Results

The treatment with the preparation provided gradual relief in pain and swelling of the joints. The patients showed significant improvement of swelling and pain of the joints within 2-3 weeks of treatment though complete relief has taken further treatment whenever it has been achieved. There is reduction in E.S.R. and improvement in functional capacity of patient, with the improvement in reduction of pain, swelling and tenderness of the joints. The overall effect of the treatment is quite significant. Since almost all of the patients who completed the treatment were relieved though complete relief was observed only in 28 per cent of cases. The effect of treatment was directly related to chronicity. The treatment appears to be more effective in less chronic cases and relatively less effective in more chronic cases. The efficacy of drug compares well with the conventional approach to Ayurvedic treatment and newer preparations reported earlier. The easy availability of its ingredients is likely to make it more popular in practice.

The large dosage of the ingredients i.e. 25 gms. of each may also be responsible for the efficacy. The anti-inflammatory and anti-rheumatic and Kapha Vata Samaka effect of Nirgundi and Rasona may also contribute to the clinical efficacy. The drugs have also shown effect in treatment of Gridhrasi (Sciatica).

Clinical Study on the Treatment of Amavata with Compound Ayurvedic Preparation: M.N.S. Namboodiri, K.S. Sethu, P. Madhavankutty, N.P. Vijaya, and P.K.N. Namboodiri. (*JRAS*: V: 1-4: 1984).

The study was conducted on 83 patients in three groups. Analysis of the result showed that the disease can be controlled by Ayurvedic drugs like Dasamularishta, Pippalyasava and Vettumaran Gutika. Reduction of ESR values was highly significant in all the three groups.

The cases were investigated thoroughly and complete information pertaining to Ama lakshanas samanya and visesa lakshanas as described in Ayurveda was recorded in a pro forma and the progress noted daily, in addition to the standard symptom evaluation in modern medicine. Patients were divided into three groups randomly as given below and the drugs were administered. (Table 2.3)

Group I—Vachadi, Dasamoolarishta, Pippalyasava, Indukanta Ghrita, Dasamoolaksira

Group II—Haridadi, Vettumaran gutika, Shatpala Ghrita, Dasamoolaksira

Group III—Dasamoolarishta-Pippalyasava, Vettumaran gutika, Indukanta Ghrita, Dasamoolaksira.

Table 2.3

Medicines	*Reference*	*Dose*
A. Vachadi B. Haridadi	Churana as described in Ashtanga Hridaya	3 gm powder, 4 times a day with hot water.
C. Dasamularishta-Pippalyasava	As described in Sahasrayoga	20 ml 3-4 times a day
D. Vettumaran gutika	As in Sahasrayoga	1 pill 3-4 times a day
E. Shatpala ghrita	As in Ashtanga Hridaya	20 gm twice a day
F. Indukanta ghrita	As in Sahasrayoga	20 gm twice a day
G. Dasamoolaksira	As in Ashtanga Hridaya	100 ml twice a day.

Ghrita and Dasamoolaksira were given after the disappearance of Ama lakshanas such as srotorodha etc.

Result

20 per cent of the cases in group I, 26 per cent group II and 28 per cent in group III got complete relief, 36 per cent, 30 per cent and 56 per cent in group I, II and III respectively showed marked improvement. Mild improvement was noted in 32 per cent of the cases in group I, 39 per cent in group II and 12 per cent in group III. 4 per cent of the cases in group I, II and III respectively did not show any improvement.

Laboratory investigations revealed that E.S.R. was highly elevated in most of the cases initially. Twenty-four cases showed E.S.R. levels varying from 100 mm/1st hr. Reduction of E.S.R. Values was highly significant in all the three groups (P 0.001)

Marginal increase in Haemoglobin percentage was more in group I. The difference in total and differential counts was negligible. Uric acid levels were within normal limits. R.A. test was positive in twenty-one cases. This became negative after treatment in two cases in group III. V. D.R.L. test was negative in all the cases.

Discussion

Amavata is a disease caused by improper food and activities. Ama is the main etiological factor and hence treatment is to be designed in such a way as to bring amavasta to nirama stage. When the ama stage is overcome, the next step is to treat the vitiated vata. Drugs which possess tikta, katu and dipana qualities are useful for amapacana and to increase agnibala. Tikta and katu rasa drugs have vedana samana (analgesic) and sothaharana (anti-inflammatory) properties, Vacadigama and Haridradigna along with Saindhava are two compound preparations said to be effective in amavata. The ingredients in these two preparations are useful for amapacana and sothaharana and sothaharatwa. Vettumaran gutika containing hingula and vatsanabhi also has the above properties and in addition is effective in jvara. Besides having these properties Dasamoolarista and Pippalyasava are useful in general debility and for removal of srotorodha. Satpala Indukanta Ghrita which contains satpala is also effective in this condition. These two ghrita preparations are used as snehana (oleation) therapy for vitiated Vata. Indukanta ghrita contains Dasamoola which is havaing vedana haratwa and sothaharatwa properties in addition to vatasamana.

The result of the study was analysed on the basis of improvement in clinical signs and symptoms, laboratory investigations and return to normal function. The response to the treatment was encouraging in all the three groups.

The better improvement noted in the third group might be due to the srotorodhaharatwa and vedanaharatwa (analgesic and antiinflammatory) properties of Dasamoolarista + Pippalyasava and Vettumaran gutika. This combination was found to be more effective in the very acute stage of the condition when there is a wide range of symptoms like fever, malaise and gastro-intestinal disturbances besides swollen and painful joints. It is also palatable as compared to Vacadi and Haridradi gana churans which occasionally cause vomiting sensation. By virtue of the properties of the ingredients, it alleviates vata and kapha and hastens srotovisodhana. These aristas possess tonic properties also. An average of ninety days' treatment was required to obtain satisfactory improvement. Time taken for disappearance of Amavasta varied from patient to patient and it ranged from twenty to thirty days.

The chances of recovery was good in cases diagnosed as rheumatic fever especially where the duration of illness was less.

Analysis of E.C.G. and X-ray findings did not give any encouraging results. However, improvement in the clinical signs and symptoms was corroborated by laboratory findings (E.S.R. level and Hb per cent).

OSTEOARTHRITIS (SANDHIGATA VATA)

Essential Features

1. A degenerative disorder without systemic manifestations.
2. Pain relieved by rest.
3. Articular inflammation minimal.
4. *Aetiology*: Degenerative joint disease either primary or secondary.
   Ayurveda: Vitiated vata dosha.
5. *X-ray findings*: narrowed joint space, osteophytes, increased density of subchondral bone, bone cysts.
6. Commonly secondary to other articular disease.
7. *Differential diagnosis*: Rheumatoid arthritis (soft tissue swelling, and involvement of metacarpophalangeal joints), Neurogenic arthropathy of charcot (X-ray and neurological examination). Especially exclude metastatic neoplasia, osteoporosis, multiple myeloma, or other bone disease in any joint particularly spine.

8. *Management*: Non-specific.
9. *Prognosis*: No permanent cure. Proper treatment may greatly relieve symptoms and thereby improve function. Although marked disability is less common than in rheumatoid arthritis, symptoms may be quite severe and limit activity considerably. This is especially true on involvement of the hips, knees, and cervical spine.

Management

Degenerative joint disease is a chronic progressive arthropathy characterised by degeneration of cartilage and by hypertrophy of bone at the articular margins. Inflammation is usually minimal and thus the popular term osteoarthritis is inappropriate. Hereditary and mechanical factors may be variably involved in the pathogenesis. Primary disease can affect any joint; but usually it is secondary to other articular disease, resulting from either intra-articular (including rheumatoid arthritis) or extra-articular causes. The injury may be acute, as in a fracture; or chronic as that due to overweight, bad posture, occupational over use of a joint, or metabolic diseases (e.g. hyperparathyroidism, hemochromotasis, ochronosis).

The disease usually occur in middle and later life. In females especially domestic workers, the knee joints are most commonly affected. Clinically the disease is characterised by pain, stiffness and at times swelling of joints. Examination of affected joint may reveal tenderness and crepitus. There is no systemic involvement of distant organs. There is no ankylosis, but limitation of motion of the affected joint or joints is common. The disease is compared with Sandhigatavata described in Ayurveda.

Ayurveda

There is very brief description of the disease Sandhigatavata in ancient Ayurvedic literature and the disease entity has been described in reference to the description of diseases caused by vitiated vata dosha known as vatavyadhi. According to Acharya Charaka, there is swelling of joints which on palpation resembles an airfilled bladder with painful and restricted movements. Acharya Sushruta has mentioned that alongwith pain and swelling, the joints are completely deformed leading to impairment of joint functioning.

Aggravated vata is the main aetiological factor of the disease Sandhigata vata which is aggravated due to its aggravating factors and produces the disease process. These factors include obesity, trauma, abnormal strain and due to faulty posture, fatigue, overwork, sleeplessness, and toxic influences. All these are supposed to aggravate the vata dosha. This is a disease of middle age or late middle age which is again the period of vata predominance.

Treatment

For general treatment, see under Rheumatic Diseases.

Clinical Report

A Preliminary Clinical Trial of Trikushta Guggulu in the Treatment of Sandhigata Vata (Osteoarthritis): B.N. Sannd and Krishnakumari. (*Sachitra Ayurved*: 46: 10: 1994).

A combination of Guggulu (Commiphora mukul) and Kustha (Saussurea lappa) named as Trikushata Guggulu has been prepared to evaluate its therapeutic efficacy in the treatment of Sandhigatavata of knee joints. A comparative study was carried out by dividing the total 60 patients in two groups consisting of 30 patients each. A regular and periodic examination was carried out to observe the effect of drug. The duration of treatment was 60 days and at the end of treatment encouraging results in patients treated with Trikushata Guggulu were obtained.

Kushta is katu, madhur and tikta in rasa, usna in veerya and alleviates vata dosha. It is one of the important drugs available in Himalayan belt of Kashmir. Its roots are widely used by the people of Jammu and Kashmir for the treatment of joint pains as folk medicine.

Guggulu, the oleogum resin of C. mukul is an important drug of indigenous system of medicine. It is katu, tikta, kashayam and madhur in rasa, usna in veerya and alleviates all the three doshas. It is a known and experimentally proved anti-inflammatory and anti-rheumatic drug which is widely used for the treatment of obesity, joint pains and other vatik disorders by Ayurvedic physicians.

Dosage

Group A: A herbal combination of purified guggulu and kushta root powder in the tablet form weighing 500 mgm each and named as Trikushta guggulu tablets in the doses of two tablets thrice a day.

Group B: Capsulated glucose as placebo one capsule thrice a day.

Method of Preparation of Drug

1. Trikushta Guggulu—Guggulu was purifed in trifala kvath as per method prescribed in classical texts. It was mixed with finely powdered kushta root powder in the ratio of 2:1 respectively and made into tablets weighing 500 mgm each.
2. Glucose—Commercial glucose available in the local market used as 500 mgm capsules weight.
3. Patra Pinda Sweda with Nirgundi (Vitex nigundo) leaves were applied locally to the patients of both the groups.

Results

The study reveals the predominance of disease incidence among females in both the groups i.e. 63.3 per cent in Gr. A and 90 per cent in Gr B; Age—41 to 60 years ie. 60 per cent Gr A and 90 per cent in Gr B.; Obesity—66.7 per cent in Gr A and 60 per cent in Gr B; H/o trauma in 23.3 per cent in Gr A and 13.3 per cent in Gr B.; Total 10 per cent cases (in both the groups) gave the family history of the disease. Majority of the patients i.e. 93.3 per cent in Gr A and 80 per cent in Gr B were having bilateral involvement of knee joints. Haematological investigation i.e. Haemoglobin percentage, ESR, were within the normal range. Rheumatoid factor was negative and routine urine and stool tests did not show any abnormality. Osteoarthritic changes were found to be positive in all the patients treated under both the groups on X-ray examination.

Clinical improvement was noticed among the patients treated under Gr A. Stiffness, pain, swelling, tenderness was improved obviously within a period of 2 to 3 weeks and joint movements also became less painful depending upon the severity of disease. After 60 days of the treatment marked reduction in average body weight was also noticed.

Total 10 per cent cases got complete relief, 13.4 per cent got marked relief, 50 per cent showed moderate relief, 20 per cent got mild relief and 6.7 per cent of cases got no relief. Whereas, total of 70 per cent of cases treated in Gr B remained unchanged or showed marginal improvement of pain. This insignificant improvement may be due to local application of patrapinda sweda. The severity of disease increased in 30 per cent of cases.

Conclusion

To conclude, as the disease Sandhigata vata (Osteoarthritis) is considered to be a pathological condition which is caused by vata; hence its treatment measures include to ensure the state of equilibrium of vitiated vata by vatahar drugs. The herbal combination of guggulu and kushta showed very encouraging results in present trial. Though Guggulu is a renowned and experimentally proved anti-inflammatory and anti-rheumatic drug including for weight reduction, Kushta has not shown any anti-inflammatory activity experimentally. It shows the importance of validity of Rasa Panchaka Siddhanta of Ayurveda in drug selection.

On the other hand, despite of observing the same dietary measures i.e. easily digestible nutrious diet and patra pinda sweda application with Nirgundi patra leaves, patients treated under placebo group did not significantly improved. Clinically severity of disease increased on 30 per cent of cases.

Hence the combination of Guggulu and Kushta is proved as an excellent herbal remedy for the treatment of Sandhigatavata

(Osteoarthritis). Again it is very safe for long term use without any side effect.

Note: Under both the groups maximum cases i.e. 12 (40 per cent in Gr A) and 14 (46,7 per cent) in Gr B were recorded with duration of disease less than one year.

In both the groups onset of disease was found to be insidious among majority of patients i.e. 28 (93.3 per cent in Gr A) and 26 (86.7 per cent in Gr B).

(Non-specific measures: Rest, Light diet, local heat)

Orthopaedic measures: Correction of developmental anomalies, deformities, disparity in leg length, and severely damaged joint surfaces.

ANKYLOSING SPONDYLITIS

Essential Features

1. A chronic inflammatory disease of the joints of the axial skeleton, manifested clinically by pain and progressive stiffening of the spine.
2. Chronic low backache in young adults.
3. Progressive limitation of back motion and of chest expansion.
4. Transient (50 per cent) or permanent (25 per cent) peripheral joint involvement in-distinguishable from peripheral rheumatoid arthritis.
5. *Diagnostic X-ray changes in sacroiliac joints*: Erosion and sclerosis of the sacroiliac joints; later, involvement of the apophyseal joints of the spine, ossification of the annulus fibrosus, calcification of the anterior and lateral spinal ligaments, and squaring and generalised demineralisation of the vertebral bodies; the term bamboo spine has been used to describe the late findings. Peripheral joint changes are also seen.
6. Uveitis in 20-25 per cent.
7. Raised ESR and negative serologic tests for rheumatoid factor.
8. HLA-B 27 positive.
9. *Differential diagnosis*: Rheumatoid arthritis-involves cervical spine, small joints of the hands and feet, presence of

subcutaneous nodules, positive serologic tests for rheumatoid factor.

History and physical findings of ankylosing spondylitis serve to distinguish this disorder from other causes of low back ache, degenerative disc disease, osteoporosis, soft tissue trauma and tumors. Important sign is involvement of sacroiliac joints in Ankylosing spondylitis. Also exclude brucellosis and fluoride poisoning in certain areas.

10. *Treatment*: Similar to rheumatoid arthritis.
11. *Prognosis*: Spontaneous remissions and relapses are common and may occur at any age. In general, the functional prognosis is good unless the hips are seriously and permanently involved.
12. *Ayurvedic management*: See under Rheumatic Diseases.

FIBROMYALGIA

Fibromyalgia is a relatively common form of non-articular rheumatism. The condition is characterised by diffuse musculoskeletal aching associated with multiple tender points in soft tissues. It affects chiefly women in the sixth decade of life. Associated symptoms include morning stiffness, fatigue, headache, neck pain, and sleep disturbances. Laboratory tests are noncontributory. Although fibromyalgia usually occurs in the absence of any other disease (primary form), it may accompany rheumatoid arthrits, osteoarthrits, or hypothyroidism (secondary form). Attention to the sleep disorder often leads to improvement in the symptom complex.

Ayurvedic Management: See under Rheumatic Diseases.

CONCEPT OF VATAVYADHIS AND THEIR MANAGEMENT

Introduction—General

Vatavyadhis are a group of diseases caused by the vitiated vata dosa and are generally considered to be 80 in number. It is also said that these diseases because of their complex nature are mostly incurable. All Ayurvedic classics without any exception have dealt various aspects of Vatavyadhis such as Etiology, Pathology, classification and management. Though a few differences of opinion have been put forth by the authors of these texts it is generally accepted that this group is a major group of diseases involving the vitiation of vata and that these diseases are the most difficult ones to be get rid of even by a most competent physician, using most powerful medicines.

In the modern terms Vatavyadhis include major neurological problems prevalent in those times. In addition a few GIT problems and a few psychoneurological problems and a few diseases of musculo-skeletal system have also been included. To be more precise Ayurvedic vata system is a broader classification involving many systems as classified in current text books of medicine.

Introduction—Specific

Charaka in his illustrious text Charaka Samhita, has classified the diseases into two major groups—Nanatmaja and Samanyaja groups—based on the involvement of dosas either singularly or in combination.[1] Nanatmaja Vyadhis which are caused by the vitiation of single dosa are again divided into three groups—Vataja, Pittaja and Kaphaja,[2] Vataja diseases are said to be 80 in number and other two are 40 and 20 in number respectively.[3] These are Vataja Nanatmaja Vyadhis and not Vatavyadhis. The diseases the author describes under vatavyadhi[4] in Chikitsa Sthana are in variance with the description made earlier (Ca. Su.20/10) both in number and nomenclature. All the other texts have mentioned only Vatavyadhis and the terms Nanatmaja is not found in any text other than Charaka Samhita. Kasyapa[5] and Sarangadhara[6] have also mentioned about 80 diseases under Vatavyadhis and this infect is a selective/judicious mixture of those diseases mentioned by Charaka in Sutra and Chikitsa Sthana. Sushruta[7] and Vagbhata[8] have also described Vatavyadhis but the number is far less (less than 50). But this number is approximately equal to the number of diseases which Charaka described in Cikitsa 28th Chapter.

Thus we have two sets of Vatavyadhis which are roughly similar in number and nomenclature. The first group comprises of those diseases which are mentioned by Charaka in Sutra 20/10 (Vata Nanatmaja) and those mentioned by Kasyapa and Sarangadhara under the head Vatavyadhis. The second group includes those which are discussed in Charaka Cikitsa 28 and those described by Vagbhata[9] and Sushruta.[10] Thus any discussion related to Vatavyadhis is difficult in the absence of clarification with reference to vatavyadhi and vatananatmaja vyadhi. This in itself is a topic for a separate discussion and hence the author does not wish to go into the details of this aspect. Hence the discussion that follows is generally based on the common conventional lines that Vatavyadhis and Nanatmaja Vatavyadhis are not dissimilar.

Vatavyadhis—Definition

Various definitions have been offered by different authors for this terms.

1. Vata Eva Vyadhih Vatavyadhih[11]
2. Vatatvyadhih Vatavyadhih[12]
3. Vikruto Dhukhakari Vato Vatavyadhih[13]
4. Vikruto Vatajanito Vyadhih Vatavyadhih[14]
5. Vikruta Vatajanito Asadharano Vyadhih Vatavyadhih[15]

1. Vata in itself cannot be a disease because it is present even in healthy individuals.

2. It is true that Vatavyadhi is caused by vata but all diseases by Vata cannot be called Vatavyadhis.

3-4. These definitions though do not give complete picture of Vatavyadhi are certainly more comprehensive.

5. This is the most appropriate definition available inasmuch as it makes out that difference between Vatavyadhi and other diseases where Vata is involved—the usage Asadharana is the key term.

Madhava, author of Madhava Nidana while defining Vatavyadhi has made some interesting observations, as to why only Vatavyadhis and not pittavyadhis and kaphavyadhis are being considered for elaboration. 'Vayu is most powerful of all and produces the disease instantaneously. Vatavyadhis are of very serious nature and need contradictory approaches for management and incurable in general. Besides they often cause medical emergencies.'[16]

Vatavyadhi group of diseases is also considered among Ashta Mahagadas[17]—8 major diseases which are extremely difficult to be cured.

Basavarajiyam a south Indian treatise on Ayurveda has described a number of new diseases under Vatavyadhi which are not found in any Ayurvedic text.

'Vatavyadhi' is used as a synonym for the sage Uddhava in Kautilya's Arthasastra.[18&19]

The definition of Nanatmaja Vyadhi on the other hand has two components: 1. Ekadosa Janya—only one dosa should be involved in the genesis of the disease. 2. Na Anatmaja—Na Anyena Jatah—the disease could never be produced by dosa other than the concerned dosha.

Number

Vatavyadhis are said to be innumerable[21] but most commonly manifested 80 disease conditions have been enumerated by Charaka.[22] Though the number is fixed at 80 a few editions have counted 81 and a few even 79. Referring various editions of the text, the total number is found to be 86. Kasyapa Samhita and Sarangadhara Samhita, the two other texts which have enumerated 80 Vatavyadhis, have enlisted many conditions which are not found in Charaka Samhita, but also have omitted a good number of diseases from Charaka's list. If all these three lists are to be clubbed the number swells to 160.

In Charaka Cikitsa 28, the author has discussed only 26 diseases. Out of this only 10 diseases are those which have already appeared under Nanatmaja variety (Sutra 20/10) (Table 2.5). Other diseases come into the group o Ghatavatas or Avarana Vatas.' Sushruta Samhita (48) and Ashtanga Hridaya (39) also have not discussed all the eighty diseases. If one keeps aside the chapter on Nanatmaja Vyadhis (Ca. Su. 20) (most of the diseases mentioned here are only symptoms) there is much similarities in number, nomenclature and management of Vatavyadhis in all these three Samhitas (Table 2.4). The minimal omissions and commissions can be attributed to the variance of time, region the authors belonged to, and also due to the prevalence of the disease conditions. For example conditions such as Viswachi, Apabahuka are not mentioned in Charaka but are explained by both Sushruta[23] and Vagbhata.[24] Similarly the disease 'Khalli' is not explained by Sushruta but is mentioned by both Charaka[25] and Vagbhata.[26] The disease Urusthambha is counted among vatavyadhis by Sushruta[27] and Vagbhata[28] but not by Charaka. These are but a few examples and the details are not being discussed here.

Etiology

Those qualities of food, mind and activity which are in concomitance with those of Vata are responsible for the causation of the diseases of Vata. Thus foods which is ununctous, cold etc., the mind which is angered, feared etc., and activities like excessive sexual indulgence, night vigil would aggravate Vata to produce Vatavyadhis. All the common etiological factors mentioned by Charaka can be grouped into two categories, which also represent the two different pathologies involved in the manifestation of a vata disease[29] (Table No. 2.6).

1. The causes which induce Dhathukshaya
2. The causes which produce Margavarana.

Pathogenesis

As said earlier pathology involved in the genesis of the disease is twofold—Dhatukshya and Margavarana. But it is desirable to identify the components of Pathogenesis.

Site of origin: Both vayu[30] and diseases of Vayu[31] have been said to originate from pakwasaya (large bowel).

Dosa-Vata

Dushya—Seven Dhatus, Three Malas, Ama, Kandara, Sira, Snayu: All these dushya are not involved in all the disease conditions. But one or more Dhusyas may be involved in a disease.

Srotas—Vatavaha Srotas

The very term Vatavaha Srotas has not been used by any Ayurvedic text. However Charaka[32] has given an indirect reference towards existence of such srotas for vata. The Vatavaha Srotas probably has two components in Ceshtavaha Srotas and Samjnavaha Srotas. The former represents motor activity while the latter is related to sensory system. The term Samjnavaha Srotas has appeared in Charaka Samhita.[33] But the former is missing. In vatavadhis both these srotas are involved in respective disease conditions.

Site of Pathology—This varies according to the disease which is concerned.

Site of Manifestation—This again is different, to different disease conditions. The two types of Pathogeneses can be summarised as under.

1. Vatavridhikara or Dhatukshayakara | Nidana → Srotorikatata → Entry and accumulation of Vayu at the site of Pathology → Vatavyadhi

2. Amotpadaka Nidana → Amasanchaya in Srotas → Srotovarodha → Trapping of Vayu leading to Avarana → Vatavyadhi

In the first instance, the foods, activities and psychological factors, whose qualities are in concomitance with those of Vata produce roughness, emptiness, lightness in the organs, and naturally when Vata reaches such organs/channels it settles there and when the conditions become favourable produces Vatavyadhis.[34] In the latter, when Ama collects and obstructs the flow of Vata which gets vitiated and moves around in different directions producing different Vatavyadhis. Ama true to its definition can be any waste material[35] which is formed at different places in the body and which is the root cause of all diseases.

The pathology leads to increment or inhibition in the activity of Vayu—Vatakarma Vridhi or Vatakarma Kshaya as in case of Akshepaka and Pakshaghata respectively.

Thus all these aspects of Pathogenesis can be represented as under:

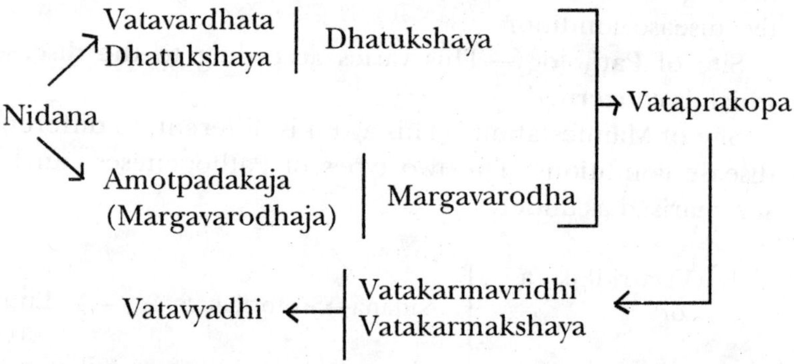

Premonitary Symptoms

The premonitary symptoms of Vatavyadhi are said to be invisible (Avyakta)36. That means to say the disease can be identified only in its manifested state. The only other disease whose premonitary symptoms are said to be invisible is Urakshata.[37]

Symptomatology

Three terms[38] have been used in relation to common symptomatology of Vatavyadhis.

Atma Rupa—This refers to symptoms that are produced after the manifestation of the disease. This is not specific.

Apaya—Refers to absence (Abhava) or instability/remission (Asthiratva). True to the nature of Vata the symptoms produced are said to be unstable. Further remissions are said to be common in conditions like Ardita etc.

Laghuta—Lightness—The organ which is affected becomes light in keeping with the light nature of *Vata.*

The interpretation *'Apayo-laghuta'* is also considered by a few lightness (laghuta) or amelioration of the symptoms is indicative of absence (Apaya) or the cure of the disease.

In addition to the above Charaka has listed some symptoms[39] most of which are enumerated by him in Charaka Sutra 20/10 where he calls them as *Nanatmaja Vatavyadhis.*

Classification

Initial attempts at classification appear to have been made by *Bhela Samhita.* He has mentioned two groups—*Ekanga Roginah* and *Sarvanga Roginah*[40] and has listed a few diseases under each group. Sushruta also has used the terms *Ekanga sthitha* and *Sarvanga Sthitha*[41] *Vyadhis.* The more pronouncing classification by Sushruta, himself is categorising *Vatavyadhis* in to *Vatavyadhi* group and *Mahavatavyadhi* group, for which he has allocated separate chapters in *Cikitsa Sthana.* However more classifications can be done based on different criteria.

(Table 2.7, 2.8, 2.9).

A. *Clinical*

1.	Maha Vatavyadhis	e.g. Ardita
	Vatavyadhis	e.g. Amasayagata Vata
2.	Sarvangagata	e.g. Sarvangavata
	Ekanga gata	e.g. Vatakantaka
3.	Sula Pradhana	e.g. Viswaci
	Kampa Pradhana	e.g. Kampavata
	Akarmanyata Pradhana	e.g. Pakshaghata
	Sosa Pradhana	e.g. Bahusosa
	Sthamba Pradhana	e.g. Dandaka
	Sotha Pradhana	e.g. Kroshtuka shirsha.

B. *Etio Pathological*

Dhatukshayaja	e.g. Pakshaghata
Margavarodhaja	e.g. Avritavata
Samsrushtaja	e.g. Kaphanugata

An attempt has been made to group the diseases under the above heads one should note that over lappings are common when more than one group is made. For example disease like *pakshaghata* can be caused by *Dhatukshaya* as well as *Margavarana.* Similarly *Gridhrasi* is both *Suddha vataja* and *Samsrushtaja.*

Complications and Prognosis

Vatavyadhis in general are either incurable or curable with difficulty. It is said that the cure can be effected only by Daiva— the Supernatural all powerful entity and a Physician treats hoping only to manage the condition.[42]

However Vatayadhi when it is new, devoid of complications and has affected a patient who has strong will and physique can be managed.[43]

Among the complications are such simple symptoms as anorexia and loss of appetite and such a serious ones like anaesthesia, unconsciousness etc.,[44] Charaka has mentioned some complications which are produced by Avrita vata. All these have been tabulated separately (Table No. 2.10).

Principles of Management (Table 2.11 to 2.13)

Principles of management of a Vatavyadhi revolve around Vata Dosa inasmuch as it is solely responsible for the manifestation of disease. The drugs, the diet and therapeutic procedure should be aimed at alleviating this dosha. Further it is essential to identify the changes in the attributes (Guna) of the dosa and also to quantify them. For example when Vata is aggravated it is important to know whether the aggravation is due to Roughness or coldness, and should be treated with unctousness or hotness respectively. Further quantification of the attributes-increase normalcy, and decrease (Vridhi Sthana-Kshaya) of these qualities should be asserted and treatment should be aimed at bringing back normal state.

Further, the site of origin of Vata and Vatavyadhi being Pacvasaya, the treatment should be aimed at this very level of origin. It is needless to say that the removal of the causative factor is as important as others.

The principles of management of vatavyadhi have been laid down by Charaka in a singular verse:

Kevalam nirupasthambam adou snehairupacaret (Ca.Ci.28/75)

Commenting on this verse Cakrapani, the renowned commentator of the text *Charaka Samhita* observes

Kevalamiti asamprushtam nirupasthambamiti anavritam

Kevalam refers to *Vata* which is not associated with either *Pitta* or *Kapha*. *Nirupasthamba* is synonymous with *Anavrita* which denotes *Vata* is not enclosed by other components of pathogenesis (Dosha, Dushya etc.)

Thus we evolve three major approaches to the management of *Vatavyadhi.*[45]

1. Treatment of *Shuddha Vatavyadhi*
2. Treatment of *Samsrushta Vatavyadhi*
3. Treatment of *Avrita Vatavyadhi*

Treatment of Shuddha Vatavyadhi

Treatment here mainly aims at alleviating Vata by inducing opposite qualities. Therapy is mainly palliative and oleation as sudation play a major role. The approach has 3 stages—each stage having further divisions (Table No. 2-11).

Stage I

When the disease is in its initial stage or when it is of mild nature only two treatment procedures Snehana and Swedana would suffice to effect a cure. The same procedures are also useful in the later two stages of management, but there they play only a supporting role.

Snehana: This is the best treatment for *Vata* because the most pronounced quality of vitiated *Vata* is ununctuousness (Ruksha)[46]—which is exactly opposite to unctuousness (Sneha). Further *Suddha Vatavyadhi* is characterised by wasting of tissue elements (Dhatukshaya) and loss of strength (Balakshaya) for which Sneha is said to be most effective.[47] Among the *Snehas, Taila* is the most suitable, because its attributes are exactly opposite to those of *Vata.*[48]

Snehana further, should be done in the following phases.

(A) Initially any one of the four Snehas (Taila, Gritha, Majja, Vasa) should be administered in Acchapana procedure (pure state).[48]

(B) Snehaklanta should be allowed rest for a period of few days during which he should be advised such diet and regimen, as is suitable to the condition of the patient.[49]

(C) Sneha should again be administered but this time in the form of Vicarana by mixing it with milk, salt, meat etc. or in the form of preparations like Yusa etc.[50] External use of Sneha in any form (Sirovasti etc.) can be done depending on the condition.

Swedana: The treatment of *Vatavyadhi* is never complete without *Swedana*, but *Swedana* in case of *Shuddha vata* should always be preceded by *Snehana*—in the form of *Abhyanga*. Procedures to be followed for Swedana should always associate with *Sneha* in any form.[51] Among the various types of *Sweda, Tapa* variety is to be avoided.[52] *Sneha* and *Sweda* should be repeatedly administered until the symptoms such as pain, rigidity, inflammation are relieved and opposite qualities of *Vata* such as unctuousness, softness and hotness are deployed in the body and in such circumstances *Vatavyadhis* cannot manage to retain their hold over the body.[53]

Stage II

When therapy as cited in stage I fails, or to supplement the therapy at Stage I, the following management should be advocated.

(A) Procedures followed during stage I should be repeated.

(B) *Visodhana*—Because of the excessiveness of vitiation of *Vata* the disease is not alleviated with *Snehana* and *Swedana*, one should resort to *Visodhana*.[54]

Visodhana in general terms is a synonym of *Samshodhana/ Shodhana* and is composed of *Vamana* and *Virecana*. However as *Vamana* in general is contraindicated for *Vatavyadhi*,[55] *Visodhana* in this context implies only *Virecana*. This *Virecana* should be in the form of *Anulomana*[56] and should be associated with unctuousness.[57]

The word *Sadosatwa*, according to Cakrapani refers to the accumulation of waste material, *mala*, as a consequence of use of the food and medicine used during *Snehana* and *Swedana*. The word *Sadosa* is not related to *Vatadosha* as such but is related to the *Vatahara* therapy.[58]

Niruhana: In a weak patient where *Virecana* is contraindicated *Niruhana* is advisable.[59]

Both *Visodhana* and *Niruhana* in this stage (II) are aimed to relieve constipation or expel the accumulated waste as a result of *Sadosha*. However the purpose and meaning of *Niruhana* is entirely different during stage III, which would be discussed later.

Stage III

For the sake of proper understanding a simple modification has to be effected in the sequence of events described by Charaka in relation to general principles of management. However, there is no compromise on principles. This course of therapy should be administered (A) When the therapy at Stage I and II fails or B) to supplement the above therapy for complete remission and to prevent recurrence.

This should be done in following phases.

(A) Repeat of therapy as in Stage I and II.

(B) *Niruhana*—*Niruhana* generally refers to *Asthapana* type of *Vasti* which is devoid of *Sneha*. (*Sneha* is negligible). This is given in alternation with *Anuvasana Vasti* (*Sneha vasti*) in all *Vatavyadhis*. *Vasti* in itself is a complete treatment for *vata* diseases[60] and hence *Niruhana* at this reference should be considered synonymous with *Vasti*. Charaka while enumerating different therapies for *Vatavyadhis* at a later place has used the word *Vasti* and has avoided the term *Niruha*.[61] This *Vasti* has two major objectives:
1. Expulsion of *mala* (*Asthapana* type)
2. Alleviation of *Vata* (both type)

(C) Agni Sandhukshna—A purificatory procedure should always be followed by *Samsarjana* to augment the digestive fire.

(D) *Snehana Swedana*

(E) Visesha Ahara

Food which is predominantly unctuous, hot, sweet, sour and saltish should be taken.[62]

(F) *Rakta Mokshana*

Keeping with the general principles of treatment, when the diseases of *Vata*[63] or any *dosa* for that matter is not amenable to *Snigdha/Ruksha, Sita/Usna* type of treatment, blood letting in any form should be done.

Procedures like *Nasya* and *Dhumapana* can be adopted during any of these stages as per the need in desired forms (*Snehayukta*).

Management of Samsrushta Vatavyadhi

Samsrushta refers to the association of *Pitta, Kapha* or *Rakta* in a *Vatavyadhi*. Though *vatavyadhis* are caused by *Vata* alone association by any other *dosha* is not uncommon during the course of a disease.

1. When *Vata* is associated with *Kapha, Pitta* or *Rakta,* such therapy should be employed which is not contradictory to other *dosha*.[65]
2. When both *Kapha* and *Pitta* are associated with *Vata, Pitta* should be treated first.[66]
3. When only *Kapha* is associated, it should be treated by *Anuvasana* type of Enema which is prepared by ingredients with hot quality and it should be mixed with cow's urine before administration.[67]

   When the associated *Kapha* is seated in stomach, *Vamana* should be administered,[68] and when it is seated in large bowel it should be treated with either purgation[69] or enema therapy.[70] When *Kapha* enters the head, errhines or smoking therapy should be administered.[71]
4. When *Pitta,* is associated with *Vata, Niruha* type of enema mixed with milk should be administered.[72]

When this *Pitta,* is seated in large bowel it should be treated with enema,[73] and if it has spread all over the body, purgation therapy should be administered.[74]

Management of Avrita Vatavyadhi

Different therapies and approaches have been advocated for different *Avarnas* by *doshas, dhatus* and *malas*. However, the following are the general principles of management.

1. The drugs which are *Anabhishyandhi, Srotoshodhaka* and *Snigdha* but which are not antagonistic to *kapha* and *pitta*, should be administered.[75]
2. Procedures like *Samsrana, Vatanulomana, Yapana Vasti, Anuvasana Vasti,* should be resorted to.[76]
3. Shilajit and Guggul with milk should be given.[77]
4. Chyavanaprasha lehya with milk should be administered.[78]
5. Rasayana therapy in general and specific rasayana preparations mentioned in Abayamalaki section of Rasayana chapter of Charaka Samhita should be administered.[79]

These general principles which are discussed as related to three types of *Vatavyadhis* cover all *vatavyadhis* mentioned under different categories. Treatment mentioned for Type I (*Shuddha Vataja*) can be applicable to all diseases, including those which come under Type II (*Samsrushta*) and Type III (*Avritaja*). However, in these two types (Type II and Type III) initial treatment should be employed as directed under their own categories, and once *Samsrushta dosa* is pacified or *Avarna* is cleared, treatment mentioned under Type I should be followed.

In case of the individual diseases, the therapy should be considered basing on the type of the disease, stage of the disease and other factors.

Do's and Don'ts

The attributes, tastes, foods, activities, psychological factors and others which are in concomitance with those of *vata* in general are to be avoided and those opposite should be practiced (Table No. 2.12).

Last Word

In the presence of many confusing and contradictory statements it is difficult to arrive at conclusions on many aspects of *vatavyadhis.* If some of the descriptions are vogue at times, it is either too little or totally missing in many instances. Add to this is the difference of opinion among the authors of various texts on various aspects of this disease group. Inadequacy in classifications and absence of specific instructions in the management for different categories of diseases which come under this group poses a major problem in treating these diseases. The author has made an attempt, hopefully, successful to answer some of the problems.

Table 2.4: *Vatavyadhis in Brihattrayee*

Charaka Samhita	*Sushruta Samhita*	*Ashtanga Hridaya*
(1)	*(2)*	*(3)*
Dhatugata (7)	Dhatugata (7)	Dhatugata (7)
Srotradigata	Srotradigata	Srotradigata
Amasayagata	Amasayagata	Amasayagata
Pakwasayagata	Pakwasayagata	Pakwasayagata
Siragata	Siragata	Siragata
Snayugata	Snayugata	Snayugata
Sandhigata	Sandhigata	Sandhigata
Sarvangagata	Sarvangagata	Sarvangagata
Shirogata	Shirogata	Shirogata
Manyasthambha	Manyasthambha	Manyasthamba
Hanusthambha	Hanusthambha	Hanusthamba
Ardita	Ardita	Ardita
Pakshaghata	Pakshaghata	Pakshaghata
Akshepaka	Akshepaka	Akshepaka
Gradrasi	Gradrasi	Gradrasi
Avrita vata	Avrita vata	Avrita vata
Khalli	Vatarakta	Khalli
Bahirayama	Manyagata	Bahirayama
Dandavata	Vastigata	Dandaka
Koshtagatavata	Apatanaka	Apatanaka
Gudagatavata	Apatantraka	Apatantraka
Kubjatawata	Vatashtila	Vranayama

(1)	*(2)*	*(3)*
Ekangavata	Apabhahuka	Apabhahuka
	Viswaci	Viswaci
	Khanja	Khanja
	Pangu	Pangu
	Kalayakanja	Kalayakanja
	Kroshtuka Shirsha	Kroshtuka shirsha
	Urusthambha	Urusthambha
	Vatakantaka	Vatakanta
	Pada daha	Pada daha
	Pada harsha	Pada harsha
	Tuni	Hanusramsa
	Parati Tuni	Jihwa sthambha
	Admana	Siragraha
	Pratyadmana	Sarvanga roga
	Ashtild	
	Pratya Shtila	
	Karnasula	
	Bhadiryd	
	Mukaminmind Gadgada	

Table 2.5: *Diseases Mentioned Both at Charaka Sutra (20) and Cikista (28)*

Ardita
Pakshavadha
Gridrasi
Akshepaka
Manyasthamba
Dandaka
Kubjatwa
Ekanga vata
Sarvanga vata
Pangulya

Table 2.6: *Etilogical Factors in Vatavyadhis*

For Dhatukshaya				*For Avarana*
Food	*Activity*	*Psychological Factors*	*Others*	
Ruksha	Vyayama	Cinta	Dososrava	Amadosa
Sita	Vyayaya	Soka	Raktasrava	Divaswapna
Laghu	Jagarana	Krodha	Dhatukshaya	Vegavarodha
Alpa	Langhana	Bhaya	Rogajakshya	
Abhojana	Plawana		Abhighata	
	Patana		Marmaghata	
	Advagamana			
	Visama Sayya			
	Visama Asana			
	Visamopacara			

Table 2.7: *Classification of Vatavyadhis*

Shuddha Vataja	*Margavarodhaja*	*Samsrushthaja*
(1)	*(2)*	*(3)*
Sthana gata vatas	Anyonya Avarana (20)	Paksha Ghata (p.k.)*
Akshepaka	Dosaja Avarana (12)	Griarosi (k)
Apatantraka	Dnatwa varana (7)	Ardita (k.p.)
Apatanataka	Sarva Dhatwavarna (1)	Padadaha (p)
Khalli	Vidavarana (1)	Padaharsha (k)
Kubjatwa	Mutravarna (1)	Bhadirya (k)
Apabahuka	Annavarna (1)	Mukaminmina Gadgada (k)
Viswaci	Amavarna (1)	Urusthambha (k)
Khanja		Vata Rakta (R)
Kalayakhanja		Kroshtuka Sirsha (R)
Pangu		Dandasatanka (k)
Vatakantaka		Akshepaka (k.p.)
Karnasula		Manya Sthambha (k)
Dandavata		Pratyadmana (k)
Hanusthambha		Vranayama (pk)
Manyasthambha		Siradgraha (R)
Pakshaghata		Dandaka (k)
Gridrasi		
Bahirayama		
Tuni- Prati Tuni		
Admana		
Astila		
Pratyashtila		
Vatashtila		
Jihwa Sthamba		
Sarvanga Roga		

*k = Kapha Samsrushta
p = Pitta Samsrushta
R = Rakta Samsrushta

Table 2.8: *Classification of Vatavyadhis*

Ekanga gata	*Sarvanga gata*
Sthanagata	Dhatugata
Gridrasi	Sira, Snayu, Sandhigata
Kroshtaka Shirsha	Sarvanga gata
Vatakantaka	Pakshaghata
Pada daha	Ardita (Charaka's type-I)
Pada harsha	Akshepaka
Khalli	Apatanka
Viswaci	Apatantraka
Bahu Sosa	Dandavata
Hanusthambha	Dandaka
Manya Sthambha	Vatarakta
Khanja	Bahirayama
Kalayakanja	Antarayama
Pangu	Vranayama
Urusthambha	Siragradha
Tuni-Pratituni	Hanusamsra
Ashtila Pratyashtila	Kubjatwa
Vatashtila	Kampavata
Admana Pratyadmana	
Ardita	
Karna Sula	
Bhadirya	
Muka Minmina Gadgada	
Jihwa Sthamba	
Kampavata	

Table 2.9: *Classification of Vatavyadhis*

Sula Pradhana	*Sthamba Pradhana*	*Akarmanyata Pradhana*	*Kampa Pradhana*	*Sotha Pradhana*	*Sosa Pradhana*	**Anya*
Gridrasi	Manyasthamba	Paksha Ghata	Kampavata	Kroshuka Shirsha	Bahusosha	Padadaha
Viswachi	Hanusthamba	Khanja	Apatanaka	Vata Rakta	Apabahuka	Padaharsha
Khalli	Urusthambha	Kalayakhanja	Akshepaka			Bhadisya
Tuni	Jihwasthamba	Phangu				Apatantraka
Pratithuni	Dandavata	Viswaci				Ashitla
Ardita	Dandaka					Vatashtila
Karna Sula	Antarayama					Kubjatwa
Kroshta Sirsha	Bahirayama					Muka Minmiha Gadgada
Vatakantaka	Vrdnayama					
Sarvangagata						
Vatarakta						
Admana						
Pratyadmana						
Pratya Shtila						
Siragraha						
Sthanagatavata						
Dhatugata vata						

* These diseases cannot be included in any of the above group.

Table 2.10: *Complications of Vatavyadhis*

Samanyaja			*Avaranaja*
Aruci	Kasa	Prana Kshaya	Hridroga
Avipaka	Swasa	Mamsa Kshaya	Vidhradhi
Trishna	Hikka	Sosa	Pliha
Chardhi		Murcha	Gulma
Atisara		Jwara	Atisara
Admana		Sopha	
		Bhagna	
		Kampa	
		Sula	
		Sthamba	
		Visarana	
		Sankocana	
		Supti	

Table 2.11: *Stages of Therapy in Vatavyadhis*

		Suddha Vataja	*Samsrushta Vataja*	*Avrita Vataja*
Stage—I	Snehana	Acchapana Visrama Vicarana	I. Treatment for Somsrushta dosa. II. Treatment for Snuddha vata	I. Treatment for Avarana II. Treatment for Snuddha vata
		Abhyanga		
	Swedana	Swedana		
Stage—II	Stage I. Visodhana Niruhana Stages I & II			
	Niruhana	Niruhana		
		Anuvasana-Ashapana		
Stage—III	Agni Sandukshna Snehana Swedana Visishta Ahára Rakta Mokshana			

Table 2.12: *Do's and Don'ts in Vatavyadhis*

	Pathya	*Apathya*
Foods		
Rasa	Madhura Amla Lavana	Katu Tikta Kasaya
Guna	Snigdha Usna Ghana Mridu	Ruksha Sita Laghu, Abhishyandi
Grains	Raka Sali (Old) Masa Kulaththa Godhuma	Kalaya, Cana, Nivara, Yava Mudga Syamaka, Kuruvinda
Vegetables	Kushmanda Vartaka Brihati, Karuvallaka Patola Shighru Vasthuka Kasạmarda Mundi Mulka Surana Punarnava	Mrinala, Tundi, Urvaru, Kandas
Fruits	Dadima, Draksha, Badara Amral, Parushaka	Jambu, Udumbara, Kramuka
Meals	Aja Aswad Gaja Garadhabha Hamsa Cakravaka Kukkuta Mayura, Bheka Cataka Tittira Nakra Shilindra, Krudisa Jangala Mamsa	Anupa, Bilesaya Prasaha-Mamsa, Matsya
Drinks and Foods	Usnajala, Dugda, Ghrita, Narikela Jala Kshara, Asava Sura, Kilata, Dadhi Kurcika	Udamantha, Madha, Tadaga Tala Tatini Jala
Activities	Upaveshtana, Unmardana, Mridu Sayya-Asana Hemanta Ritu Carya	Ativyavaya, Ativyayama, Vega dharan Jagarana, Srama, Cankramana
Psychological Factors	Vitrasana Vismarana, Vismapana	Cinta Udvega

Table 2.13: *Some Important Drugs/Procedures Useful in Vatavyadhis*

Ekadravya	*Kwatha/Arishta*	*Taila*	*Ghritam*	*Guggulu/Rasayoga*	*Upakrama*	*Gana*
Taila	Maha Rasnadi K.	Narayana T.	Dasamooladi	Yogaraja G.	Vasthi	Vatasamsamana
Rasna	Masabaladi K.	Mahamasa T.	Aswagandhadi	Trayodasanga G.	Snehna	(Su.Su.39/7)
Lasuna	Rasna Dasamoola K.	Prasarini T.	Brihatchagaladi	Sadasiti G.	Swedana	Vata Prasamaka
Guggulu	Balarishta	Bala T.	Citrakadi	Dwatrimsat G.	Vamana	(As.Su.14/10)
Bala	Dasamoolarishta	Dhanwantara T.	Dasamooladi	Rasnadi G.	Virecana	Vatanasaka
Bilva	Aswagandharishta	Sahacharadi T.	Majja Sneha		Anulomana	(Cakradatta)
Eranda		Amritadi T.	Dasamooladi	B. Vatacinta-	Niruhana	
			Vasasneha	mani R.		
Guduci		Rasnadi T.	Triphaladi	Rasaraja R.	Anuvasana	
			Catusneha			
Hingu		Aswagandhadi T.		Yogendra R.	Nasya	
Kushta		Mulakadi T.		Cintamani R.	Raktamokshana	
Amlavetasa		Satavari T.		Laghnananda R.	Dhumapana	
Prishniparni		Rasona T.		Khanjana Kari R.	Sirovasti	
Ghrita		Swadamstra T.		Vasari R.	Gandusa	
				Mallasindhura	Upanaha	
					Unmardhana	

REFERENCES

1,2,3	Caraka Samhita Sutra Sthana	20-10
4	Caraka Samhita Cikitsa Sthana	28
5	Kasyapa Samhita Sutra Sthana	27-10
6	Sarangadhara Samhita—Madhyama Khanda	7-105
7,10	Susruta Samhita, Nidana–I and Chikitsa 4&5	
8,9	Asthanga Hridaya, Nidana 15 and Chikitsa 21	
11 to 16	Madhava Nidana (Madhukosa)	22-1
17	Susruta Samhita, Sutra Sthana	22/4-7
18,19	Kautilya Artha Sastra (Amatyotpatti Prakarana)	
20	Caraka Samhita, Sutra Sthana (Cakrapani)	20-11
21,22	Caraka Samhita Sutra Sthana	20-11
23	Susruta Samhita Nidana Sthana	1-75
24	Asthanga Hridaya Nidana Sthana	15-44
25	Caraka Samhita Cikitsa Sthana	28-37
26	Ashtanga Hridaya Nidana Sthana	15-54
27	Susruta Samhita Cikitsa Sthana	5-32
28	Ashtanga Hridaya Cikitsa Sthana	28-59
30	Ashtanga Sangraha, Sharira Sthana	6
31	Caraka Samhita Vimana Sthana (Cakrapani)	6-3
32	Caraka Samhita Vimana Sthana	5-6
33	Caraka Samhita Cikitsa Sthana	24-25
34	Caraka Samhita Sutra Sthana	12-7
35	Madhava Nidana (Madhukosha)	22-1
36, 38	Caraka Samhita Cikitsa Sthana	28-19
37	Madhava Nidana	10-29
39	Caraka Samhita Cikitsa Sthana	28-20
40	Bhela Samhita, Sutra Sthana	25/34-39
41	Susruta Samhita Cikitsa Sthana	4-20
42	Yoga Ratnakara Vatavyadhi Chikitsa	
43	Caraka Samhita Cikitsa Sthana	28-74
	Susruta Samhita Suthra Sthana	24/4-7
44	Susruta Samhita Cikitsa Sthana	5-6
	Caraka Samhita, Cikitsa Sthana	28-236
45	Susruta Samhita Cikitsa Sthana	5-29
46	Caraka Samhita Sutra Sthana (Cakrapani)	1-59
47	Caraka Samhita Cikitsa Sthana	28-81
48 to 51	Caraka Samhita Cikitsa Sthana	28/76-78
52	Susruta Samhita Cikitsa Sthana (Dalhana)	4/14-15
53,54,57	Caraka Samhita Cikitsa Sthana	28/82-83
55	Ashtanga Hridaya Sutra Sthana	18/3-5
56	Caraka Samhita Cikitsa Sthana (Gangadhara)	28-85
58	Caraka Samhita, Cikitsa Sthana (Cakrapani)	28-83

59	Caraka Samhita Cikitsa Sthana	28-84
60	Susruta Samhita Cikitsa Sthana	4-20
61	Caraka Samhita Cikitsa Sthana	28-104
62	Caraka Samhita Cikitsa Sthana	28-88
63	Caraka Samhita Sutra Sthana	24-17
64	Gadanigraha	19-9
65	Susruta Samhita Cikitsa Sthana	4-12
66 to 74	Caraka Samhita Cikitsa Sthana	28/188-193
75-79	Caraka Samhita Cikitsa Sthana	28/239-43

VATAVYADHI VIS-A-VIS VATANANATMAJA VYADHI
A Critical Conceptual Analysis

Introduction

Caraka has classified the diseases into *Nanatmaja* and *Samanyaja* groups basing on the involvement of the *doshas* either singularly or in combination.[1] Kasyapa and Sarangadhara too seem to have been influenced by this classification though the very terms *Nanatmaja* and *Samanyaja* have not been used.[2 & 3] Interestingly enough Vagbhata, a true follower of Charaka, and also Sushruta donot subscribe to this classification. However all the above classics and other extant texts have dealt in detail about *Vatavyadhis*. The general consideration is that the terms *Vatavyadhi* and *Nanatmaja Vatavyadhi* are synonymous. Cakrapani, too seems to have subscribed to this view. However it appears that there is something more to it than that merely meets the eye. The present article probes in depth about this aspect and endeavours to offer some clarifications.

Vatavyadhi

Various definitions have been offered by different authors for this terms:

1. *Vata Eva Vyadhih Vatavyadhih*[4]
2. *Vatat Vyadhih Vatavyadhih*[5]
3. V*ikruto Dukhahkari Vato Vatavyadhih*[6]
4. *Vikruta Vatajanito Vyadhih—Vatavyadhih*[7]
5. *Vatajanito Asadharanovyadhih Vatavyadhih*[8]

1. *Vata* itself cannot be a *vyadhi* because it is present even in healthy individuals.

2. It is true that Vatavyadhi is caused by *Vata* but all diseases caused by vata cannot be considered as Vatavyadhis.

3 & 4. These definitions, though do not give a complete picture of what a *Vata Vyadhi* is, certainly are more appropriate than the earlier ones. They make three points clear.

(i) The *Vata* should be *Vikruta*
(ii) The disease should be *Vatajanita*
(iii) The condition should be painful.

5. This definition is the most complete definition available. The additional trust given by "*Asadharana*" makes all the difference.

Thus for a disease to be termed Vatavyadhi it should be (1) *Vikruta Vatajanita* (2) It should be *Asadharana.*

Madhavakara while defining Vatayvyadhi has made some interesting observations as to why only '*Vatavyadhis*' and not *Pitta Vyadhis* and *Kaphavyadhis* are being considered for elaboration. He observes[9]—"*Vayu* is the most powerful of all and causes the disease instantaneously. The diseases are very serious and need contradictory approaches at times and in general are incurable. Besides they often cause medical emergencies."

Thus *Vatavyadhis* are a group of diseases caused by vitiated *vata* and almost difficult to be got rid of even by a most competent physician, using the most powerful medicines. At times they cause medical emergencies and become incurable.

Nanatmaja Vatavyadhi

Charaka has classified the diseases into 2 groups namely *Samanyaja* and *Nanatmaja* with reference to the involvement of *doshas,*[10] either singularly or in combination.

However he does not define these two terms. The division of *Nanatmaja* into *Vataja, Pittaja* and *Kaphaja* helps one to presume that probably these diseases are caused specifically by these *doshas.* Cakrapani's observations are useful to some extent, though the clarity is still lacking.[11] He says that Samanyajas are those that are caused by *doshas* in combination (by more than one dosha) while *Nanatmajas* are caused by individual *doshas* without the involvement of other *doshas*. This is applied to mean that any disease if it is caused by a single *dosha* can be a *Nanatmaja* disease of that particular *dosha*. Thus for example '*Pandu*' if caused alone by *vata* can be *Vataja Nanatmaja* or if caused by *Pitta* or *Kapha* it can be *Pitta Nanatmaja* or *Kaphaja Nanatmaja*. Madhava Nidhana issues a statement clarifying such *doubt*.[12] He says '*Nanatmajas* are always *Ekadosajanya*. For example *Akshepa* etc., are caused only by *vata* and can never be caused by either *pitta* or *kapha*. Similarly *cosa* etc., by pitta alone and not by vata or Kapha; Tripti etc. by *kapha* alone and never by *vata* or *pitta*. He adds further—*samanyajas* are caused by a combination of three or two doshas.

There are a few diseases which are mentioned in both the groups. For Charaka includes *Urusthamba, Gridrasi* and *Hikka*[13] in both *Vata Nanatmaja* and *Samanyaja* Groups. Similarly *Raktapitta* and *Kamala* the two *Pittaja Nanatmaja* diseases are also counted among *samanyaja* diseases.[14] Charaka even included *Vatarakta* among *Pittaja Nanatmaja* (though mentioning it in *Samanyaja* Group) raising many an eye brow. For, *Vata Rakta* is counted among by *Maha Vatavyadhis* by Sushruta[15] and even Charaka says that the name '*vatabalas*' is given because *vata* here is most important. Similarly Charaka devotes a separate chapter (just before the chapter on *Vatavyadhis*) for *Urusthamba* though he counts it among *Nanatmaja Vata vyadhis*. This probably may be due to the fact that the therapeutic approach for *Urusthamba* is in variance with that of *Vatavyadhis*. Cakrapani however gives clarification about including *Gridrasi Urusthamba* and *Raktapitta* in both the groups. He says[16]

1. The term *Gridrasi* in vatavyadi only refers to *Gridrasi Sula*
2. In *Urusthambha* only *Sthambha* should be considered. Sthamba is a pathognomonic condition of *Vata*.
3. *Shudha Pittajanya Rattapitta* alone should be considered among *Nanatmaja* variety.

However nothing is said about *Hikka, Kamala* and *Vatarakta*. It is difficult to justify the inclusion of Hikka into *Nanatmaja* group because the following statements do not quite agree with this proposal.

1. *Kapha vatatmakavetau* (Hikka and Swasa) *Pitta Sthana Samudbhavau*—Ca. Ci. 17/8.
2. *Vayuh Kaphenanugatah Pancakitkam Karotihi*—Su.Ut. 50.

However some justification may be made with regard to the other two diseases *kamala* and *vatarakta*. Though *Kamala* is generally due to *pitta* alone vitiation of Kapha in *Sakhasrita kamala* has been explained inclusion of *kamala* among *samanyaja vyadhis* should be viewed from this angle. Similarly *Pittadika Vatarakta* may be considered among the *Nanatmaja* variety while the rest of the varieties may be counted among *Samanyaja* group. Except *Hikka*, other diseases somehow fit into both the groups.

Thus it becomes apparent *Nanatmaja* refers to those diseases which are caused by a single *dosha*. Further the disease can be caused only by that particular dosha. And never because by other *doshas*. For example *Pakshaghata* is a *Nanatmaja* disease caused by *Vata*. It can only be caused by *vata* and never by *pitta* or *kapha*. The exact meaning of the term '*Nanatmaja*' should be properly understood. '*Na*'—*Anatmaja* = *Atmaja* i.e., it is always *atmaja* (self-generated) and can never be *Anatmaja* (not generated by other dosha). However once again *pakshagata's* division into *Shudda vataja, Vatakaphaja* and *Vatapittaja* induces confusion and warrants a clarification. The description/ discussion follows would help diffuse the confusion.

'*Na-Anatmaja*' means self-generated, singular involvement. More than the involvement, it is the 'level/stage' at which the 'involvement' takes place that actually distinguishes a *Nanatmaja* disease from a *Samanyaja* disease. For a disease to be called *Nanatmaja* it should satisfy two conditions:

1. *Ekadosa Janya*—only one dosha should be involved in the 'genesis' of the disease.
2. *Na-Anyenajatah*—*Na-Anatmaja*—No *dosha* other than that particular dosha should be able to cause that particular disease.

Sometimes during the course of a *Nanatmaja* disease of a particular *dosha*, symptoms of other *doshas* are also seen. The symptoms that appear during the course are *anubanda lakshanas* and *doshas, anubanda doshas.* Thus '*doshanubanda*' should not be confused with '*Samsarga,*' which is a characteristic feature of a *Samanyaja* disease. Inclusion of *Urusthambha, Gridrasi, Kamala, Raktapitta* and *Vatarakta* if viewed from this angle do not cause any confusion. The case of *Hikka,* also should be understood on the same lines.

So much so about 'not so controversial' aspect of *vatavyadhis* and *Nanatmaja Vatavyadhis.* The million dollar question is, whether these two terms—Vatavyadhi and Nanatmaja vatavyadhi are synonymus. The simple answer is 'yes,' but it is not so simple because it requires thorough analysis before one finally arrives at an acceptable answer. It appears that Cakrapani has accepted the two terms synonymous. For, while commenting upon the very first verse in *Vatavyadhicikita*—Ca. Ci. 28, he has issued a statement to this effect.[17]

'One should not comment as to why the management of *Vatananatmaja vyadhis* is being considered, though it is necessary that even *pittaja* and *kaphaja nanatmaja* diseases be treated. As *pitta* and *kapha nanatmaja* diseases are not that important as those of *Vata,* the treatment for only those *vata nanatmaja* diseases mentioned earlier is being considered. Management of *Kaphaja-Pittaja, Nanatmaja* diseases which have been mentioned earlier should be done with the help of *vamana* and *virecana* which are the alleviators of *kapha* and *pitta.*'

The above statement having come at the beginning of the chapter on *Vatavyadhis,* only confirms that Cakrapani did not see any difference between *vatavyadhi* and *vata-nanatmaja vyadhi.* Though we do not get any direct reference denouncing the above statement, there are many factors, which contradict this new point.

The most important factor however is that the diseases detailed in the chapter on *Vatavyadhi* by Charaka are different from those which are enumerated under *Nanatmaja vatavyadhis.*

One has to give a careful look to the Table No. 2.13, 2.14, 2.15 to digest the following discussion.

It is very obvious that in the very beginning there is a gross difference in number. It also becomes clear that very few number 11 of diseases, are common in both the groups. Further it appears that a good number of the disease conditions mentioned under *Nanatmaja* group can be termed symptoms and most of those mentioned under *vatavyadhis* are found to be diseases comprising of many symptoms. Many of these are difficult to cure (a few of them mentioned under *Nanatmaja* are also difficult to cure) and need multiple approaches in management, the basis of Madhava's observations. Digressing a bit from the table, one really has to understand the importance of *samanyaja* and *nanatmaja* classification.

As far as *Nanatmaja* is concerned specific diseases/pathological conditions belonging to three body systems *Vata* system, *Pitta* system and *Kapha* system have been enumerated. This classification clearly identifies the *dosha* involved and treatment becomes easier. This in one way an oversimplication of the therapeutic procedure, as the dosha becomes very specific. Thus principles of treatment are never contradictory, because approaches are never multiple. This is more so in case of *vata* because *vata* has no '*Roopa*' and '*Rasa.*' Further the 'actions' and 'qualities' of vata help identify diagnose the disease early, easily and correctly. However *pitta* and *kapha* because of the presence of *Rasa* and *Rupa* lead to more complicated manifestations and hence cause difficulty in both diagnosis and management. However vatananatma vyadhis are said to be incurable or curable with difficulty because of special inherent qualities of vata which have been discussed by Madhava. (This has been discussed earlier). However *nanatmaja* diseases of *pitta* and *kapha* are easily diagnosable and curable as compared to *samanyaja* diseases. Looking at Madhava's description of the importance of *vatavyadhi* where he terms them serious, complicated, untreatable and incurable, one is convinced that *vatavyadhis* and *vataja nanatmaja vyadhis* are not similar.

Getting on to the table 2.16 again one should appreciate Sharangadhara's approach. His list of *vatavyadhis*[19] is a judicious mixture of *vataja nanatmaja vyadhis* and *vatavyadhis*, mentioned by Charaka. He has picked up 80 important diseases from 80 nanatmaja vyadhis mentioned in Charaka Sutra and a lesser number of vata vyadhis mentioned in Charaka Cikitsa. Interesting/confusing aspect is that he does not use the term Nanatmaja but fixes the number at 80—Equal to the number of nanatmaja mentioned by Charaka. Thus the word *Asiti* (80 Eighty) tempts one to think that they are *nanatmaja* and the usage *vataja* rogah and non-usage of the term '*nanatmaja*' presses one consider them vatavyadhis. It is probable that Sharangadhara too did not differentiate '*vatavyadhis*' and *Nanatmaja Vatavyadhis.* Kasyapa too has followed Charaka,[20] but has not used terms *Samanyaja* and *Nanatmaja.* The diseases are enlisted under vataja (80) pittaja (40) and kaphaja (20) rogas are similar with those mentioned by Charaka under *Nanatmaja* in Charaka Sutra with minimal omissions and commissions. Even Madhavakara who has made such relevant observations to differentiate *Nanatmaja* and *Samanyaja Vyadhis*, does not discuss this sensitive aspect. '*Akshepa kadayo Vatadanati bhinna rupa Nanatmajah Tena Vatavikarah Prithagucyante Natu Kaphapitta Vikara iti*'[21] makes it clear that Madhava did not differentiate the *vata-nanatmaja* and *vatavyadhi.*

Charaka himself has stated in Cikitsa 28/13, 14 that now he is detailing the diseases, mentioned earlier in *Sutrastana.*

The question now arises as to why so much of discussion when all these commentators do not find anything different. The author's contention is that these two are different is based on the following observations.

1. All the diseases mentioned under *Nanatmaja* are not discussed in *Vatavyadhi* chapter, with a gross difference in the number of diseases mentioned in these two chapters.
2. Most of the diseases detailed in chapter on *Vatayavyadhi's* are not mentioned among *Nanatmaja vatavyadhis.*

3. Only Eleven diseases are common to both the groups.
4. Most of those mentioned in nanatmaja group are very simple pathological conditions which can easily be cured which is in contrast to the nature (incurability) of *vatavyadhis.*

It is clear now that *Vatavyadhis* and *Nanatmaja vatavyadhis* are not synonymous. But the question is that where exactly lies misunderstanding.

It is accepted fact that Charaka Sutra was the original contribution of Charaka himself, while Charaka Cikitsa (17th chapter onwards) was redacted by Dridabhala. This may be the reason why the diseases mentioned in the two chapters are different. Further later authors like Sarangadhara and Madhava who were puzzled by variance of descriptions adopted a comprise formula.

There seems to be some difference about the number of *nanatmaja* vyadhis too. Though Charaka has stated it is eighty, the number is not exactly the same. A few editions have counted 81 and a few 79. Referring to the various editions of the text, the number is found to be Eighty-six should we consider the diseases mentioned by Sharangadhara and Kasyapa too as *vata nanatmaja* diseases, then the number swells to 160 (Table 2.16).

There is one more interesting aspect Sushruta classifies *Vatavyadhis* into *vatavyadhis* and *mahavatavyadhis,* devoting separate chapters for these two in Nidana Sthana. However the management aspect is dealt in only one chapter in Cikitsa. Further Sushruta includes *Vataraktc,* among *Mahavatavyadhis.* Charaka does not make any such divisions, but in Cikitsa 28 he has considered a few diseases as *viseshavatavyadhis.*[22] It is interesting to note that Charaka who does not describe *vatarakta* in *vatavyadhis* chapter (it is dealt in a separate chapter in Ca, Ci, 29) has mentioned it among *visesha-vyadhis.* Bhela has divided the patients afflicted with vatavyadhis into No. 1. Sarvanga Roginah (2) Ekanga Roginah.[23] However the details are not available, the extant text being incomplete.

Thus to conclude Ayurvedic description of *vatavyadhis* has many salient features. There are differences of opinion among the scholars about the number, division and subtler aspects of classification. Caraka has mentioned different sets of diseases under *Vatananatmajavyadhis* and *Vatavyadhis*. There is a gross difference in number and nomenclature. Only a minimal number of diseases are found in both the groups. No commentator has however touched this aspect. The author feels they are different. It is worth a thorough discussion like this.

Table 2.14: *Vata (Nanatmaja) Vyadhis Mentioned in Caraka Samhita*

Vatavyadhis *(Cikitsa—28)*	*Nanatmaja Vata Vyadhis* *(Sutra—20)*
(1)	*(2)*
1. Pakshavadha	1. Pakshavadha
2. Sarvangaroga	2. Sarvangaroga
3. Ekanga Roga	3. Ekanga Roga
4. Ardita	4. Ardita
5. Manyasthamba (Antarayama)	5. Manyasthamba (Antarayama)
6. Grivasthambha	6. Grivasthambha
7. Akshepaka	7. Akshepaka
8. Dandaka	8. Dandaka
9. Kubja	9. Kubja
10. Pangu	10. Pangu
11. Gridhrasi	11. Gridhrasi
12. Hanusthamba (Bahirayama)	12. Nakhabheda
13. Hanuygraha	13. Vipadika
14. Angasosha	14. Padasula
15. Kuncana	15. Padabhramsa

(1)	*(2)*
16. Khudavata	16. Padasuptata
17. Khalli	.17. Vatakhuddata
18. Adyavata	18. Gulphagraha
19. Sthamba	19. Pindikodvestana
20. Sandhichyuti	20. Janubheda
21. Kashtagatavata	21. Januvislesa
22. Amasayagatavata	22. Urustamba
23. Pakwasayagatavata	23. Urusada
24. Gudagatavata	24. Gudabhramsa
25. Indriyagatavata	25. Gudarti
26. Sarvangagatavata	26. Vrsanaksepa
27. Snayugatavata	27. Sephastambha
28. Siragatavata	28. Vankasananaha
29. Sandhigatavata	29. Sronibheda
30. Jwagasritavata	30. Vidbheda
31. Raktasritavata	31. Udavarta
32. Mamsasritavata	32. Khanjatva
33. Medasritavata	33. Srama
34. Astyasritavata	34. Vamanatva
35. Majjasritavata	35. Trikagraha
36. Sukrasritavata	36. Prsthagraha
37. Raktavrutavata	37. Parsvavamarda
38. Mamsavrutavata	38. Udaravesta
39. Medasavruta (Adhyavata)	39. Hrnmoha
40. Asthyavruta	40. Hyddrava
41. Majjavruta(Vinama)	41. Vaksauddharsa
42. Sukravruta	42. Vaksauparodha
43. Annavruta	43. Vaksastoda
44. Mutravruta	44. Bahusosa
45. Purishavruta	45. Unmada
46. Kaphavruta	46. Khalli

(1)	(2)
47. Pittavruta	47. Kanthoddhvamsa
48. Anyonyavruta	48. Hanubheda
	49. Osthabheda
	50. Aksibheda
	51. Dantabheda
	52. Dantasaithilya
	53. Mukatva
	54. Vaksanga
	55. Kasayasyata
	56. Mukhasosa
	57. Arasajnata
	58. Ghrananasa
	59. Karnasula
	60. Asabdasravana
	61. Uccaibruti
	62. Badhirya
	63. Vartmastambha
	64. Vartmasamkoca
	65. Timira
	66. Aksisula
	67. Aksivyudasa
	68. Bhruvyudasa
	69. Sankhabheda
	70. Lalatabheda
	71. Siroruk
	72. Kesabhumisphutana
	73. Parusya
	74. Syavarunavadhasata
	75. Asvapna
	76. Anavasthitacittatva
	77. Akshipaka
	78. Sandya
	79. Tama
	80. Bhrama

(1)	(2)
	81. Vepathu
	82. Jrmbha
	83. Hikka
	84. Visada
	85. Atipratapa
	86. Rauksya

Table. 2.15: *Vatavyadhis in Brihatrayee*
(Ca—Ci—28, Su-N1-1, Su—Ci 4 & 5, A.H.N. 15-16, Ci 21, 22)

Sl. No.	*Disease*	*Charaka*	*Sushruta*	*A.Hridaya*
(1)	*(2)*	*(3)*	*(4)*	*(5)*
1.	Pakshavadha	+	+	+
2.	Sarvangaroga	+	+	+
3.	Ekanga Roga	+	+	+
4.	Ardita	+	+	+
5.	Manyasthamba (Antarayama)	+	+	+
6.	Griva sthambha	+	+	+
7.	Akshepaka	+	+	
8.	Dandaka	+	+	+
9.	Kubja	+		
10.	Pangu	+	+	+
11.	Gridhrasi	+	+	+
12.	Hanusthamba (Bahirayama)	+	+	+
13.	Hanugraha	+		
14.	Angasosha	+		
15.	Kuncana	+		
16.	Khudavata	+	+	+
17.	Khalli	+		+
18.	Adyavata	+		+
19.	Sthamba	+		

(1)	*(2)*	*(3)*	*(4)*	*(5)*
20.	Sandhichyuti	+		
21.	Koshtagatavata	+		
22.	Amasayagatavata	+		+
23.	Pakwasayagatavata	+		+
24.	Guda gatavata	+		
25.	Indriyagatavata	+	+	
26.	Saruangagatavata	+		
27.	Snayugatavata	+	+	
28.	Siragatavata	+	+	
29.	Sandhigatavata	+	+	
30.	Twagasritavata	+	+	
31.	Raktasrita vata	+	+	+
32.	Mamsasritavata	+	+	
33.	Medasritavata	+	+	
34.	Astyasritavata	+	+	
35.	Majjasritavata	+	+	
36.	Sukrasritavata	+		
37.	Raktavrutavata	+	+	+
38.	Mamsavrutavata	+		+
39.	Medasavruta (Adhyavata)	+		+
40.	Asthyavruta	+		+
41.	Majjavruta (Vinama)	+		+
42.	Sukravruta	+		+
43.	Annavruta	+		+
44.	Mutravruta	+		+
45.	Purishavruta	+		+
46.	Kaphavruta	+	+	+
47.	Pittavruta	+	+	+
48.	Anyonyavruta	+		+
49.	Apatantraka		+	+
50.	Vishwachi		+	+
51.	Kroshtukasirsha		+	+
52.	Khanja		+	+

(1)	(2)	(3)	(4)	(5)
53.	Kalayakhanja		+	+
54.	Padadha		+	+
55.	Padaharsha		+	+
56.	Avabahuka		+	+
57.	Vatakantaka		+	+
58.	Badhirya		+	
59.	Karnashula		+	
60.	Muka		+	
61.	Minmina		+	
62.	Gadgada		+	
63.	Tuunee		+	
64.	Pratituunee		+	
65.	Adhmana		+	
66.	Pratyadhmana		+	
67.	Ashteela		+	
68.	Vatashteela		+	
69.	Vastigatavata		+	
70.	Skandagatavata		+	
71.	Trikagatavata		+	
72.	Manyagatavata		+	
73.	Vakshagatavata		+	
74.	Urusthambha		+	+
75.	Vranayama			+
76.	Siragraha			+
77.	Sirogatavata			+
78.	Nabhigatavata			+
79.	Hritstavata			+
80.	Jihwa Stambha			+

Table 2.16: *Vata (Nanatmaja) Vyadhis according to Different texts*
(Cu.—Su.—20/11, Ka.-Su 27/20-29, Su.-Pu.-7/105-114)

	S.No.	*Disease*	*Charaka*	*Kash-yapa*	*Saran-gadhara*
	(1)	*(2)*	*(3)*	*(4)*	*(5)*
(C.K.S.)	1.	Ardita	+	+	+
	2.	(Athi) Pralapa	+	+	+
	3.	Urusthambha	+	+	+
	4.	Vamanatwa	+	+	+
	5.	Gridhrasi	+	+	+
	6.	Jrumbha	+	+	+
	7.	Pakshavadha	+	+	+
	8.	Rouksha	+	+	+
	9.	Kubjatwa	+	+	+
(C.K.)	10.	Akshishula	+	+	
	11.	Udavarta	+	+	
	12.	Udaraveshta	+	+	
	13.	Ucchaihishruthi	+	+	
	14.	Urusada	+	+	
	15.	Oshtabheda	+	+	
	16.	Kantodhwamsa	+	+	
	17.	Keshabhumis-putanam	+	+	
	18.	Karnashula	+	+	
	19.	Kashayasyatha	+	+	
	20.	Greevasthambha	+	+	
	21.	Gudabhramsa	+	+	
	22.	Gudarthi	+	+	
	23.	Ghrananasa	+	+	
	24.	Janubheda	+	+	
	25.	Januvislesha	+	+	
	26.	Timira	+	+	

(1)	*(2)*	*(3)*	*(4)*	*(5)*
	27. Nakhabheda	+	+	
	28. Padashula	+	+	
	29. Padabhramsa	+	+	
	30. Padasuptata	+	+	
	31. Pangulya	+	+	
	32. Prushtagraha	+	+	
	33. Pindikodweshta	+	+	
	34. Bahusosha	+	+	
	35. Badhirya	+	+	
	36. Bhrama	+	+	
	37. Bhruvyudasa	+	+	
	38. Vankhananaha	+	+	
	39. Vakshodgharsha	+	+	
	40. Vakshoparoda	+	+	
	41. Veksharthoda	+	+	
	42. Vartamasankocha	+	+	
	43. Vatakhuddata	+	+	
	44. Vishada	+	+	
	45. Vepadhu	+	+	
	46. Vrishnakshepa	+	+	
	47. Ekangata (Ekangaroga)	+	+	
	48. Vipadika	+	+	
	49. Shrama	+	+	
	50. Shronibheda	+	+	
	51. Sankhabheda	+	+	
	52. Shandya	+	+	
	53. Shiroruk	+	+	
	54. Shephastha-mbha	+	+	
	55. Shyavaaruna bhasatha	+	+	
	56. Hrinmoha	+	+	

	(1)	*(2)*	*(3)*	*(4)*	*(5)*
	57.	Hridrava	+	+	
	58.	Trikagraha	+	+	
K.S.	59.	Nidraparikshaya		+	+
	60.	Parswashula		+	+
	61.	Mukatwa		+	+
	62.	Vatakantaka		+	+
	63.	Vidgraha		+	+
(C.&S.)	64.	Anavasthita Chittatwa	+		+
	65.	Akshepaka	+		+
	66.	Arasagnata	+		+
	67.	Khalli	+		+
C.	68.	Manyasthamba	+		
	69.	Parswavamarda	+		
	70.	Dhanta Bheda	+		
	71.	Asabdasravana	+		
	72.	Vartmasthambha	+		
	73.	Vaksanga	+		
	74.	Hanubhedha	+		
	75.	Aswapna	+		
	76.	Hikka	+		
	77.	Unmada	+		
	78.	Akshibheda	+		
	79.	Vidbheda	+		
	80.	Gadgadatwa	+		
	81.	Akshvyudasa	+		
	82.	Gulfa Graha	+		
	83.	Sarvanga Rodha	+		
	84.	Tama	+		
	85.	Mukhasosha	+		
	86.	Danta Bheda	+		
	87.	Danta Shaitilya	+		
	88.	Dandaka	+		
(K.)	89.	Anavasthana		+	

(1)	(2)	(3)	(4)	(5)
	90. Pratishyaya		+	
	91. Asabdata		+	
	92. Anilagraha		+	
	93. Vishtamba		+	
	94. Asyasosha		+	
	95. Vudasa		+	
	96. Dantachala		+	
	97. Vandhyatwa		+	
	98. Dandakshepaka		+	
	99. Vatagulfa		+	
	100. Glani		+	
	101. Vaggraha		+	
	102. Swasa		+	
	103. Vidgada		+	
(S.)	104. Antarayama			+
	105. Apabahuka			+
	106. Apatanaka			+
	107. Apatantraka			+
	108. Durbalatwa			+
	109. Jihwasthambha			+
	110. Tuunee			+
	111. Toda			+
	112. Drishtikshayam			+
	113. Pratituunee			+
	114. Padaharsha			+
	115. Pratyashteela			+
	116. Pratyadhmana			+
	117. Prasupti			+
	118. Balakshaya			+
	119. Baddhavitkata			+
	120. Bahyayama			+
	121. Bheerutwa			+
	122. Vatapravritti			+
	123. Vranayama			+

(1)	*(2)*	*(3)*	*(4)*	*(5)*
124.	Virasasyata			+
125.	Viswachi			+
126.	Syavatha			+
127.	Shiragraha			+
128.	Shirapurana			+
129.	Athyudgara			+
130.	Ashteelika			+
131.	Angapeeda			+
132.	Angabheda			+
133.	Angabhanga			+
134.	Angasosha			+
135.	Angashula			+
136.	Adhmana			+
137.	Angavabhramsa			+
138.	Anthrakujana			+
139.	Katigraha			+
140.	Kroshtaseersha			+
141.	Kalayakhanjata			+
142.	Kallana			+
143.	Kampa			+
144.	Karshya			+
145.	Katinya			+
146.	Kandu			+
147.	Khanjatwa			+
148.	Ganvashakha			+
149.	Dandapatanaka			+
150.	Sheetata			+
151.	Shabdagnata			+
152.	Shukratipravritti			+
153.	Shukrakshaya			+
154.	Sankocha			+
155.	Sthambha			+
156.	Sphurana			+

(1)	*(2)*	*(3)*	*(4)*	*(5)*
157.	Swedanasa			+
158.	Retonasha			+
159.	Romaharsha			+
160.	Hanugraha			+

REFERENCES

1.	Caraka Samhita Sutra Sthana	20/10
2.	Kasyapa Samhita	
3.	Sharangadhara Samhita Purva Khanda	7/105
4. & 5.	Caraka Samhita Cikitsa Sthana—Cakrapani	28/2
6. to 9.	Madhava Nidana—Madhukosa	22/1
10.	Caraka Sutra Sthana	20/10
11.	Caraka Sutra Sthana—Cakrapani	20/10
12.	Madhava Nidana Madhukosa	22/11
13.	Caraka Samhita Sutra Sthana	19/3 & 20/11
14.	Caraka Samhita Sutra Sthana	19/3 & 20/14
15.	Susruta Samhita Nidhana Sthana	5/
16.	Caraka Samhita Sutra Sthana—Cakrapani	20/11, 14
17.	Caraka Samhita Cikistsa Sthana	28/
18.	Madhava Nidana Madhukosa	22/1
19.	Sharangadhara Samhita Purvakanda	7/105
20.	Kasyapa Samhita	
21.	Madhava Nidana Madhukosa	22/1
22.	Caraka Samhita Cikitsa Sthana	28/72-74
23.	Bhela Samhita	

Clinical Report

Preliminary Clinical Trial of Hingutriguna Taila in Vatavyadhis: M.M. Padhi, N.S. Tewari and Prem Kishore (*JRAS*: II: 1: 1981)

Summary

Vatavyadhis considered to be difficult of prognosis have been taken up for clinical studies. In order to evolve a simple herbal treatment for these diseases, Hingutriguna taila has been selected and preliminary clinical studies have been taken up in 32 different cases of vatavyadhis. This preliminary observations indicates definite efficacy of this preparation Hingutriguna taila in the treatment of vatavyadhi. The effect is found to be more pronounced in the patients suffering from Gridhrasi and Pakshagata.

Introduction

Vata, one of the tridosha, plays an important role in the regulation of the vital functions of the body and also in the causation of various diseases. But certain specific diseases caused by only Vatadosha, mostly of neurological and rheumatic origin, come under the group of Vatavyadhis. The prognosis of these diseases is considered to be difficult. The diseases like Pakshagata (Hemiplegia), Gridhrasi (Sciatica), and Katisula (Bachache), are more frequent in this area and are due to various dietetic and climatic factors. In common practice, Guggulu preparations are prescribed for the treatment of these diseases. With a view to finding out an alternate and more efficacious treatment and to popularise it in practice, the formulation Hingutriguna taila (Ashtanga Hridaya, Gulma Chikitsa) was taken up for clinical evaluation in certain types of vatavyadhi. This preparation has been selected considering the potent Vatashamaka properties of its ingredients., i.e. Hingu, Saindhava, Rasona and Eranda. The utility of this preparation in the treatment of rheumatism has also been reported recently by Nadkarni (1976). The present communication deals with the study of the effect of Hingutriguna taila on 32 cases of Vatavyadhis.

Method of Study

Out of a total of 32 cases taken up for study, 8 were of Pakshagata, 11 of Gridhrasi, 6 of Katisula and one each of Ardita and Visvaci, 3 of Sarvangavata and 2 cases of the other Vatavikara. The selection and diagnosis of the cases were made on the basis of cardinal clinical features of the respective diseases as described in Ayurvedic texts. The drug was administered orally in the dosage of 5 ml 2-3 times daily with warm water. Simultaneously, Abhyanga was given with Kshirabala taila or Mahanarayana taila followed by sweda. The diet provided to the patients consisted of Rice, Atta, Dal, Suji, Milk and vegetable curry. The assessment of the results has been made on the basis of changes observed in clinical features and objective tests. The results were classified into four groups: complete relief (100 per cent relief), partial relief (50 per cent relief), no relief (including marginal improvement) and drop out.

Table 2.17: *The Results of Treatment in Various Types of Vatavyadhis*

Diseases	*C.R.*	*P.R.*	*N.R.*	*D.O.*	*Total*
1. Pakshagata	2 (25%)	5 (62.5%)	–	1 (12.5%)	8
2. Gridhrasi	6 (54.54%)	3 (27.27%)	–	2 (18.18%)	11
3. Katisula	1 (16.66%)	5 (83.83%)	–	–	6
4. Ardita	–	1 (100%)	–	–	1
5. Visvaci	1 (100%)	–	–	–	1
6. Sarvangavata	–	2 (66.66%)	–	1 (33.3%)	3
7. Others	–	1 (50%)	1 (50%)	–	2
Total	10 (31.25%)	17 (53.12%)	1 (3.12%)	4 (12.5%)	32

Results

The overall results of the treatment indicate fairly good response, i.e. 31.25 per cent complete relief and 53.12 per cent partial relief. The effect is relatively more pronounced in the cases of Gridhrasi. Nine cases of this disease who completed the course of treatment of 3-4 weeks duration showed very good response. The effect of this formulation in the cases of Pakshagata was also found to be fairly good who were given the treatment for a period ranging from 37 to 99 days. In other diseases taken up for trial, the effect of this formulation was found to be relatively less.

Comments

The efficacy of the treatment could be ascribed to the known vatahara properties i.e. Snigdha, Guru, Tikshana and Ushnavirya—the Sareera gunas of all these ingredients are opposite to the Sarira gunas or Vatadosa which could also be the cause of the efficacy of this formulation. The effect in the cases of Pakshagata has also been relatively better as compared to the effect of certain other types of treatment. Considering the difficult prognosis of these diseases, the results obtained so far in the studies suggest that Hingutriguna taila may prove to be an useful drug for the treatment of Vatavyadhis.

HEADACHE

Headache is such a common complaint and can occur for so many different reasons that its proper evaluation may be difficult. Although underlying structural lesions are not present in most patients presenting with headache, it is nevertheless important to bear this possibility in mind. About one-third of patients with brain tumors, for example, present with a primary complaint of headache.

The intensity, quality, and site of pain and especially the duration of the headache and the presence of associated neurological symptoms may provide clues to the underlying cause. The onset of severe headache in a previously well patient is more likely than chronic headache to relate to an intracranial disorder such as subarachnoid-haemorrhage or meningitis. Headaches that disturb sleep, exertional headaches, and late-onset paroxysmal headaches are also more suggestive of an underlying structural lesion, as are headaches accompanied by neurological symptoms such as drowsiness, visual or limb problems, seizures or altered mental status.

Chronic headaches are commonly due to migraine, tension, or depression, but they may be related to intracranial lesions, head injury, cervical spondylosis, dental or ocular disease, temporomandibular joint dysfunction, sinusitis, or hypertension and a wide variety of general medical disorders.

All patients should be examined fully for these and other neurological and medical problems. Depending on the initial clinical impression, the need for such investigations as CT scan of the head, electroencephalography, and lumbar puncture must be assessed on an individual basis. The diagnosis and treatment of primary neurologic disorders associated with headaches should be considered separately.

TENSION HEADACHE (SHIRAH SHOOLA)

Patients frequently complain of poor concentration and other vague non-specific symptoms, in addition to constant daily headaches that are often tight in quality and may be exacerbated by emotional stress, fatigue, noise, or glare. The headaches are usually generalized, may be most intense about the neck or back of the head, and are not associated with focal neurologic symptoms. In addition to drug therapy such as simple analgesics and tranquillizers, techniques to induce relaxation are also useful and include massage, hot baths, and biofeedback. Psychologic counselling to explore underlying causes of chronic anxiety is often rewarding.

Treatment

See Clinical Report on Psychogenic headache.

For dyspeptic headache, give soda water tablet every four hours till relieved. If headache is also due to constipation, give Samudrak Virechan Churna or Shivkshar Pachan as a laxative.

If headache commences shortly after a meal, Madanadi Vaman Churna will relieve it.

When the liver or bowels are most in fault give Eliyadi Guti at night and Samudra Virechak Churna in the morning.

References: S.U. Ch 25; Ch. Chi. Ch. 26.

Clinical Reports

Controlled Study on Role of Ksheerabala Taila in Psychogenic Headache (Vataja Shirah Shoola): M.G. Ramu et al (*JRAS*:1:2:1980).

The term 'Psychogenic Headache' most commonly refers to those categories of headache where the influence of emotional factors is apparent and significant. Generally treatment for such conditions are through sedatives such as barbiturates and analgeics which offer only a temporary relief. Further more, the side effects curtail their prolonged use.

Detailed description of headache i.e. Shirah shoola is available from Charaka's time (3000 to 500 B.C.). Twelve varieties of Shirah shoola (shiro-roga) have been described in Ayurvedic classics.

Of the ninety-four symptoms of shirah shoola, fifteen symptoms have been ascribed to vataja variety of headache. Treatment for each type has been suggested in detail.

In the preliminary study, 131 patients suffering from different types of shirah shoola were successfully treated with various Ayurvedic medicines on the basis of Doshasthithi. It was noted that Ksheerabala taila was the principal medicine used.

Ksheerabala taila consists of milk and root of Bala (Sida cordifolia). It is vatahara and has been recommended in all vata vyadhies (Sahasrayoga Tailaprakaranam). Vata gets provoked by emotional factors like kama (desire), shoka (grief), and bhaya(fear). Shoola (pain) is due to vatashuddhi (vitiation of vata) (Charaka Chi. 3). In vataja shirah shoola, involvement of vata is more obvious).

With the above facts in view, it was proposed to screen the effectiveness of Ksheerabala taila in patients suffering from vataja shirah shoola (psychogenic headache) in the present study.

Material and Method

Patient's fulfilling the following criteria were included for the study: (i) Those who were the residents of Bangalore with headache as chief complaint; (ii) Those without any organic condition to account for their headache and; (iii) Those who were diagnosed as vataja shirah shoola.

Treatment

Ksheerabala taila was used in the form of Nasya, Pana and Abhayanga for the treated group. Ksheerabala ordinary (once medicated) was used for Abhayanga and Ksheerabala—41 (41 times medicated) for pana and nasya. Placebo group was supplied with coloured capsules filled with sugar. Duration of the treatment was six weeks.

Table 2.18: *Shows the Mode of Administration of Dose and Time Ksheerabala Taila*

Mode of Administration	*Dose*	*Time*
Abhayanga	15-25 ml.	Before breakfast
Pana	1-2 ml.	After dinner at bedtime
Nasya	6-12 ml.	Before sunset

Table 2.19: *Shows Type of Administration* of *Kshirabala-Weekwise*

Week	*Abhayanga*	*Pana*	*Nasya*
First	+	+	–
Second	+*	+	+*
Third	+*	+	+*
Fourth	+*	+	–
Fifth	+	+	–
Sixth	+	+	–

* indicates that Abhayanga and Nasya done on alternate days.

Detailed assessment was done on modern scientific methods.

Results

56 patients completed the six weeks of treatment, out of 106 patients (in two groups of treatment consisting of 28 patients each). Distribution of sex, age, marital status, duration of illness and socio-economic status of the patients in both the groups were almost similar.

Intensity of headache was compared for six weeks from initial assessment. In all the six weeks of assessment, the proportion of improvement in Ksheerabala group was better than that of Placebo group.

In the Ksheerabala treatment group, 11 patients showed signs of anxiety, 5 patients showed signs of depression, and 8 showed signs of both in their personality whereas 4 showed none on Rorschach.

In the Placebo treatment group, 12 patients showed signs of anxiety, 5 patients showed signs of depression and 8 showed signs of both, in their personality, whereas 3 showed none on Rorschach. Some of the features seen on the personality profile of the male and female patients are:

1. They are ruled by immediate need for gratification than the long range goals.
2. There is presence of tension, too powerful to permit the use of one's own inner resources for constructive solution of every day problems.
3. They show a severe need for affection which is so acute so as to swamp the whole personality.
4. The other features in the female group seen was weak emotional control and a tendency to act out their reactions.
5. Many of the anxiety patients have high aspirations but maladjustment or anxiety itself interferes in achieving them.

Discussion

"Severity of headache" was reduced in Ksheerabala treated group during all the six assessments than that of Placebo group. However, the difference between the two groups was not statistically significant during 1st, 2nd, and 5th weeks. Influence of emotional factors is apparent and significant in psychogenic headache. Vata gets provoked by emotional factors like kama (desire), shoka (grief), bhaya (fear). Always the pain is due to vata dosha (vitiated). Due to its vatahara quality Ksheerabala taila might have reduced vata dushti thereby resulting in the reduction of severity of headache. Hence the difference in severity of the headache in both the groups is expected.

It is observed that there was no significant difference in both the groups as regards to headache days.' The probable reasons for this may be (i) limited duration of treatment and (ii) chronicity of illness (more than 50 per cent of the samples were of the chronicity between 2 to 10 years).

The emerging picture on the Rorschach Ink Blot test of the anxiety patients includes an immediate need for gratification and affection, and also presence of powerful tensions.

There was significant reduction in anxiety syndrome in treated group at the end of six weeks but no significant difference was observed in the depression syndrome. The 'anxiety' syndrome appears to be vata predominant, whereas depression syndrome seems to be kapha pradhana from Ayurvedic point of view. Ksheerabala taila is well known for its usefulness in vatavyadhis; hence the reduction in anxiety syndrome and non-reduction in the depression syndrome was as expected.

APASMARA (EPILEPSIES OR CONVULSIVE DISEASES)

Definition (Nirvachana)

Apasmara is a disease, where there is a loss of Smarana

(memory) due to deviation of Buddhi and Manas. The patient cannot recollect the happenings occurred during the course of disease and experiences vigorous movements of all parts of the body.

General Considerations (Vichara)

Apasmara is a dreadful disease and it is included in 8 Maharogas (deeprooted diseases). Human population is suffering from it since the time of Daksha Yajna. It affects almost 2 per cent of the population of all age groups and both sexes equally. It is a chronic disease with an occasional family history and needs a long-term treatment. In modern medicine, epilepsies are described as a group of disorders due to chronic recurrent paroxysmal changes in neurologic function caused by abnormalities in the electrical activity of the brain.

Pathogenesis (Samprapti)

According to Charaka, in persons with perverted mind Doshas (Vata, Pitta, Kapha, Rajas and Tamas) being carried by vessels to Hridaya (Heart) afflict it and as such, the patient becomes stupified with wandering mind and then the disease appears. In modern medicine, electrical activity generated at a point (focal) or in the entire area (generalized) spreads and creates a neurological dysfunction there by causing seizures or convulsions.

Aetiological Factors (Roga Karana)

In the evolvement of Apasmara disease, the following factors may be held responsible, which lead to the pathogenesis. These factors help in a proper diagnosis and assessment of the state of the disease. Without knowing the proper Roga Karana, we cannot put forward even a step, in the management of the disease.

1. Vitiation of Manas by Rajas and Tamas, where Sattwaguna is totally inhibited.
2. Excess accumulation of Sariraka Doshas i.e. Vata, Pitta and Kapha.

3. Consumption of contaminated and impure food material.
4. Improper adoptation of treatment methods like Panchakarma.
5. Misused and improperly adopted rituals which impact the psyche.
6. Sleeping, sitting and travelling in irregular postures which cause stress and strain physically and mentally.
7. Excess emaciation or loss of weight due to malnutrition or intentional avoidance of food.
8. Unidentified factors which include head injury or congenital abnormality.
9. Alcoholism and withdrawal from alcoholism.

(According to the modern medical observations, a familial tendency is also observed where siblings exhibit some sort of manifestations. A growth in the brain or an infection may precipitate an attack.)

Classification

According to the predominance of doshas, Apasmara is classified into 4 types.

1. Vataja
2. Pittaja
3. Kaphaja
4. Sannipataja

The doshic classifications mostly depend upon the prodromal symptoms that are experienced and remembered by the patient even after recovery and also upon the nature or individual prakriti of that patient. This classification indicates the time taken to recover completely.

Clinical Manifestations (Lakshana Vichara)

Apasmara manifests clinically in a typical manner. The patient looks like a normal person and behaves like a normal person and poses no sociological problems. The clinical picture is almost similar in all types. In some cases, prodromal symptoms or Aura appear a few minutes before the actual commencement of the disease; such as sensory halucinations, vertigo and temporary loss of vision. Not all the patients complain the same thing and few may not even completely show any aura.

In the initiation of an attack, the patient abruptly falls on the ground due to complete loss of motor control. Then commences convulsions or Akshepaka. We can find an invulantary rotation of eye balls. Then he starts weeping suddenly and frothes from his mouth. The colour of the froth varies according to the Doshas. In vatic type it is light coloured, in paittic type yellow coloured and in Kaphaja variety pure white in colour. He emits certain specific sounds or cry. There is a sensation of having experienced different moving objects with varying colours. Then the patient recovers completely and goes to normal sleep or to his routine. The total time of an attack is mostly 3-4 minutes and in rare cases the time taken may be 5-6 minutes.

By observing the above said description of Apasmara, we can understand that our ancestors could record mainly the cases of complex partial seizures and generalized Tonicclonic seizures. The other types of seizures though they are not given place here, are described in other chapters like Vata Vyadhis under the heading of Akshepaka vata and others. So, the treatment elaborated in the following pages also aims at treating the said condition only. But as the pathogenesis behind all the types of seizures is generation of impulses in the brain, the same treatment can be extended to other types of seizures also with care.

Diagnosis (Nidana)

The disease itself is called Apasmara and the patient can not present before us any history about his disease except about few prodromal symptoms if present. So, the physician has to depend completely upon the close observers surrounding him. The description of symptoms described above will give us a precise knowledge of the disease. So, a careful enquiry about the duration, periodicity and other symptoms should be made and recorded. The knowledge of doshic classification is acquired by knowing the colour of the froth and the colour of the objects he has experienced before, if he remembers.We can make a symptomatic diagnosis by a correct clinical picture. To confirm our diagnosis, we can take the help from the modern diagnostic methods like E.E.G., Ultrasound,Computerized Tomography, M.R. Imaging etc.

Differential Diagnosis (Visleshana)

Not all convulsive diseases come under Apasmara. A detailed history of the attack, onset, periodicity and duration is to be acquired both from the patients and their relatives. If the patient is a child or infant, relying information is obtained from the parents. The following diseases may mimic Apasmara in certain aspects.

1. *Tetanus or Dhanustambha:* A previous history of injury somewhere or a bite of an animal is present. The attack lasts for longer period. The patient is almost conscious. Presence of lock-jaw will give a clue. Usually no frothing is present.
2. *Poisoning:* A sudden onset without previous history other symptoms of poisoning like vomiting, feeble pulse, tachycardia are present.
3. *Uraemia:* In uraemic convulsions, a definite history; is there about anuria or scanty micturition. A smell of urine is there on expiration. Blood urea levels are measured in case of doubtful history.
4. *Hysteria:* There is no periodicity or frothing. Tremor if present is relieved by grip. A highly emotional patient with disturbed thought is presented before the physician.

Management (Chikitsa)

In treating a case of Apasmara, the foremost principle is to eliminate the cause if found. But unfortunately, in most of the cases, the physician is not in a position, how precise, the exact cause is. So, a general methodology of treatment is to be adopted. If the patient is under continuous convulsions he should be brought back to consciousness. Then the patient must be protected from having further attacks without interfering with normal intellectual functions. He should be managed for any psychosocial consequences and complications.

After making a thorough diagnosis, the treatment regimen should be commenced at once. If the patient is found unconscious irritant nasal drops should be used. According to the doshic type, Vastikarma should be undertaken in vatic type, Virechana in Paittic type and Vamana in Kaphaja type. In all the Ayurvedic texts, the basic form of using most antiepileptic drugs is ghee preparation. Cow ghee is processed with decoction and powders of different plant and animal material and is prescribed to the patient to be used orally.

Use of old cow ghee in Apasmara is heavily praised, In Charaka Samhita, it is enlisted under the best Medhya drugs (Brain Tonics) and is very much useful in all psychiatric conditions. It is proved by modern researches also that, Ketogenic diet plays an important role in the treatment and control of convulsions, probably by interfering the levels of GABA. (Gamma-amino-butyric acid)

The following are some of the important and clinically useful compounds that are in common usage. These are classified basing on the form of preparation. The main ingredients of these compounds are put in a table form.

I. *Ghritas*

These are compounds of processed old cow Ghee. The normal adult dosage is 15-20 ml, 2 times a day. Hotwater or Hot milk should be taken after taking these drugs.

1. Panchagavya Ghrita
2. Brahmi Ghrita
6. Kalyanaka Ghrita
7. Lasunadi Ghrita

3. Vacha Ghrita
4. Hinguvadi Ghrita
5. Siddharthaka Ghrita
8. Kushmandaka Ghrita
9. Maha Satavari Ghrita

II. *Tailas*

Jyotishmati Tailam

1 gram of Tailam once or twice a day with hot milk.

III. *Choornas*

1. Musta Choorna—2-3 grams 2 times a day with honey and Ghee.
2. Vacha Choorna—2-3 grams 2 times a day with honey and Ghee.

IV. *Rasa Oushadhas*

1. Smriti Sagara Rasa	200 mg 2 times a day with Ghee
2. Rasa Raja Rasa	100 mg 2 times a day with Ghee
3. Rasa Sindoora	100 mg 2 times a day with Ghee
4. Tamra Bhasma	100 mg 2 times a day with Ghee

Besides the above said medications, some less popular methods are also seen in texts. These are:

1. Urine of female donkey and male goat
2. Fumigation with hairs, nails and bones of some animals like, dog, cat and fox.
3. Anjana or ophthalmic applications with Talaka, Manassila and Pepper.

These are practised here and there by physicians with good success. But just because of lack of scientific statistical data and lesser acceptability, these preparations though authenticated by Charaka and Sushruta are not in much vogue.

Time Factor

The physician has to choose one or two or three preparations depending upon the age, doshic type and severity of the disease. Then the treatment should be continued for 2-3 years after the complete disappearance of an attack. To achieve this goal, drugs are to be continued from 6 months to 5 years. So, the total period of treatment may extend upto 8 years. The patient and their relatives must be educated that, such a long term therapy is required to avoid relapse.

Prognosis (Sadhya-Sadhyata)

As described by Charaka, Apasmara is a grave disease and is very difficult to cure. If the patient is too old and is highly emaciated, the chances of cure are not so good. But if the patient is physically strong, and of younger age group and with no other complications, the time taken to cure the disease is minimum and the rate of relapse is also very low. It may be impossible to cure such cases with a history of Head injury or brain tumour or a definite organic lesion with medicines alone.

Clinical and Experimental Reports

1. Mehta, A.K. and Singh R.H.: Studies on the Psychotropic Effect of the Medhya Rasayana Drug Samkha Pushpi, Ph. D. Thesis from Banaras Hindu University.
2. Rai, N.P. and Chaturvedi, G.N.: Clinical and Experimental Studies on Epilepsy with Special Reference to Its Management with Aswagandha, Ph.D. Thesis from Banaras Hindu University.
3. Dixit, S.P. and Tiwari P.V.: Effect of Certain Indigenous Drugs in Convulsions in Children, Ph.D. Thesis from Banaras Hindu University.
4. Singh, R.H. and Mishra, B.K.: Clinical and Experimental Evaluation of Medhya Rasayana, Ph.D. Thesis from Banaras Hindu University.
5. Sitaram B. and Chunekar, K.C.: Anti-convulsive Effect of Different Sankha Pushpis. An Experimental Study, M.D. (Ay) Thesis from Banaras Hindu University.

Table 220: *Drugs Used Individually or in Compounds in Apasmara*

Plant Origin:

S. No.	*Name*	*Botanical Name*	*Part Used*	*Form of Usage*	*Dose/ Day*
(1)	*(2)*	*(3)*	*(4)*	*(5)*	*(6)*
1.	Sankha Pushpi	Convolvulus pluricanlis Choicy	Whole plant	Paste or Juice	20 g
2.	Brahmi	Centella asiatica (Linn) Urban	Whole plant	Paste or Juice	20 g
3.	Yashmi	Glycerrhiza glabra Linn	Root	Powder	10 g
4.	Guduchi	Tinospora cordifolia (willd) Miers	Stem	Juice	30 ml
5.	Vacha	Acorus calamus Linn	Rhizome	Powder	5 g
6.	Jatamamsi	Nardostachys jatamamsi DC	Rhizome	Hot infusion	50 ml
7.	Jyotishmati	Celastrus paniculatus willd	Seed	Oil expressed	2 g
8.	Satavari	Asparagus racemosus willd	Root	Powder	15 g
9.	Aswagandha	Withania sommifera Dunall	Root	Powder	10 g
10.	Aragvadha	Cassia fistula Linn	Fruit	Pulp paste	2 g
11.	Hingu	Ferula northex Boiss	Latex	Powder	1 g
12.	Arimeda	Acacia lengophlola willd	Heart wood	Decoction	20 ml
13.	Guggulu	Balasmodendron mukul Hook. ex stocks	Latex	Powder	5 g
14.	Choraka	Angelia glauca Edgw.	Root	Powder	5 g
15.	Durva	Cynodon dactylon (Linn) pers	Whole plant	Juice	20 ml

16.	Saptaparna	Alstonia scholaris R.Br.	Bark	Powder	5 g
17.	Kakodumbara	Ficus hispida Linn.	Fruit & Bark	Powder	5 g
18.	Bharangi	Clerodendron serratum spreng.	Root	Powder	10 g
19.	Pushkara Mula	Inula racemosa Hook. f.	Root	Powder	10 g
20.	Kushta	Saussirea leppa C.B. Clarke	Rhizome	Powder	10 g
21.	Vidari	Pueraria tuberosa D.C.	Tuber	Powder	20 g
22.	Lasuna	Allium capa Linn.	Bulb	Paste	10 g
23.	Devadaru	Cedrus deodara (Roxb.) Lond.	Heart wood	Hot infusion	30 ml
24.	Sirisha	Albizzia lebbeck Benth	Bark	Decoction	30 ml
25.	Siddhartha	Brassica species	Seeds	Powder	10 g
26.	Mundi	Sphaeranthus indicus Linn.	Whole plant	Distilled extract	40 ml
27.	Vandaka	Vanda roxburghie R.Br.	Root	Powder	5 g
28.	Kushmanda	Benincasa urifera Savi	Fruit	Paste	50 g
29.	Vidanga	Embelia ribes Burm.	Fruit	Powder	20 g
30.	Haridra	Curcuma longa Linn.	Rhizome	Powder	10 g
31.	Musta	Cyperus rotundus Linn.	Rhizome	Powder	10 g

Mineral Origin

1. Rasa	–	Mercury	2. Gandhaka	–	Sulphur
3. Talaka	–	AS2 S2	4. Manassila	–	AS2 S3
5. Tamra	–	Copper			

REFERENCES

1. Agnivesa: Charaka Samhita, Revised by Charaka and Dridha Bala, Comm. by Chakrapanidatta, 4th edn. (1981), Munshi Ram Manoharlal Publishers Pvt. Ltd., New Delhi
2. Bhavamisra: Bhava Prakash, Vol. II Comm. by Brahma Sankara Misra, 5th edn. (1993) Chaukhamba Sanskrit Bhavan, Varanasi.
3. Harrison: Principles of Internal Medicine Vol. II International Edition, 12th edn. (1991), McGraw-Hill, Inc. Health Professions Division, New York.
4. Madhavakara: Madhava Nidana, Comm. by Vijaya Rakshita and Srikantha Datta, Part I and II, 23rd edn. (1994), Chaukhamba Sanskrit Bhavan, Varanasi.
5. Sushruta: Sushruta Samhita, Translation by Kunjalal Bhishagratna, 4th edn. (1991), Chaukhamba Sanskrit Series Office, Varanasi.
6. Vagbhata: Ashtanga Hridaya, Comm. by Aruna Datta and Hemadri, 7th edn. (1982), Chaukhamba Orientation, Varanasi.

MEDHYA RASAYANA THERAPY IN THE MANAGEMENT OF APASMARA VIS-A-VIS EPILEPSIES

Epilepsy is a common neurological disease associated with periodic attacks of typical fits occurring more often in children. In a major proportion of patients the cause of such fits is not known, however organic causes like head injury, encephalopathies, intracranial tumours and cerebrovascular disorders are known to be responsible in several cases. The overall treatment of epilepsy is not very satisfactory. With the advent of barbiturates and other anticonvulsive drugs it has become possible to control the epileptic fits in large number of patients. However, the ideal drug for the treatment of epilepsy is still to be searched.

It is interesting to note that the disease and the syndrome of Epilepsy is vividly described in Ayurvedic classics in terms of *Apasmara.* A number of drugs mostly of herbal origin have been described for the management of *Apasmara.* A critical study of the drugs used in the treatment of *Apasmara* indicates that Medhya Drugs have been used very frequently for this purpose. Hence it was decided to evaluate the effect of common preparations of Medhya Rasayana Drugs in cases of Apasmara.

A series of 75 cases of epilepsy were registered consecutively during the years 1984-86. An epidemiological break up of 75 patients showed that majority of patients were below the age of 20 years. Vata Prakriti was dominant. Only 70 per cent patients showed positive EEG changes. Average duration of illness in the series was 2.5 years.

All the 75 patients of the above series were randomly put on trial with the following schedule of treatment: 1. Medhya Vati (0.5) two vatis, three times a day, 2. Saraswatarista 20 ml twice a day and 3. Ashwagandha Choorna 6 gm once a day at bed time. The treatment was continued for one year and patients were called for follow-up every month. After one year, treatment was stopped and the patients were kept under follow-up. The overall observations indicate that over 75 per cent patients responded significantly in terms of reduction of frequency of fits, severity of fits and complete absence of fits wherever observed. The drugs were found completely free from toxicity and side effects.

Introduction

Epilepsy is a fairly common disease of psychoneurological origin encountered mainly in children and adolescents belonging to rural areas, and low socio-economic conditions, though it is observed in all the age groups, and all types of habitat and population. Etiology of the disease is not much clear, though vascular lesions, trauma, space occupying lesions, inflammatory diseases and degenerative conditions like presenile dementia, besides common causes like fever, teething and helmenthic infestations especially in children have all been attributed to the onset of this disease. Modern treatment has not been very much satisfactory and a single, universally effective drug regimen is yet to be searched out.

The disease is well-known in Ayurveda as *Apasmara* and a substantial material in the way of *Nidana, Laksana, Samprapti,*

Bheda and *Cikitsa,* is available in almost all Ayurvedic classics and Samgraha texts.

In view of the common occurrence of the disease in rural masses and in light of the fact that Modern treatment is not fully satisfactory mainly because of the toxicity hazards of drugs and less so because of the failure of these drugs to eradicate the disease in some of the cases; it was considered useful to launch a preliminary study on the effect of some Ayurvedic preparations. Some Medhya Rasayana drugs were chosen because of their extensive use seen in the Ayurvedic texts and also to examine the attractive claims made by Ayurvedic physicians.

Methods and Materials

A series of 75 cases of Apasmara were registered consecutively from the out-patients of Kayacikitsa department, S.S. Hospital, B.H.U., during the year 1984-86. The diagnosed patients who agreed to undergo the treatment were interviewed for the collection of demographic data, details regarding the medical illness, family history and the past history of the illness. A thorough physical examination was done to exclude the possibilities of organic illnesses which would need different approach altogether. These included the recordings of pulse, blood pressure, body weight and height and determination of the Prakrti.

All these 75 patients were put on trial treatment which consisted of the following drugs:

1. Medhyavati (BHU) 2 pills t.d.s.
2. Saraswatarista 20 ml b.d.
3. Aswagandha Choorna 6 gm once at bed time.

The treatment was continued for 1 year and the patients were called for follow-up every month. The patients remained under observation and follow-up.

Relevant investigations like Routine blood, stool and urine examinations, and V.D.R.L were carried out in each case. E.E.G. could be done only in 24 cases and X-Ray skull in 38 cases. The purpose of course was to exclude the organic disease which would have been the cause for the manifesting symptoms.

Observations and Results

The Table No. 2.21 shows age incidence in 75 cases of Apasmara. It is evident that the maximum number of patients (42) were in age group 11-20 years followed by 12 in the age group 1-10 years and 10 in the age group 21-30 years. However, least number of cases (2) were seen in the age group 51-60. Duration of the manifesting symptoms varied from 2 months to 16 years.

Table 2.21: *Age Incidence in 75 cases of Apasmara*

Age Group	*No. of Patients*	*Percentage*
1-10	12	16.00%
11-20	42	56.00%
21-30	10	13.33%
31-40	05	06.66%
41-50	04	05.33%
51-60	02	02.66%

Minimum age—3 years, Maximum age—60 years.

Table 2.22 shows the sex incidence and habitat distribution in the present series of patients. The disease was seen more prevalent in males (68 per cent) as compared to females. Rural population (74.66) was observed to be three times more affected than the urban population.

Table 2.22: *Sex Incidence and Habitat Distribution in 75 Cases of Apasmara*

Sex/Habitat	*No. of Patients*	*Percentage*
Male	51	68
Female	24	32
Rural	56	74.66
Urban	19	25.33

Incidence of different types of Epilepsies in 75 cases of Apasmara have been recorded in Table No. 2-23. As is evident Grandmal Epilepsy (GME) was seen in maximum number of patients (86.66 per cent). Focal Epilepsy was seen in 12 per cent of patients. A case of Grandmal Epilepsy of organic origin (traumatic) was also recorded.

Table 2.23: *Incidence of Types of Epilepsies in 75 Cases of Apasmara*

Type of Epilepsy	*No. of Patients*	*Percentage*
Grandmal Epilepsy	65	86.66
Focal (Jacksonian) Epilepsy	09	12.00
Organic (GME type) Epilepsy	01	01.33

Electro Encephelography (EEG) could be done in only 24 cases because of the technical difficulties encountered, in the present series of patients. Only 18 patients (75 per cent) recorded positive EEG changes, while Four patients (16.66 per cent) had normal EEG recordings. Two patients (8.33 per cent) showed border-line changes in EEG. X-Ray skull could be had in 38 patients and no abnormality was detected in any one of these cases.

Table 2.24: *Incidence of EEG +ve Cases of Epilepsy in the Present Series of Apasmara*

S.No.	*Observations*	*No. of Cases*	*Percentage*
1.	Total cases investigated	24	
2.	E.E.G. positive	18	75%
3.	E.E.G. negative	04	16.66%
4.	Borderline EEG	02	8.33%

The effects of Medhya Rasayana therapy have been

summarised in Table 2.25. It should be noted that only 34 patients out of the total number of 75 cases treated, came for follow-up study and hence the clinical observations on therapeutic trials could be made only in these 34 cases.

Quite a good number of patients recorded improvement. The improvement was recorded in terms of reduction in the frequency of attacks of fits (64.7 per cent) and complete absence of fits after one year of treatment (25.53 per cent). In a few cases (5.88 per cent) this complete absence of fits was associated with return of EEG records to normalcy. Two cases did not show any improvement with the treatment.

Table 2-25: *Pattern of Effect of Medhya Rasayana Therapy in 34 Cases of Apasmara Kept Under Trial*

S.No.	*Observations*	*No. of Cases*	*Percentage*
1.	Reduction in frequency of fits	22	64.71%
2.	Complete absence of fits after one year of treatment	08	23.53%
3.	Absence of fits and return of EEG to normalcy	02	05.88%
4.	No relief	02	05.88%

Discussion

General observations on 75 cases of Apasmara reveal that the disease is predominantly seen in the age groups 11-20 years and is more common in males than in females and also that majority of the sufferers are from rural population. The cause for the predominance of this disease in adolescents could not be traced out. However in good number of patients the onset could be traced back to early childhood and in many no definite history was available. The cause for the common occurrence of the disease in rural masses was, again obscure and may only be attributed to improper hygienic conditions, negligence, inadequate health care measures, mostly due to low socio-economic conditions. Types of Apasmara as described in Ayurvedic texts could not be identified because of the insufficient data that could be collected from the patients. It was also a fact, that in many patients who were interviewed no such symptoms as described by Ayurvedic classics could be observed. As far as the major investigations are concerned, the Negative recording of EEG in clinically diagnosed cases of Epilepsy only demonstrates the importance of clinical observation and exposes the inadequacy of the technological diagnostic measures adopted by the Western scientists. However, in spite of some shortcomings EEG still remains a major diagnostic aid for the diagnosis of GME.

The effect of trial treatment has been recorded in terms of prolongation of remission periods, reduction in the severity of the attacks and also complete absence of seizures in some cases. It was interesting to note that the abnormal EEG could be rendered normal after one year of treatment in two cases.

A look at the ingredients of the preparations used for the trial reveals that the drugs were basically of Medhya nature, having Katu, Tikta, Rasa, Laghu, Ruksa, Guna, Katu, Vipaka and Usna Virya. Few were having Madhura Rasa, Madhura Vipaka, Sita Virya besides being Balya and Rasayana. Some drugs are Deepana and Pacana in nature. So one can think of the possible mechanism of action based on these facts. The overall improvement in the physical health may be due to the better digestion and absorption of nutrients effected by these drugs. Besides due to specific action as being Rasayana and Balya a few ingredients may have also helped in improving physical standards. Influence of Medhya drugs on Sadhaka Pitta which has subduing effect on Tamasa and Rajasa Gunas may also be considered. The Medhyá drugs are already known to possess significant anxiolytic and anticonvulsive effect. Possibly due to their general restorative and adaptogenic effect and anxiolytic and anticonvulsive effect the Medhya drugs of Ayurveda appear to be very safe and beneficial remedies for patients of Epilepsy.

Comments and Conclusions

The present study cannot be considered flawless because there were unavoidable limitations to this study which impair it's scientific perfection. As far as the clinical evaluation was concerned, symptoms should have been graded and monthly assessments in terms of shift of grades would have proved more objective. Psychological evaluation would have contributed to the clarity. However, in spite of these limitations and short comings the study has a lot to contribute to the Ayurvedic management of Apasmara in present times. An attempt has been made to treat the cases of Apasmara with a comprehensive regimen, for a specific period and the oveall observations show that over 75 per cent of the patients responded favourably. It can be a first step in the standardization of the Ayurvedic management of Apasmara but further studies are warranted before a standard therapeutic procedure can be finally arrived at.

A CRITICAL ANALYSIS OF THE AYURVEDIC CONCEPT OF GRIDRASI (SCIATICA)

Abstract

Gridrasi, a diseased condition explained in Ayurvedic texts has a clear resemblance to a clinical condition called Sciatica, mentioned in the current textbooks of Medicine. Though Westerm Medicine identifies many etiological factors based on the underlying pathology, both Ayurveda and Modern Medicine agree'Vataprakopa' in the form of degenerative changes as the most common of all the causes. There is a lot of similarity in the symptomatological aspects as well. Terms like 'Sakti Utkshepa' and 'Sakti Kshepa' available in Ayurvedic texts appear to be the primitive forms of S.L.R. (Straight Leg Raising) and Lesegue Signs. Ayurvedic management measures seems to be more satisfactory because of their simplicity, applicability, easy availability, and cost effectivity.

Introduction

Gridrasi is a clinical condition characterised by severe pain starting from the low back region and radiating down along the course of the leg. This is a common entity encountered in clinical practice. The terms 'Gridrasi' and 'Sciatica' can be termed synonymous inasmuch as they refer to singular similar presentation—pain along the course of the leg, irrespective of the etiological variations. While Ayurveda limits itself to call Vata prakopa (Vata prakopa in turn can be due to many reasons) as the cause of this condition, Western medical science probes further to identify different possible causes for such a presentation and also tries to explain the underlying pathology in terms of structural and functional changes. However the commonest cause for such type of pain is degenerative changes effected in the lumber spine, which probably was what is meant by Vata-prakopa in simple terms. Nevertheless Ayurvedic management is more satisfactory inasmuch as the medicines are more effective, easily available and many a times cost almost nothing to the patient in terms of monitary involvement. The present write up elaborates on all these aspects. Besides a unique attempt is made to glean all the related literature from the extant texts and compose them under different heads for the benefit of the science and scientists as well.

Definition

1. Spikpurva Katiprishtoru Janu Jangha Padam Kramat Gridrasi . . . . (Ca. Ci. 28/56)
2. Parsni Pratyangulinam Ya Kandora Marutardita Sakthnah Kshepam Nigruhnhati . . . . (Su. Ni. 1/74)

Gridrasi refers to the pain originating in the low back region, radiating towards toes.

Etiology

Low back aches and pain radiating down the leg has been termed as Lumbago-sciatic syndrome. Multiple causes have been implicated for such a condition.

- Disc Prolapse (L4-L5 or L5-S1)
- Trauma (Spinal)
- Tuberculosis (Spine)
- Tumours of the spinal cord
- Malignancy in the pelvis
- Ankylosing spondylitis
- Diabetic Neuropathy
- Cauda Equina Syndrome
- Spondylo-Listhesis
- Spinal stenosis.

Of the above, Disc-prolapse is by far the commonest etiological factor; causes for this disc prolapse may be many. Degenerative changes (old age), Trauma, lifting heavy weights. Postural changes, psychological causes, so on and so forth.

Ayurveda does not mention any specific etiology for Gridrasi, but the common etiological factors for Vatavyadhi have been attributed to this diseased state also. Thus Vatavriddhi due to old age (degenerative changes), Abhighata (Trauma), Bharavahana, Ativyayama (lifting heavy weights), Visama Sayya, Visama Ceshta (Postural changes), besides many Vataprakopaka causes can produce Gridrasi.

Thus while Ayurveda restrict itself to call Vataprakopa as the etiology for Gridrasi, Western Medical science identifies many causes based on the underlying pathology. Nevertheless both Ayurveda and Western medicine agree that the most common cause is Vataprakopa in the form of degenerative changes. However, for an Ayurvedist it becomes necessary, to give a thought about all the etiological factors mentioned above, before treating the condition as Gridrasi.

Classification

Two types of Gridrasi have been explained based on the association of different symptoms related to Vata and Kapha doshas viz., Shuddha Vataja and Vatakaphaja. Gridrasi is mentioned among Vata Nanatmaja Vyadhis, and involvement of Kapha, naturally needs clarification. Nanatmaja—'Na-Anatmaja' means involvement of a singular dosha. More than the involvement, it is the level/stage at which 'involvement,' takes place, is the one which distinguishes a Nanatmaja Vyadhi from a Samanyaja Vyadhi. For a disease to be called Nanatmaja it should satisfy two basic conditions.

1. Only one dosha should be involved in the genesis of the disease.
2. No dosha, other than that particular dosha, should be able to cause that particular disease.

Sometimes during the course of a Nanatmaja disease of a particular dosha, symptoms of other doshas are also seen. The symptoms that appear during the course of a disease, are termed Anubandha Lakshanas and can be seen in any kind of a disease. Thus classification of Gridrasi into Shuddha Vataja and Vatakaphaja is justified.

Symptomatology

Symptoms mentioned in different texts are enumerated in Table 2-26.

Shuddha Vataja

Symptoms — Sthamba
Ruja
Toda
Spandana
Deha Vakrata
Janu Kati, Uru
Sandhigata— Sula, Spurana, Sthabdata

Vatakaphaja

Tandra
Gowrava
Arocaka
Agni Mardava
Mukha Praseka
Bhaktadevesha
Sthaimitya

Pain radiating down the leg is common in both of these varieties. Sushruta does not classify the disease, but says along with the pain 'Sakti-Kshepa' Nasa would be present. Vagbhata follows Sushruta, but uses 'Sakti-Utkēpa' Nasa. These two terms need further elaboration as it leads to a very interesting situation.

'Kshepa' means prasarana (Dalhana) meaning extension. Utkepha means elevation/raising. Thus in Gridrasi, there would be difficulty/inability in raising the leg as well as extending the leg. Very interestingly, raising/elevation (Utkepha) and Extension (kshepa) have been considered as two important parameters for arriving at the diagnosis and measuring the progress of the disease by the Western Medical Science while S.L.R.—Straight Leg Raising test measures elevation, Lesegue sign tests the extension. Thus it appears, the seedlings had long been sprouted for the development of S.L.Rs and Lesegues.

Management

Ayurvedic texts, with the exception of the classics have given a detailed account of the management procedures. (Table 2.27).

Charaka has advised Siravyadha (venous puncture) and Agnikarma (cautery) while Sushruta has advocated only siravyadha. Vagbhata has not mentioned any treatment procedure. However Bhela Samhita, written much earlier has prescribed specific measures in the form of internal and external use of medicated oil; Medicated Enema (vasti) and Blood letting (Rakta Mokshana). Later texts like Cakradatta, Sarangadhara Samhita, Bhavaprakasa and Yoga Ratnakara, have given quite a substantial account of therapeutic procedures. Surprisingly much later works like Vaidyacintamani, Gadanigraha and Basava Rajiyam have not given much details. All panchakarmas with the exception of Nasya have been mentioned. A number of drugs both single and compound, herbal and mineral are advocated. Many of them are common to all these texts, are simple and found to be very handy and effective in clinical practice. Decoction of leaves of sephalika (Viter Nigenda or N. Arborstristris) is one which is extensively used, with fair amount of success. Internal use of cow's urine with castor oil is also found to be quite useful.

In a About 25 cases in which author has tried these combinations, the results have been highly encouraging. Various therapies found in the literature can be summarised as under.

Purificatory Procedures (Panchakarmas)

Application of oil (Snehana) and sudation (Swedana) should be done first in the affected limb. This should be followed by measures to augment the digestive fire (Dipana and pachana). Induction of Emesis (Vamana) and purgation (Virecana) should be done as per the need. Medicated Enema (Basti) should be undertaken only when the patient has undergone the purificatory procedures and his appetite is good. Basti, administered without satisfying the above conditions will only prove futile. Blood letting (Raktamokshana) should also be employed, (at the site of the ankle joint) as and when found needed/useful surgical techniques like cautery (Agnikarma) is also advocated by some texts. A special technique of excision of a part of Gridrasi (? Sciatic nerve) near the ankle and following it up the cautery is also mentioned. However it is quite difficult to understand the procedure as the description is quite vague and the information, insufficient.

Palliative Measures (Samana Cikitsa)

Internal use of castor oil with cow's urine for Vataja Gridrasi and addition of pippali to this combination for Vatakaphaja Gridrasi is advocated by Cakradatta, Bhavaprakasa and Yoga Ratnakara. Brihat Rasnokalka prescribed by Sharangadhara is one of the most useful and highly effective measure in the management of Gridrasi and many diseases of Vata system including Hemiplegia, Facial palsy etc. Dasamoola Kasaya mixed with Ginger (dry) and castor oil has been advised by many of the texts for internal use in this disease Entity. Maha Rasnadi Quatha, Vataga Jankasha Rasa and Rasna Guggulu are highly specific combinations advised. Paste of Gunja seeds for local application is highly praised. Reknowned oil preparations like Sahạcharadi Tailam, Maha Masha Tailam, Maha Narayana Tailam are also useful. Table gives a summarised account of the drugs used in this condition.

Table 2.26: *Symptomatology in Various Texts*

Texts / *Symptoms*	*Charaka*	*Sushruta*	*Vagbhata*	*Bhava Prakasa*	*Gadanigraha and Vaidya Chintamani*	*Bhela, Cakradatta, Sarangadhara, Yoga, Ratnakara, and Basavarajiyam*
Kati, Prishta, Uru, Janu, Jangha, Pada						
Ruk	+	+	+	+	+	Not mentioned
Toda	+	–	–	+	+	
Sthamba	+	–	–	+	+	
Saktikshepa	–	+	–	–	–	
Saktyutkshepa	–	–	+	–	–	
Deha Vakrata	–	–	–	+	+	
Arocaka	+	–	–	+	+	
Agnimandya	–	–	–	+	+	
Bhakta Dwesa	–	–	–	+	+	
Mukha Praseka	–	–	–	+	+	
Gaurava	+	–	–	+	+	
Staimitya	–	–	–	+	+	
Tandra	+	–	–	+	+	

Conclusion

Gridrasi, is a disease condition characterised by severe radiating pain down the leg. It is counted among the disease of vata system. Sciatica a clinical Entity, which is described in Western Medical texts, has a striking resemblance to the Symptomatology of Gridrasi. Sciatica has varied origin, but the commonest cause is the prolapse of the disc signifying degenerative changes. Vata represents degeneration and thus there are Etiological, Pathological and Symptomatological Correlates for Gridrasi explained in Ayurvedic texts and Sciatica mentioned in Western texts. Ayurvedic managment revolves around a good number of combinations which are very simple, easily available, highly effective and have no untoward effects and this makes the approach more comprehensive.

Table 2.27: *Management of Gridrasi—Break-up*

Dravya	*Yoga*	*Karma*
Ardraka	*Kalka*	
Bala	Rasona Kalka	Deepana
Bilwa	Mahanimba Kalka	Pacana
Brihati	Tagarasipha Kalka	Snehana
Eranda	*Choorna*	Swedana
Guduchi	Ajamodadi C	Vamana
Gomutra	*Kwatha*	Virechana
Kantakari	Rasna Saptaka K	Vasti
Masha	Dasamoola K	Rakta Mokshana
Matulanga	Rasna K	Agni Karma
Nimba	*Guggulu*	
Paribadra	Rasna Guggulu	
Rasna	Pathyadi Guggulu	
Sunti	*Taila*	
Sephalika	*Internal*	
(Nirgundi/ Parijatha)	Mashadi Taila	

Trivrit Eranda Taila

External

Arkadi Taila

Both

Bala Tailam

Moolaka Tailam

Sahachara Taila

Satavaryadi Taila

Narayana Taila

LOW BACKACHE SYNDROME (KATISULA)

Low back pain or ache may be associated with a variety of causes, and careful history and physical examination of such a patient may yield important clues regarding the site and cause of the disorders. Such a patient may be subjected to a large number of laboratory X-ray and diagnostic procedures with ambiguous or unrevealing results. This may inturn reflect inadequate clinical evaluation and failure to fully utilize information obtained from properly conducted physical examinations.

Differential Diagnosis

The cause of back pain may often be established by correlating the findings of a carefully elicited history with a thorough physical examination. When findings suggest physical injury or diseases requiring specific treatment, X-rays of the involved area of the spine are often required for diagnostic and legal purposes. X-ray findings may provide a convenient basis for the differentiation of the causes of back pain.

A. Disorders of the Spine without Essential Radiographic Findings of the Spine:
   1. Musculotendinous strain.
   2. Herniated nuceosus pulposus.
   3. Ankylosing spondylitis.
   4. Rheumatoid·arthritis of the spine.
   5. Osteomyelitis
   6. Neoplasma.

B. Disorders of the Spine with Special Radiographic Findings of the Spine:
   1. Spondylosis
   2. Osteoarthritis
   3. Spinal stenosis
   4. Spondylolysis and Spondylolisthesis
   5. Facet tropism
   6. Unilateral transitional vertebra
   7. Compression fractures
   8. Untreated scoliosis
   9. Osteoporosis

C. Other Disorders with Normal Radiographic Findings of the Spine:
   1. Abdominal aneurysm
   2. Thrombotic occlusion of the terminal aorta
   3. Gastrointestinal disorders
   4. Genitourinary disorders
   5. Anxiety reaction with back pain
   6. Hysterical reaction with back pain
   7. Malingering with back pain
   8. Compensatory back pain.

Clinical Reports

The Role of Sodhana Therapy in Gridhrasi—P. Ramachandran Nair et al.-*JRAS*:1:4:1980.

The pain origination at kati (lumbo-sacral region) and gradually radiating towards the feet due to the vitiation of vata is the main complaint in Gridhrasi (Sciatica) (Charaka Chikitsa:XXVIII:56-57). Two types of Gridhrasi—Vataja and Vatakaphaja have been described and in both, vitiated vata is the main cause of the disease (Sushruta Nidana:1:74). Snehopachara (Oleation) internally and externally, is considered the best treatment for vata diseases (Vagbhata Nidana XV:54). Treatment is classified as Sodhana and Samana (Charaka Chikitsa:XXVIII:56-58), in brief. The disease will not relapse if relieved by sodhana measures (Vagbhata

Chi. XXI-1-8). Moreover complete purification of the body through sodhana processes makes the body immune to other diseases.

The present study aims at a comparison of the efficacy of Samana with Sodhana cum Samana treatment in Gridhrasi.

Nirgundi (Vitex negundo) and Guggulu (Commiphora mukul) were taken up for the trial as these drugs are well known for their anti-inflammatory and anti-arthritic effects. Nirgundi is suggested as an effective drug for Katyasrita vata (Charaka Chi. XXVIII:75-82).

Materials and Methods

Sixty-six patients in the age group of 12 to 70 years belonging to either sex, suffering from Gridhrasi were selected from the out-patient departments of the Institute for the study. All the selected patients were divided into two blocks at random—one receiving Sodhana cum Samana and the other Samana treatment, alone. The maximum duration of illness was fixed as two years. Patients having full expression of signs and symptoms of Gridhrasi tenderness over the sciatic nerve and pain during "straight leg rasing test" were taken for the study. Radiological examination of lumbosacral region was done initially to find out any organic lesions, and wherever such lesions were noted, the examination was repeated at the end. Detailed investigations were also done before and after the trial. Serum cholesterol estimation was done after Snehana in Sodhana block to study the changes influenced by the large quantity of sneha intake.

Assessment was done on the basis of clinical improvement. The parameters evolved and accepted by Nair et al in their previous work (1978) were adopted for assessment.

Treatment

Ghrita and taila prepared with Nirgundi (whole plant) administered for snehapana, Basti and Abhyanga respectively. Nirgundi Kashaya was used for Niroha basti and for internal consumption. Guggulu was purified by steam generated from

Nimba leaf (Azadirachta indica) and Ardraharidra (Curcuma longa Linn.) kwatha.

The treatment was designed as follows:

Block I

1st to 7th day	Snehapana with Nirgundi Ghrita
8th to 10th day	Bashpa sweda
11th day	Vireka with Nirgundi Eranda Taila
12th to 13th day	Samsarjana
14th to 18th day	Samana treatment with Nirgundi Ghrita 10 ml with Nirgundi Kashaya 60 ml at 6 a.m. Suddha Guggulu 1 gm with Nirgundi Kashaya 60 ml at 12 p.m. and 6 p.m. Nirgundi Taila for Abhyanga.
19th to 26th day	Yoga Basti. Anuvasana with Nirgundi Taila. Nirooha using Nirgundi Kashaya.
27th to 45th day	Same as for 14th to 18th day.
46th day	Discharge.

Block II

Samana treatment	Same Samana treatment as in Block I from the first day onwards for 45 days.

Diet

During Snehapana and Basti periods in Block I, light diet was given. During the remaining days in Block I and the whole period of treatment in Block II all the patients were kept under the following diet:

Morning	—	Milk 200 ml + Rava 75 gm., 10 gm Sugar.
Lunch	—	Rice 200 g + Vegetable 250 g
Evening	—	Milk 150 ml and 10 g sugar
Supper	—	Rice Kanji 200 g and Green gram 25 gm.

Results and Discussion

Maximum number of cases were reported in the age group of 51-60 years (17) and the minimum number in the age group of upto 20 years (7). Male patients were more in both blocks. Majority of patients belonged to Hindu relegion. The disease is more prevalent in persons doing heavy work. Majority of the patients treated have middle school education. The study shows that habits like alcohol, chewing, smoking, etc. are not main responsible factors for Gridhrasi. 44% of the patients were free from such habits. Pathological and biochemical estimations of blood did not show any significant change. However, decrease in eosinophil count in the age group of 41-50 years in block I was significant. Blood sugar in the age group of 61-70 years increased significantly. Reduction of lymphocytes in the age group of 41-50 years. and increase in the age group of 61-70 years were significant in Block II. Serum protein showed significant lowering in the age group of 61-70 years in block II. In the block I Sodhana, wherein large quantity of sneha was given as Snehapana, did not affect serum cholesterol level.

Radiological examination revealed osteoarthritis of lumbar spine in 7 cases in block I and 9 cases in block II. Ankylosing spondylitis in one case in block I and two in block II. Scoliosis in one in block I. Bony erosions in 4 cases in block II. Bone displacement in 2 cases in block II and sacralisation of vertebrae in one in block II. The X-ray taken after completion of the treatment did not show any change.

Result

The treatment in both the blocks was very effective. 76 per cent of the patients were completely cured and 26 per cent got moderate relief on block I. In comparison, 64 per cent were completely cured, 30 per cent got moderate relief and 3 per cent mild relief in block II. The duration of illness did not have any impact on the degree of improvement.

Conclusion

Clinical improvement in both blocks was highly encouraging. Even then, the result in Sodhana and Samana block (I) presented a better result than Samana block (II). Nirgundi (whole plant) and Guggulu have been proved as effective drugs for Gridhrasi and the result is much better in Sodhana followed by Samana treatment.

A CRITICAL ANALYSIS OF AYURVEDIC CONCEPT OF ARDITA (BELL'S PALSY)

Abstract

Ardita has been described by almost all Ayurvedic texts and is counted among *Maha Vatavyadhis* by Sushruta. While all the other classics restrict *Ardita* to mean paralysis of one half of face alone, Charaka has put forth a concept which is much different from the rest. Ardita according to him is of two types—one involving the face alone (one half) and the other involving the face (one half) and the body (one half). In this division Charaka seems to have conceived the concept of Supra and Infra Nuclear types (Bell's type) of facial paralysis. Comments offered by Cakradatta and Vijaya Rakshita have only contributed to the confusion already created by Vagbhata who says that *Ardita* can involve lower half of the body (paraplagia?) and that it is also called *Ekayama* (Monoplegia?).

Though Ayurvedic management revolves around limited number of *Yogas* they are very simple, easily available and highly effective.

Introduction

Paralysis of one half of the face is quite a common presentation in clinical practice. Facial palsy as it is commonly known, the clinical condition has varied presentations based on the site of the pathology in the course of the Facial Nerve. The simplest and the commonest mode of presentation, however, is in terms of Bell's palsy resulting from the inflammation of facial nerve in the facial canal within the stylomastoid foramen. Complicated varieties include Supra Nuclear Facial Paralysis associated with Hemiplegia, and a pontine lesion involving the Ipsilateral facial palsy associated with Contralateral Hemiplegia (Millard Gubler's Syndrome). Depending upon the level of the lesion facial paralysis may be associated with deafness, hyperaccusis, loss of taste, sensation over the anterior 2/3 of the tongue, and other related symptoms.

Among these two varieties stand common—Bell's palsy involving only facial paralysis and Supra Nuclear Facial Paralysis in which facial palsy is associated with Hemiplegia. *Ayurveda* seems to have conceived the above two conditions in 'Ardita,' much of the credit going to Charaka for the concept he has putforth, much different from the rest. The present writeup is aimed at giving a detailed account of the disease entity '*Ardita.*' It also discusses it's relevance in the present times. However, the most important contribution the author feels, is the reference data. The entire literature related to '*Ardita*' has been gleaned from the extant texts starting from *Bhelasamhita* ending up with *Baishajya Ratnavali.*

Ardita is a 'Vata Vyadhi' of Nanatmaja variety. Sushruta puts it under *Mahavatavyadhi* category—showing the importance it enjoys among the incurable diseases. (*Vatavyadhis* are generally considered incurable). The fact that almost all texts including Samhitas and Sangraha Granthas have described the disease is in itself a documental evidence for the importance given by the seers to this clinical entity.

Chronology

The most eloborate description of '*Ardita*' as related with the facial palsy is available in *Bhela Samhita,* where exactly $21\frac{1}{2}$ verses have been devoted to describe the Etiopatho genesis, Symptomatology clinical variant, and treatment of the disease. However, it is Charaka who clinches the issue, by giving the essential 'twist.' He describes and differentiates two types of *Ardita*—one involving the face only, and the other involving the half side of body including the face. This is again to Modern of classification of Supra Nuclear (UMN) and Intra Nuclear types (LMN) of Facial Paralysis, the former being comparable to LMN variety and the latter to UMN type.

Arde Tasmin Mukharde Va Kevale Syat Tadarditam.

Ca.Ci 28/42

Vagbhata follows suit and endorses the views putforth by Charaka. But as is his wont Vagbhata draws himself into controversy and puts everyone into confusion by stating that the condition may also involve the lower half of the body suggestive of paralysis of the lower limbs akin to paraplegia (?). He also states the *Ardita* is called *Ekayama* (Monoplegia) by some scientists.

Jatrorudwam ruja tivra sarirarde-adharepiva
Tamahurarditam kecidekayamama thapare.

(A.Hr.Ni. 15/-36-37)

Sushruta restricts *Ardita* to mean only Facial Paralysis mentions a few etiological factors, which have not been mentioned hitherto. Besides Sushruta mentions Romaharsa, Vepathu and Avilanetrata as premonitary symptoms.

Madhava's description is a direct copywright from Sushruta.

Sodhala in his *Gada Nigraha* classifies the disease based on Doshic predominance. He mentions three types of Ardita—*Vataja, Pittaja* and *Kaphaja.* Description regarding the Etiology Pathogenesis and symptomatology are as mentioned in Sushruta.

Bhavamisra's description is similar to that of Sodhala.

Basavarajiyam says '*Vakrita Vaktrarditah.*' It also mentions '*Mukhavata*' among *Vatavyadhis,* but this seems to be a different condition altogether.

The other texts (*Sharangadhara Samhita,* and *Vaidya Cintamani, Yoga Ratnakara, Baisagya Ratnavali* have limited themselves to deal with the therapeutic aspect of the disease.

Etymology

The meaning of the word *Ardita* (*Ardayati = Pidayati*) is referred to as to afflict, to torment, to distress, to hurt or to strike. Thus in general sense any disease can be '*Ardita*' because all diseases, hurt and torment the individual and 'distress' is the common factor to all diseases. In other words '*Vividam Dukham Adadati iti Vyadhih.*' Thus the word *Ardita* as such does not accord any special meaning with reference and the disease entity called '*Ardita.*' *Ardita* is the term given to a disease which afflicts/ torments half side of face or half side of the body including the face.

Etiopathogenesis

It has earlier been said that Charaka's (and Vagbhata's) concept of *Ardita* includes the involvement of half side of the body too, where as rest of the seers have restricted the term to indicate only facial palsy. Thus etiology for two of these types should be different. However, Charaka mentions only *Vatavriddhi* as the etiological factor for this disease entity. *Vatavriddhi* can be due to many reasons which Charaka has mentioned at the beginning of the chapter on *Vatavyadhi*'s. Rest of the authors including Bhela have specified *Ardita* as facial palsy. The etiological factors mentioned by various authors have been tabulated in (Table 2.28). Broadly these can be grouped under two heads.

I. Those which directly affect the face and its organs.
II. Those which affect the body in general.

Group I includes:

Sirasa Bharaharana
Uccha Vyaharana
Ati Vyaharana
Ati Hasya
Jhrumbha
Abhughata
Khathina Padartha Carvana
Jihwa Nirlekhana
Netrakarna Nasa Vigharshana
Vranapaka
Siravyadhana
Marma Sanchedhana
Visama Sayana
Visama Asana

Group II includes:

Kashtaprahara
Nityavyayama
Vegadharana
Patana
Diwa Swapna
Ati Maithuna
Karaghata
Dhanushasca Vikarshana

Chardhana
Langhana
Tikshna Madyasava pana
Vyadhijanita Karsya

It is apparent from the (Table 2.28) that the etiological factors mentioned by Bhela are those which are generally considered as *Vataprakopaka* factors. The causes mentioned by Bhela for *Ardita* are almost similar to those mentioned by Charaka while dealing with common etiological factors of *Vatavyadhis.* Thus Bhela and Charaka talk of common etiological factors, though they differ in the conceptual aspect of the disease. Thus the causes mentioned by Charaka and Bhela should be considered non-specific and those mentioned by rest should be considered specific as far as 'Ardita' (Facial Palsy) is considered. Yoga Ratnakara has mentioned both of these factors.

The etiological factors aggravate *Vayu* which travels upwards, enters different parts of the face producing facial paralysis. According to Charaka the vitiated *Vayu* also travels one half of the body producing the paralysis of one half of the body including face.

Cerebro vascular accidents (Haemorrhage, Thrombosis and Embolism) are considered as etiological factors for Supra Nuclear Facial Paralysis in the current practice of medicine. While *Asrik Sravana* and *Dhatukshaya* represent Haemorrhage, *Srotovarodha* indicates obstructive pathology comprising of Thrombosis and Embolism. Inflammation of facial nerve develops due to exposure to cold and chill leading to Bell's palsy. In Ayurvedic term *Vataprakopa* occurs due to *Sita Martura Samsparsa.* Current medicine does not consider 'Specific factors' mentioned earlier among the etiological factors for Bell's palsy). Comparison made above does not mean to say the ancient seers meant C.V.A. or exposure to cold air, while mentioning *Asrik Kshaya* etc. One do not know what exactly they meant then, but today such an approach has become a necessity for better understanding of the Ayurvedic concepts.

Symptomatology (Table 2.29)

For *Ardita* afflicting the face alone, Ayurvedic texts have mentioned many symptoms related to changes—both structural and functional—effected above the Clavicle (*Jatrordwa*). They can be systematised/summarized as below

Head	Sirah Soola Sirahcalati Kampate Murdha
Forehead	Lalata Vakrata
Temporal & Malar Regions	Shankha/vedana Ganda/vedana
Eye-brows	Bhru Vakrata
Eyes	Netra Vakrata Sthabda Netrata Avila Netrata Akshi Vedana Ekasya Akshnoh Nimilanam
Ear	Sravana Vedana Srutihani Badyeta Sravanau
Nose	Nasavakrata Gandhas jananam
Mouth	Vakram Vrajatyasye Bhojanam Mukha Vakrata
Teeth	Danta Vedana Caladanta
Lips	Ostha Swayathu
Mandibles	Hanugraha Hanu Vakrata Cibuka Vedana Cibuka Namana
Neck	Griva Vakrata Griva Vedana Griva Kampa Manya Graha Manya Vedana

	Jatroh Urdwa Ruja
Skin	Twak Supti
Swara	Swara Bramsa
	Swara Bheda
Vak	Vak Sanga
	Dina
	Jihwa
	Samutkshipta
	Kala Sajjati—Vak
Kshawathu	Nirodha
Smriti	Smriti Moha
Constitutional	Vepathu
	Trasa
	Supti
	Romaharsa
	Parswa Nishtivana

When we talk about *Ardita* meaning paralysis of one half of face, it should be stated at first that the ancient texts have meant paralysis involving both upper and lower halfs of the face. Western medicine has identified this condition as Infranuclear facial paralysis. Many types of Infranuclear paralysis have been described basing on the level of lesion—starting from site below the nucleus in the pons to the extreme periphery of the facial nerve. The most common variety however is called Bell's *palsy* resulting from the inflammation of facial nerve in the stylomastoid foramen. The signs and symptoms are:

Forehead	–	Absence of wrinkles on forehead on looking upwards or frowning.
	–	Drooping of the lower eyelid
Eye	–	Inability to close the eye or rolling of the Eye ball upwards in this attempt
	–	Affected eye is more widely open Epiphora.
Mouth	–	Sagging of the mouth
	–	Inability to move the mouth so as to expose teeth
	–	Dribbling of the saliva

	–	Food is collected between teeth and gums
	–	Absence of naso-labial fold on the affected side.
Mandible	–	Numbness and stiffness of the cheek
Speech	–	Difficulty in pronouncing pa, ba, ma,
	–	Inability to whistle.

Thus by comparison it becomes very clear that *Lalatavakrata, Netravakrata, Netrasthabdata, Avilanetrata, Vakram Vrajatyasye, Bhojanam, Hanugraha,* all have appeared among the symptomatology of Bells's palsy. A few more presentations of Infranuclear lesion can also be identified.

Deafness (*Sruti Hani*), Scanning Speech (*Sajjati ca Asya Vak*) (Site—Cerebello-pontine angle), pain in the Ear (*Sravana Vedana*) (Site—Geniculate Ganglion) can also be seen.

Notable omission in Ayurvedic texts is about the loss of taste sensation over the anterior 2/3 of the tongue, which is quite common—due to involvement of Charda tympani. Notable inclusion is *'Gandhasjnanam'* loss of sensation of smell, which has not been mentioned in any of the texts of Modern medicine.

Symptoms like *Danta Sula, Dantacala, Shankhavedana, Grivavedana, Manyavedana, Jatrordwa Raja* are frequently seen in the patients of Bell's palsy, though have not been mentioned in the texts. It may be a co-incidence, but form a part of the system at times.

Thus it becomes clear that *'Ardita'* has many things in common with the Facial paralysis of Infranuclear types. Any difference of description in an ancient and modern texts should not be considered contradictory because the time-gap elapsed between the two descriptions and also the mode of presentations based on entirely different backgrounds of etiopathogenesis have their own weightage.

There is one important aspect that is to be considered. Western texts consider two types of Facial paralysis-Infra Nuclear and Supra Nuclear. In Infra Nuclear type one half of the face is (both upper and lower half) involved. In Supra Nuclear type half side of the body including the face is involved. But here only lower half of the face is involved. Upper part is spared because of bilateral innervation.

Ayurveda too conceives two types of Ardita—one involving the face alone (whole of the face—both upper and lower halfs) and another involving the half of the body including the face. Though this classification is akin to Infra Nuclear and Supra Nuclear division, in the latter type Ayurvedic texts have not specified as to whether only lower half or both the halfs of face (including the half of the body) are involved. However, both Cakradatta and Vijayarakshita have pointed out that while in *Ardita* (that involves face alone) all the symptoms would be present in *Ardanga Ardita* (Face + Body), all the symptoms will not manifest. By this they probably meant that in *Ardanga Ardita* (Supra Nuclear Facial Palsy) many signs and symptoms of Ardita (Bell's palsy) would be absent. It's clear that they did not differentiate upper and lower halfs of the face, but they certainly identified the differences between the two types of facial paralysis, as far as the signs and symptoms related to face are concerned.

Classification

In contrast to current Anatomical classification, Ayurveda has classified Ardita based on the doshic influence.

Glimpses of an initial attempt at classification are available in *Bhela Samhita;* Bhela in fact does not make a distinct classification, but talks of '*Sleshmopashtabda*' Ardita in *Cikitsa-sthana* where he mentions some distinct symptoms for this type of Ardita. Besides he goes on to describe a different management altogether. This Ardita is said to have the following symptoms:

Murdha Manya Ganda Sosa
Bhrisa Lalasrava
Jihwa Jihmata
Kantha Niswasa
Nidradhikya
Mukata

Sodala in *Gada Nigraha* classified Ardita into three types:

Vataja	Lalatisrava
	Oshta sotha
	Kampa, Spurna Hanusangraha
Pittaja	Jwara
	Trishna
	Angapeetata
Kaphaja	Sirah Ganda, Manya—Sosa, Sthamba

Three premonitary symptoms of Ardita are mentioned by Sushruta:

Avila Netrata
Roma Harsha
Vepathu

There appears to be some confusion about a few aspects of symptomatology and classification.

Apart from the symptoms mentioned earlier Caraka has observed the following:

Hastapada Sankoca/Vedana

Janu	Sankoca
Jhanga	Vedana
Vru	Vedana

As Charaka has incorporated the concept of Supra Nuclear Facial Paralysis into *Ardita* (vide author's article under publication—J.R.E.I.M.), the symptoms he has mentioned above, relating to the extremities, are acceptable. However, Vagbhata though he followed Charaka in this concept does not mention the symptoms related to the limbs. Further, it is interesting to note that apart from Facial paralysis, Supra Nuclear and Infra Nuclear, Vagbhata includes a condition which, resembles paraplagia when he says '*Sarirarde—Adharepiva*'—while describing *Ardita*. Thus Charaka's statement '*Arde Tasmin Mukharde va Kevale Syat Tadartam*' and Vagbhata's statement '*Jatrorurdwam Rujah Tivra Sarirarde Adharepiva*' induce some amount of confusion. There is no doubt as to whether they recognised facial paralysis or not, because their description of *Ardita* resembles Facial Paralysis of Infra Nuclear type particularly Bell's palsy in all respects. However, though Charaka says 'Sarirarde' he talks only about pain and contracture in the upper and lower limbs, but does not talk about paralysis of the limbs. Similarly Vagbhata does not even talk about pain, leave alone paralysis of one half of the body or the lower half of the body. Thus it becomes increasingly difficult to analyse because general consideration and common interpretation of the Charaka's statement—'Arde tasmin Mukharde va' is that *Ardita* has two types in *Mukhavyapi Ardita* and *Sarirarda Vyapi Ardita.* Though the term *'Pakshavadha'* is not used here *Sarirarda Vyapi Ardita* is being considered as paralysis of one half side of the body including face. This in modern terminology is termed as Supra Nuclear Facial Paralysis. However, Vagbhata's statement '*Ardharepiva'* in the absence of substantiating evidence, needs be analysed further before finally calling it paralysis of lower limits (paraplegia).

Cakrapani and Vijaya Rakshita have made some interesting observations about the differentiating factors between the two types of *Ardita* mentioned by Caraka. Cakrapani says

'*Dehardevyapi Twamarditasya Tatharditena Adangasya Ko Bedhah? Bhrumah, Ardito Vegitaya Na Sarvakalam Bhavati Ardangstu Sarvakalam Vyapya Bhavati, Kim Va Yathoktha Visishta Lakshano Arditah Ardange tu Naitani Sarvani Bhavanti.*'

Thus instead of giving a clarification, Cakrapani has drawn us into confusion by dividing Ardita into '*Deharda Vyapi Ardita*' and *Ardanga Vyapi Ardita.* For, this is in contrast to Caraka's original division of *Mukhavyapi Ardita* and *Sariradavyapi Ardita.*

Thus while Charaka's description is akin to Supra Nuclear and Infra Nuclear types of Facial Paralysis, Cakrapani's division is one resembling complete and incomplete Hemiplegia. As incomplete Hemiplagia is termed as *pakshaghata* and is described separately in all Ayurvedic texts the concept of *Ardanga Vyapi Ardita* looks a bit confusing and even appears contradictory. Cakrapani's clarification regarding the two types of *Ardita* is also not satisfactory. According to him *'Ardita'* should be diagnosed when

(1) All the symptoms mentioned under *Ardita* are present

or

(2) '*Vegas*' are occasional and in between '*Vegas*' patient is alright.

Also patient will experience pain during *Vegas* only. Similarly *Ardanga Vyapi Ardita* should be diagnosed when

(1) All symptoms are not present

or

(2) Pain is constant and continuous.

It is very difficult to infer anything concrete about the differentiating factors. Even then one has to accept that Cakrapani has aimed at differentiating the two types of *Ardita* he has mentioned (*Dehardavyapi* and *Ardanga Vyapi*) and not at those mentioned by Charaka. (*Sarirada Vyapi* and *Mukhavyapi*). In spite of this the clarification he gives is inconclusive.

Vijaya Rakshita's observations however are interesting.

'Ardita Ardanga Vatayoh Kobedhah? Vegitwena Ardite Kadachitvedana Bhavavti Ardangavatetu Sarvadeveti bhedah Athava Yathokta Sarvalingoarditah Tadviparitah Ardangavata Ityahuh.'

It is apparent Vijaya Rakshita has classified *Ardita* into *Ardita* and *Ardangavata*. One really does not know whether Ardangavata means half side of the body alone (Pakshajaghata—Incomplete Hemiplegia) or half side of the body including the face (Ardita (Charaka's)—complete Hemiplegia).

Thus according to Vijaya Rakshita *Ardita* covers the concept of Facial Paralysis (*Mukhardita*) and complete and/or incomplete Hemiplegia (*Deharda Vyapi/Ardanga Vyapi Ardita*). Thus the concepts of both Charaka and Cakradutta are incorporated. Apart from this there appears to be no difference of opinion between Cakradatta and Vijaya Rakshita.

The concept of '*Vega*' discussed by both these commentators is something that is not clearly understandable. Both of them mean to say this—*Ardita* is Episodic (*Vegita*) and pain (*Vedana/Vyatha*) is present only during an Episode. It appears that this inference is based on the following statement issued by Caraka in Cikitsa 28/52.

'*Swasthah Syat Arditadinam Muhurvege Gates Gate*'

Thus the concept of Vega in *Ardita* has following components:

- Ardita is Episodic in nature.
- These Episode are quite frequent.
- The patient will have pain and other symptoms (?) during an Episode.
- Once the Episode is cleared the patient becomes healthy till another Episode sets in.

Analogous concept is not clear in Western Medicine. However, there are evidences of a patient getting more than one attack of Bell's Palsy (but rare). Many patients are afflicted by one or more attacks and in between the attacks patient is healthy. Sometimes some residual facial abnormal features remain for a quite long periods and this at times may be followed by another Episode of Bell's palsy.

Summing up different classifications, we arrive at the following:

Bhela	1. *Ardita*
	2. *Sleshmopashtabda—Ardita*
Charaka	1. *Kevala Mukharda Vyapi Ardita*
	2. *Mukharda Vyapi + Sarirarda Vyapi Ardita*
Cakradutta	1. *Deharda Vyapi Ardita*
	2. *Ardanga Vyapi Ardita*
Vijaya	1. *Ardita*
Rakshita	2. *Ardangavata*
Vagbhata	1. *Mukhardagata Ardita*
	2. *Sarirardagata Ardita*
	3. *Adhara Sariragata Ardita*
	4. *Ekayama* (?)

Sodhala's clinico pathological classification classifies *Ardita* into three types

(1) Vataja (2) Pittaja (3) Kaphaja

Prognosis

Sushruta says under the following conditions *Ardita* is incurable

Atikshēna—Severe emaciation/malnutrition

Animishakshasya—If the eye cannot be closed at all

Prasakta Aryakta Bhasanah—Inability to speak

Trivarsham—If the disease gets chronic by three years.

'*Trivarsham*' is interpreted as '*Atita Varsha Trayam*' *Athava Trayanam Mukha Nasa Cakshusham Varshah, Sravanam Yatra Tatta treyatyauhuh.*

Analogus Modern concept is that complete recovery occurs in about 80 per cent of the patients and about 5 per cent of patients may develop permanent loss of function and facial contractures. Complete recovery is virtually certain if there is any return of involuntary movement within a week after the onset and is probable of recovery of function occurs within a month. If after three months there are no signs of recovery restoration of movement may take one year and may even be impossible.

Management (Table 2.30)

Management of *Ardita* revolves around a limited number of combinations. A few of the combinations have appeared in many texts with or without minor changes in the composition. Local application of oils and medicaments has been given much importance, though all the five purification procedures (*Pancakarmas*) have been included in the management. Besides *Pancakarmas Sneha, Sweda, Upanaha Masthishkya, Sirovasti—Murda Taila Siro Dhuma* and *Karna* and *Netra Tarpana* and even *Rakta Mokshana* are prescribed. Among all these *Cikitsa Karmas, Swedana* and *Nasya* are of foremost importance. *Cikitsakarmas, Dravyas* and *Yogas* have been tabulated in (Table 2.3). Among the combinations *Mashendari* (Idli madeout of Black gram) and Navanēta (fresh Ghee) have been mentioned by most of the texts. It is said if these two are taken together for 7 days, *Ardita* is certain to be cured. The fact that the same combination has appeared in five out of seven *Sangraha Granthas* shows the utility of the combination. The author has the experience of trying this in five patients and has found the progress encouraging. Another important combination is that of *Kshira, Ghrita* and *Dasamoda ghatha,* which too has appeared in four out of seven *Sangraha* texts. Similarly Rasona kalka (Rasona, Hingu, Trikatu, Saindhava, Sauvarcala, Jiraka and Yavani) has been prescribed to be advocated with different *Anupanas* (Eranda Kwatha, Tila Taila, Navaneeta). Intake of Ghee in large quantities post prandially is another important regimen. *Bala Taila, Shairishadi Taila, Mahasneha* all have been prescribed for internal use.

A look at the above brings into one's consideration of the enormous importance given to Ghee, Milk, Oils and Mamsa. All these things have two properties in common (1) *Snehana* (2) *Brimhana.* Both these qualities are alleviators of *Vata* and *Ardita* is counted among major *Vatavyadhis.*

Among the local application of medicaments. *Navana Nasya* stands foremost. Many medicated oils have been mentioned for this purpose. *Abhyanga, Sweda* and *Upanaha* follow in the order of importance. *Sirovasti, Murdha Taila* and *Masthiskya* are different procedures of the same process which aims at oleating the organs of head. Even the procedures like *Srotra* and *Akshitarpana* have been advocated.

All these procedures mentioned above, have one thing in common—all are *Vataharas. Nasya* is said to be the best procedure for *Urdwa Jatrugata Rogas* and *Ardita* is kept under this group of diseases. Similar is the case of *Sirovasti, Murda Taila* and *Masthikya. Abhyanga, Sweda* and *Upanaha*—all are aimed at alleviating *Vata.* Local application of heat, facial exercises form the major part of the management of Facial paralysis in current practice of medicine. Ayurvedic procedure of *Sneha, Sweda* and *Upanaha* are more useful and effective forms of local heat application than facial exercises.

A careful observation of the Ayurvedic management of the disease makes one thing clear—it is aimed at treating *Mukhavyapi Ardita*—LMN Facial Paralysis of Bell's Type. Boast of a cure within seven days by many authors helps only confirm such a viewpoint. Western medicine dismisses Bells's palsy as a self-limiting entity. Recovery is sure to occur in about 80 per cent of the cases. But more than the recovery it is the time of beginning of return of involuntary movements that counts. Generally this starts within a week of onset of the disease. When it does not start even by the thirtieth day, chances of complete recovery are minimal.

Ayurvedic management certainly initiates an early recovery and in most of the cases it is complete by about four weeks of treatment. A combination of internal and external medication ensures a hundred per cent recovery in most of the cases. The Ayurvedic management is certainly more balanced. Besides being effective they are safe and many of them are so simple because they form a part of food regime of the individual.

When *Ardita* is of *Dehardavyapi* type (Supra Nuclear Facial Paralysis) the treatment would be prolonged and in such cases management should be on the lines of *Pakshaghata* and other *Vatavyadhis*.

Summary

Ayurvedic texts have given a detailed account of the disease entity *Ardita*. Caraka's concept of '*Ardita*' is different from the rest because it incorporates the concept of Supranuclear and Infranuclear Facial Paralysis. Cakrapani seems to have conceived the concept of complete and incomplete Hemiplegia. All other classes have referred *Ardita* to mean only Facial Paralysis of Infra Nuclear type.

Table 2.28: *Etiological Factors in Various Texts*

Etiological Factors	*Bhela*	*Sushruta Bava Mishra*	*Vag-bhata*	*Yoga Ratna-kara*
Abhighata				+
Ati Hasya		+	+	+
Ati Maithuna	+		+	
Ati Vyaharana		+		
Chardana	+			
Diwaswapna				+
Dhanush Vikarshana	+			
Jihwanirlekhana				+
Jhrumba		+		+
Khatina Padarta Carvana		+	+	+
Kashta Prahara	+			
Karaghata				+
Langhana	+			
Marma Sanchedana				+
Nitya Vyayama	+			
Netra Karna Nasa Vigharshana				+
Patana	+			
Siravyadhana				+
Sirasa Bharavahana		+	+	+
Tikshna Madyasavapana	+			+
Uccha Vyaharna		+		+
Vegadharana				+
Visama Sayana		+		+
Visama Asana				+
Vrana Paka				+
Vyadhijanita Karsya	+			

Table 2.29: *Symptomatology in Various Texts*

Symptoms	*Bhela Samhita*	*Charaka Samhita*	*Ashtanga Hridaya*	*Sushruta Samhita Madhava-nidana Gada Nigraha*
1	*2*	*3*	*4*	*5*
Akhi Nimilana			+	
Atinishtivana	+			
Avila Netrata				+
Avyaktavak	+	+		
Bhruvakrata		+		
Cala Danta		+	+	
Cibuka Namaha	+			
Cibuka Vedana				+
Danta Vedana				+
Dina Vak		+		
Gandasjnana			+	
Gandavedana		+		
Griva Sula	+			+
Grivavakrata				+
Hastavedana		+		
Hanugraha				+
Hanu Sula	+			
Hanu Vakrata		+		
Jihwa vak		+		
Jhanga Vedana		+		
Kshawa Graha			+	
Lalata Vakrata		+		
Manyagraha				+
Mukhavakrata	+			

1	*2*	*3*	*4*	*5*
Nasavakrata	+	+		
Netra Sthabdaṭa		+	+	
Netra Vakrata	+	+		+
Netra Nimilana	+			
Oshta Sotha	+			
Parswa Nishtivana			+	
Pada Vedana		+		
Sirah Kampa	+		+	+
Sirah Sula	+			
Shankhavedana		+		
Sravana Vedana		+		
Sruti Hani				
Swara Bhedha		+	+	
Swara Bhrmsa			+	
Samutkshipta		+		
Sajjita Vak	+	+		
Smriti Moha			+	
Supti			+	+
Uruvedana		+		
Vudwa Jatrugata Ruja			+	
Vak Sanga			+	+
Vakram Vrajatyasye Bhojanam		+		
Toda				+
Trasa			+	

Table 2.30: *Management of Ardita*

Amayika Prayoga	*Yoga*	*Karma*
1. Bala Kwatha + Kshira	*Kalka*	Vamana
2. Bhojanottara Sarpipana	Rasona	
3. Dasamoola + Kshira	*Kwatha* (KW)	Virecana
4. Dasamoola + Kshira + Mamsa	Dasamoola KW	Vasti
5. Mamsa + Ghrita + Navaneeta	Paneamoola KW	
6. Masendari + Navanita	Nidigdhika KW	Nasya
7. Matulunga Rasa + Kshira	Maha Rasnadi	
	KW	Rakta
8. Pancamoola Kwata + Kshira	Brihanmanjistadi	Mokshana
	KW	
9. Rasona Kalka + Navaneeta	Dadyaranaladi KW	Sneha
10. Rasana Kalka + Tila Taila	Eranda KW	Sweda
	Bala KW	
	Taila	Upanaha
	Bala T	Murdha Taila
	Sairisadi T	Masthito-kya
	Dadyoranaladi T	Sirovasti
	Ghrita	Siro Dhuma
	Mayura G	Srotrakshi Tarpana
	Bindu G	
	Tilwaka G	

POLIOMYELITIS
(Bala Pakshaghata)

Synonyms

Shishaveey Angaa-ghaat

Relationship

Vata vyadhis—Khanja; Pangu; Pakshaghata, Avabahuka; Amshashosha; Pakka roga.

Definition

1. In Modern Medicine, Poliomyelitis is described as an acute, infectious, and communicable disease caused by an enterovirus and principally, an infection of the alimentary tract but may affect the central nervous system resulting in paralysis.
2. In Ayurveda, the disease "Baala-pakshaaghat" has not been described directly in Ayurvedic classics. But many Ayurvedic experts are considering this disease as "Poliomyelitis."

General Considerations

Polio virus is an RNA virus of the picornal group, 8-30 um (microns) in diameter, pathogenic for humans and primates. Three antigenically distinct types of poliomyelitis virus (I, II, and III) are recognised with no cross immunity between them (i.e. infection in humans with one type does not protect against invasion by another). Under proper conditions, the virus may remain viable in water or sewage for as long as 4 months. It is not killed by ether, ethyl alcohol, low concentrations of mercury, 2 per cent tincture of iodine, or 10 min. exposure to chlorine concentration of 0.05 ppm, or freezing or drying. They remain viable at 4° C in aqueous suspension of faeces for months, but are readily destroyed by heat at 55° C for 30 minutes, potassium permanganate, and ultraviolet rays.

In India, poliomyelitis is essentially a disease of childhood and infancy; 80 per cent of total cases occur in children below 3 years and 95 per cent of cases are seen in children below 5 years. The most vulnerable population in India is the one between 6 months and 3 years. In developed countries such as USA, 25 per cent of cases occur over the age of 1-5 years. The shift in age incidence is attributed to better standards of environmental sanitation.

Males are more prone to clinical attack than females in the ratio of 3:1. Pregnant women, particularly in the last trimester are more liable to attacks than non-pregnant women of the same age group. A definite relationship has been established between trauma including fractures, intramuscular injections, operations, especially tonsillectomy and the development of paralytic polio. Inoculation with triple antigen (DPT) (combined Diphtheria, pertussiss and tetanus) vaccine has been particularly blamed, the inoculation acting as a trigger mechanism in precipitating paralytic polio. The actual incidence of post-inoculation polio is not known; but present reports indicate it to be negligible. (Basu, B.C. Ray, *Polio Clinic and Hospital for Crippled Children, Calcutta,* India—study for the Period 1967-80, *JIMA*, 84:7:1986: pp. 203-206).

Infants born of immune mothers escape infection upto the age of 6 months (because of maternal antibodies). Thereafter they become susceptible to polio; the susceptibility being the maximum in the age group of 6 months to 3 years. By the age of 5 years, over 90 per cent of children show the presence of antibody to one or more of the three types of polio virus in their sera.

Seasonal variation also play a major part in the disease occurrence. Approximately 60 per cent of cases are recorded during June to September (rainy season) in India, and also year round in the tropics and during summer and fall in temperate zones. Winter outbreaks are rare.

The case fatality rate is not easily determined because of the difficulties in diagnosis of non-paralytic cases. The rate is approximately 5-10 per cent and is higher in the older age groups.

During periods of epidemic prevalence, in both rural and urban areas, house flies and filth flies (Phormia regina, Phaenicia sericate, Sarcophage species) are contaminated with polio virus; their main role in transmission of disease is not yet clear, but virus has been found in food contaminated by flies. Although sewage is probably not a source of infection, it may serve as a source of contamination of contaminated flies of water supplies used for drinking, bathing or irrigation.

It is estimated that for every one clinical case of poliomyelitis there will be at least 100 subclinical cases. Therefore, it is the mild and subclinical cases that play a dominant role in the spread of infection. Man is the only reservoir of infection and no animal source has yet been demonstrated even though monkeys and chimpanzees can also affect with poliomyelitis virus.

Poliomyelitis is worldwide in distribution. That infection is much more prevalent than is suggested by the number of clinically recognised cases, is proved by the widespread distribution of neutralising antibody in population groups all over the world. With the introduction of polio vaccine, the disease has now become rare in most of the developed countries. In India, the first reported epidemic of poliomyelitis occurred in 1949 in and around Bombay city. Since then more epidemics were reported from different parts of India. The extent of the disease prevalence in India is not fully known.

Ayurvedic Reference

In Ayurveda, Bala Pakshagata has been described as one of the varieties of Vata-vyadhies, mostly because of paralytic symptoms. While describing vatavyadhies, all Ayurvedic Acharyas have mentioned the diseases, such as Khanja, Pangu, Avabahuka, Amshashosha, Ekangavata, Pakshagata, Sarvangavata, Phakka roga etc., but excluded Bala Pakshagata.

Throughout the country, many scholars are labelling differently the same disease poliomyelitis, as—Khanja, Pangu, Ekangavata, Bala Pakshaghata, Balavata etc.

After careful study of above mentioned diseases, we can say that all Pangu (Paraplegia), Khanja (Monoplegia), Avabahuka, Amsashosha cases, cannot be considered as poliomyelitis (Ashtanga Hridaya Nidana 15/43).

Usually polio starts with fever, then follows the paralytic stage but none of these diseases are produced with fever. In the above mentioned diseases, we will not find this symptom which plays major role in the production of poliomyelitis (see under Differential Diagnosis).

Particularly this disease occurs in late summer and in rainy season. In greeshma ritu, the vata dosha accumulates (chaya) naturally and gets excited (prakopa) in varsha ritu whereas pitta accumulates (chaya) naturally in varsha ritu and excited in sharad ritu (Ashtanga Hridaya Sutra 12/24, 25). So, normal doshic changes due to kalaswabhava in summer is vata sanchayavastha, and in rainy season it is due to vata prakopavastha, and pitta chayavastha. Therefore, the diseases must be vataja variety with pittanubandha.

Acharya Charaka clearly says that the vata jwara is kashta sadhya in varsha ritu though it is prakruta. Whereas kapha jwara in vasantha ritu (spring) and pittajwara in sharad ritu (autumn) are easily curable. Though vata jwara is kastha sadhya in varsha ritu its complications are not mentioned anywhere (Ch. Samhita Chikitsa 3/49).

Some Ayurvedic experts opined that, when vata jwara penetrates into deep dhatus such as majja, the patient may get polio (vd. Kasture, Polio and Ayurvedeeya Chikitsa Paddati, Bhishagvilas, Vol. 12, 1982, p. 4). According to Acharya Kashyapa, majja dhatu is the cause of vata dosha. Vitiated vata may disturb the majja resulting into polio. Inflammation of the whitish substance (myelin tissue, which forms the outer sheath of all nerve cell axons) as Ashtimajja which is known as Majja dhatu can be considered as vata jwara in Ayurveda.

Acharya Charaka with one of the mythological references opines that Jwara manifests due to infestation (Ch. Chikitsa 3/ 23, 24).

Acharya Sushruta further clarified that Jwara is one of the varieties of Aupasargika Vyadhies which transmit from one person to the other. (Su. Nidana 5/33/34).

Some Ayurvedic scholars are interpreting the balagrahas with virus. Balagrahas mentioned by Sushruta are also invisible and having qualities like virus. These balagrahas can be controlled by maintaining the hygenic conditions and fumigating with vata shamaka drugs (Ashtanga Hridaya Uttara 3/46) etc.

Some research scholars have described and correlated poliovirus as skandha graha as mentioned above (Shastri, C.H.S. Ph.D.). If it attacks the child, the following symptoms may develop "Stabdhangah Saswedo Baddha Musti" (Sushruta Uttara 27/8). Stiffness of the body as a whole is due to painful joints, tender and rigid muscles with light fists and sweatings. Stiffness of the spine gives rise to tripoid sign. However these features do not corroborate well with the poliomyelitis, but are in favour of Tetanus (which is a bacterial infection).

The dropping of the head when shoulders are elevated and the absence of nuchal rigidity in prone position but elicited in conventional supine position gives an appearance of stooped neck, paralysis of muscles of trunk and extremities giving rise to monoplegia or hemiplegia indicate involvement of spine.

In bulbar form of polio infection, the involvement of cranial nerves is seen. Polio encephalitis should be suspected when paralysis of some peripheral or cranial nerves is associated with signs of encephalitis, especially during epidemics. This form of infection either kills the child or leaves with permanent disability.

Pathogenesis (Samprapti)

Asthi (bone), Pakwasaya (large intestine), Kati (lumbosacral region), Saktinee (lower limbs) and Sparsanendriya—Twak (sensory organs)—(Vagbhata) are the main Sthanas (seats) of Vata doshas. Therefore, vitiation of Vata leading to the onset of a disease (Vata vyadhi) usually manifests as an impairment of these functions. Acharya Charaka has described 80 varieties of Vata vyadhies. As the disease originates at Kati due to vitiation of Vata, probably the Katyasrita vata—that is Apanavaya is involved (Vagbhata). The regulation of motor and sensory system is the main function of Vata (Charaka). Dhatuksaya (degeneration) and Margavarana (obstruction) are the two basic factors for Vataprakopa (Vagbhata). But the actual manifestation including the extent of the body affected depends upon the Dosadusyasamurchana (Vagbhata). Since the disease originates at Kati and Kukundaramarmaghata (Vagbhata) is one of main cause for this disease, the Dosadusyasamurchana can be envisaged at spinal cord—probably at Kati region (lumbosacral), or a region lesion at higher level in the spinal cord for any reason (traumatic/

neoplastic/viral/bacterial/degenerative) impairs the normal functioning of lower limbs and leads to these diseases.

Bala Pakshaghata is one of the variety of vatavyadhies with the main symptoms of fever and residual paralysis (full blown case) making the child permanently disabled. This disease occurs mostly in rainy season which is the vata prakopa period. In this ritu usually the body will have avarbhala (general debility) due to Dhatu kshaya, though it lies in visagakala. Agni is very weak and one may be prone to get all types of digestive diseases and vatavyadhies. So, one should take maximum precautions not to provoke vata dosha in varsha ritu.

Skandha graha (virus) is one of the microorganisms which enters into the stomach through the mouth, multiplies in suitable media due to weak agni in this particular ritu. In the absence of vikara vighatakara bhavas (dhatu kshaya), these skandhagrahas take shelter in kapha sthana, specially in Masthishkya Majja and produces Khavaigunyam.

Simultaneous vata dosha is provoked in Pakwashaya due to mithyaharavihara, kala swabhava, abhighata (injection or trauma) and dhatu kshaya which is the main seat of vata dosha. It deranges Samanavayu functions and produces agnimandhya resulting into Ama and Jwara. It is well-known fact that the jwara makes Santapa not only in deha but also in indriyas and manaha (senses and mind). In vata jwara, increased adravapitta and vata dosha produces rukshata in the body and results into kapha ksheenata (Tarpaka shleshma). Tarpaka shleshma gives the nourishment to all indriyas. The decreased tarpaka kapha and dhatu kshaya provocates the pranavayu which is mainly related in performing all the functions of indriyas. This provocated pranavayu localised at Masthishkya majja (kapha sthana), where already khavaigunya occurred due to skandhagrahas and deranges the function of indriyas particularly in karmendriyas. Rukshavata and shuska tarpaka kapha makes more derangement in Masthiskya majja (sthanavikrutti) and results into permanent disability. Moreover, shaithilyata takes place in all most all of the affected joints (kaphasthanashleshaka shleshma (Yadaiah P. *Concept of Balapakshaghata (Poliomyelitis) in Ayurveda, "Ayu"* Vol 10:3:1989, pp. 1-12; *Samprapti of Polio in Ayurveda, NIMA:* 1989: Sept.: pp. 9-10). Hence, in this disease, vata dosha provocates and kapha dosha decreases. Therefore, we have to plan Santarpana type of treatment, which decreases vata and increases kapha. Snehana, Swedana, Brimhana, Balya line of treatment should be advocated in this disease (see under Management).

Modern Medical Point of View

Human beings are the sole reservoir of poliomyelitis virus. Carriers with inapparent infection are the most important group in transmission of virus. A history of contact with recognised cases is uncommon. Virus can be demonstrated in the pharyngeal secretions for few days and faeces for several weeks. The intestinal tract is the main source from which virus is disseminated. Large quantities of virus is present in sewage drained from areas in which the infection is present. Poliomyelitis is thus as communicable disease as Measles and Varicella. In the 15 years and under age group, infection with or without clinical manifestation occurs in 100 per cent of household and 87 per cent of daily contacts.

The mouth is the portal of entry of the virus and primary multiplication takes place in the oropharynx or intestines. The virus is regularly present in the throat secretions and stool before the onset of illness (incubation period is 3-35 days) and it has been demonstrated in the faeces as long as 19 days prior to the onset of disease. Constitutional disturbances may be noted during its presence in the throat and faeces, and during the period of viremia, which persists for only few days. One week after onset, there is little virus in the throat, but virus continues to be excreted in the stools for several weeks even though high antibody levels are present in the blood.

Recent studies have now appear to show that the virus first multiplies in the tonsils, the lymphnodes of the neck, payers patches, of the small intestines. The central nervous system may then be invaded by way of the circulating blood. Once the organism enter the CNS, it spreads along the nerve fibres. Polio virus can spread along a zone of peripheral nerves to the CNS and there it continues to progress along the fibres of the lower motor neurons to increasingly involve the spinal cord or brain. This may occur in children after tonsillectomy (this is probably the reason why more mumber of cases of disease are seen after the tonsil removal). Polio virus present in their oropharynges may thus enter nerve fibres exposed during tonsillectomy and spread to the brain.

Polio virus invades only certain nerve cells and in process of its intracellular multiplication, it may damage or completely destroy these cells. The anterior horn cells of the spinal cord are particularly involved; but in severe cases the intermediate grey ganglia and even the posterior horn and dorsal root ganglia are often involved. In the brain the reticular formation, vestibular nucleus and deep cerebellar nuclei are most often affected. The cortex is virtually spared with the exception of the motor cortex along the precentral gyrus.

Polio virus does not multiply in muscle in vivo. The changes that occur in peripheral nerves and voluntary muscles are secondary to the destruction of nerve cells. Change occur rapidly in nerve cells, from mild chromolysis to complete destruction. Cells that lose function may recover completely. Inflammation occurs secondary to the attack on nerve cells, the focal and perivascular infiltrations are chiefly lymphocytes with polymorphonuclear cells, plasma cells and microglia.

Samprapti (Pathogenesis) of Bala Pakshaghata

—Skandhagrah—Enters through stomach—Takes shelter in Mashthishkya Majja—Khavaigunyam

Nidana—Dhatu kshya—Vikara Vighatakara abhava
—Vata Pakopa (Pakwashaya)—Samanavayu & Pachakapitta
Vikrutti
Urdhwagati Amotpatti

Reaches Murdha
Provocation of Pranavayu
Decrease in Tarpaka
and Shleshaka Kapha

Srotorodha
Jwara (Vataja)
Increased Adrava
Pitta and Vata Dosha
Rukshata in whole
body

Localisation at
Masthiskya Majja
Derangement of Indriyas
Karmendriyas

Sandhi Shaithilya

Bala Pakshaghata

Yadaiah, P. *Management of Poliomyelitis, Jaya Publications,* 1991, p. 15.

In addition to pathologic changes in the nervous system, there may be myocarditis, lymphatic hyperplasia, ulceration of payers patches, prominence of follicles, and enlargement of lymphnodes.

The most important determinant of human susceptibility to poliomyelitis is serum antibody. Previous inapparent infection and illness without invasion of CNS are common. Many children and most adults possess neutralising antibody for all three types of virus; this appears to be the reason for relative infrequency of the disease in older age groups. Infants under six months old rarely get poliomyelitis because immunity is positively transferred from the mother. Babies born to women in the acute phase of poliomyelitis can develop the disease shortly after birth. Among children, males are affected more often than females; the opposite is true in adults. Pregnancy increases the risk of clinically apparent poliomyelitis and multiparous females are more susceptible than primiparas. The disease is somewhat more frequent in the second than in the first or third trimesters of pregnancy. Menstruation or ovulation appears to heighten susceptibility. Absence of the tonsils and adenoids, regardless the time of their removal is associated with a marked increase in the incidence of bulbar poliomyelitis.

Diagnostic Features

1. Muscle weakness, headache, stiffneck, fever, nausea and vomiting, sore throat and diarrhoea.
2. Lower motor neurone lesion (flaccid paralysis) with decreased deep tendon reflexes and muscle wasting.
3. Cerebrospinal fluid shows excess cells, lymphocytes predominate, rarely more than 500 per microlitre.
4. The incubation period is 5-35 days (usually 7-14 days). Infectivity is maximal during the first week, but virus is excreted in stools for several weeks. About 80 per cent of cases occur 6-20 days after contact with the virus.

Clinical Manifestations

The infection may manifest in one of the four forms:

1. Inapparent infection without symptoms
2. Abortive poliomyelitis (mild illness)
3. Non-paralytic poliomyelitis (aseptic meningitis)
4. Paralytic poliomyelitis

I. Spinal
- (i) cervical
- (ii) thoracic
- (iii) lumbar
- (iv) any combination of (i), (ii) and (iii)

II. Bulbar
- (i) upper cranial nerve involvement III, V, VI, VII, VIII.
- (ii) lower cranial nerve involvement IX, X. XI, XII.
- (iii) involvement of cardiorespiratory centres.

III. Bulbospinal

IV. Polioencephalitis, paralytic or non-paralytic
- (i) diffuse encephalitis
- (ii) local encephalitis
- (iii) cerebellar involvement(?)
- (iv) bulboencephalitic disease
- (v) spinal encephalitic disease.

In inapparent infection without symptoms form—no clinical features are noted; bulk of infection with the virus of poliomyelitis (95 per cent) occurs in this form; virus can be demonstrated (pharynx, intestines, blood) and neutralising antibody develop.

In abortive poliomyelitis—nonspecific without clinical or laboratory evidence of CNS involvement. Virus can be demonstrated (pharynx, faeces, blood). Type specific neutralising and complement fixing antibodies developed during convalescence.

Non-paralytic Poliomyelitis (Aseptic Meningitis)

This form is similar to abortive poliomyelitis but with signs of CNS involvement (i.e. meningeal irritation, abnormal CSF findings) and usually present for several days before the onset of other signs. The tripod (patient extends arms behind back with hands on bed for support when sitting up) and hoynes sign (head falls back when with patient in supine position shoulders are elevated) can be elicited in paralytic or non-paralytic poliomyelitis but are non-pathognomonic. Nonspecific abnormalities of CSF are noted during this form resembling those of aseptic meningitis. The diagnosis of nonparalytic poliomyelitis therefore on clinical grounds alone is very difficult because the clinical features and laboratory findings are completely nonspecific. Studies have shown that less than 40 per cent of patients in whom nonparalytic poliomyelitis is diagnosed actually have the disease. The course of nonparalytic poliomyelitis is benign and disease lasts 3-5 days but meningeal irritation may persist for 2 weeks. No change in muscle and nerve function is detectable. In a small percentage of cases the disease advances to paralysis, and meningitis. In the absence of virologic diagnosis, polio virus must be suspected if the disease occurs in persons associated with paralytic patients.

Paralytic Poliomyelitis

The major illness usually follows the minor illness described above but it can also come without the antecedent first phase. The spinal fluid findings in paralytic poliomyelitis are the same as those in the nonparalytic disease. A completely normal CSF may be present initially and rarely throughout the entire course of the disease. Prodromal manifestations are often absent in paralytic poliomyelitis. In some cases the illness may show biphasic character in its presentation i.e. there is a short symptom free interlude between initial minor febrile illness and recurrence of fever culminating in paralysis. The disease starts with fever and manifestations of one of the minor illness. After several days, all the symptoms disappear; in 5-10 days there is recrudescence of fever, the development of signs of meningeal irritation and the appearance of paralysis.

Spinal Paralytic Poliomyelitis

To reach its maximum symptoms, it may take from few hours to three days and affect one muscle group or the entire body, i.e. arms, legs, trunk etc. Fever is an indication of the activity of the virus and therefore of likelihood of the paralysis, extending while it lasts. Falling temperature is an encouraging sign. Spinal cord is most frequently affected—the lower limbs being more often involved than the upper limbs especially in infants but the paralysis may have any distribution and is characteristically asymmetrical. The large muscle groups of the lower extremities (anterior tibial, the deltoid) are more often involved than small muscles. Spinal and abdominal muscles are also frequently involved. (Guntur epidemic 1960-61, Andhra Pradesh). Temporary bladder paralysis of 1-3 days duration may occur in the acute phase of the disease. Constipation is common and occasionally may be very severe.

Bulbar Poliomyelitis

The incidence varies from 6-25 per cent. About 85 per cent of patients subjected to tonsilloadenoidectomy within 30 days of onset of disease as well as others who had this operation years before develop this type of infection. It is characterised by weakness of the muscles supplied by the cranial nerves and variable "encephalitis" symptoms. Bulbar symptom include diplopia (uncommon), facial weakness, dysphagia, dysphonia, nasal voice, weakness of the sternocleidomastoid and trapezius muscles, difficulty in chewing, inability to swallow or expel saliva, and regurgitation of fluids through the nose. The most life-threatening aspect of bulbar poliomyelitis is respiratory paralysis.

Bulbospinal Form

This is a combination of the spinal and bulbar forms and occurred in 25 per cent of cases in the Guntur epidemic and 20 per cent in the Bombay epidemic.

Respiratory Form

Respiratory insufficiency occurs from nil to 16 per cent of cases and may occur from various factors acting singly or in combination.

Encephalitic Form

Here mental changes like irritability or drowsiness are found. If some peripheral muscles or cranical nerves palsy is present, the diagnosis of poliomyelitis become more justifiable. It must be remembered that respiratory insufficiency in bulbar or diaphragm involvement may produce mental changes like disorientation without true encephalitis. Lethargy or coma may be due to encephalitis or hypoxia, most often caused by hypoventilation.

Hypertension, hypotension, and tachycardia may occur. Convulsions are rare.

Course of the Disease

The course of paralytic poliomyelitis varies considerably from complete recovery of all paralysed muscles to complete loss of function in the altered groups. Each variability occurs because the early changes in the motor cells of spinal cord and brain stem may halt and the cells return to normal or proceed to irreversible destruction of the neuron. Cases with respiratory paralysis require careful follow up and treatment as recovery is slow and residual paralysis is common in the intercostal muscles and diaphragm. Bulbar poliomyelitis is more lifethreatening than the spinal form. Recorded case fatalities have varied from 3-7 per cent in different epidemics, depending on the incidence of bulbar and respiratory cases in the series. Most deaths occur during the acute stage, i.e. within the first two weeks after which period convalescence may begin and no further extension of paralysis need be anticipated. Unexpected improvement may be evident soon after defervescence and again about 6 weeks or longer, after which very little further improvement can be expected due to physiotherapy and orthopaedic measure. *Actue stage is for 40 days. Recovery stage is upto two years. Residual stage is after two years.*

Residual Paralysis and Sequalae

The muscles that have not recovered may atrophy in course of time; deformities and contractures result from such atrophy combined with the unopposed action of the healthy muscle groups. Flail limb results, from the complete paralysis of all the muscles of an extremity. Tight tendoachilles, genu recurvatum, valgus foot are some of the common residual deformities.

In poliomyelitis, initial cause of deformities may be due to muscle spasm followed by interstitial fibrosis. The exact cause of muscle spasm is unknown. However, it may be due to incoordinated involuntary contractions of surviving fibres in partly paralysed muscles. In poliomyelitis, the important cause of deformities in acute stage is muscle spasm, whereas, the growth of the limb is most important factor in almost all deformities in chronic polio. Therefore, the deformities are much worst in children than in the adults.

The imporant deformities which are seen in poliomyelitis at the chronic stage are as follows:

1. *Hip deformities*: Hip deformities in polio consists usually of a flexion-abduction deformity due to weakness of abduction and extension. Sometimes abduction deformity may lead to subluxation or dislocation of the hip.
2. *Knee deformities*: Flexion deformity is the most commonest in knee due to imbalance between flexors and extensors. Mild valgus deformity in knee is also common in polio. Genu recurvatum which is caused by the lateral rotation of the tibia or the femur, and lateral subluxation of the

knee. This deformity is more often due to early weight bearing on weak knee.

3. *Ankle deformities*: Equinus deformity is the most commonest in ankle due to weak dorsiflexors and a relatively stronger calf muscles. Valgus deformity and Varus deformity are due to imbalance of invertors and evertors.

Cavus foot is due to weak intrinsic muscles and strong flexors of the toes. Due to weak calf muscles, calcaneal deformity may occur, but this is not common.

A short leg, or a flexed hip, knee or ankle may cause the pelvis to tilt and a conpensatory scoliosis may develop in the spine. If it is not treated, severe scoliosis associated with apparent kyphosis may occur.

Diagnosis

Isolation of polio virus from the patient and demonstration of a fourfold or greater increase in the monotypic antibody in the paired sera collected from the patient confirms the diagnosis in all cases of poliomyelitis whether they be silent, abortive, nonparalytic, or paralytic. The antibody studies are important especially in areas where the infection is endemic as the virus isolated may be an associated finding rather than one of the aetiologic import. Antibody contents of the sera are determined by doing neutralization tests with serial dilutions of patients sera and the three antigenic types of polio viruses in cell cultures. Neutralising and complement fixing antibodies appear during the first or second week of illness.

Differential Diagnosis

Nonparalytic poliomyelitis is very difficult to distinguish from other forms of aseptic meningitis due to other enteroviruses. Muscle tenderness and spasm point to poliomyelitis, otherwise, the distinction is made by laboratory means. Acute infectious polyneuritis (Guillain-Barre Syndrome) and paralysis from a tick bite may initially resemble poliomyelitis but are easily distinguishable on the basis of clinical and laboratory findings. In infective polyneuritis, the paralysis or paresis is symmetrical; bilateral facial palsy and subjective sensory changes are common while meningeal signs are less noticeable. The cells in CSF are few or none but the elevated protein levels in the CSF are characteristic of the condition (cytoalbuminous dissociation). In post-diphtheritic paralysis also, the involvement of the limbs is symmetrical and consists of weakness but not complete paralysis. Cranial nerve palsies may also be seen. Demyelinating encephalomyelitis is associated with antecedent eruptive fevers, antirabies vaccination etc. The weakness is often widespread and other neurological phenomena (tremors etc.) may be present.

Conditions causing pseudoparalysis in infants like trauma, acute osteomyelitis (swelling and X-ray changes in bone) and syphilitic osteochondritis which occurs in very young infants only, have also to be kept in mind.

Ayurvedic Reference

Khanja — Vitiated vayu localised at kati (lumbosacral) region produces flaccidity and weakness in the muscles of one lower limb. (Sushruta Nidana 1/77; Ashtanga Hridaya Nidana 15/45)

Pangu — Similar to Khanja but involves both lower limbs (Sushruta Nidana 1/77)

Pakshaghata — Morbid vata takes half of the body seizing the siras and snayus producing looseness in almost all joints in the affected side, as a result patient cannot perform any function with the affected limbs (Ch. Samh. Chi. 28/53 to 55; Asta. Hrid Nidana 15/38,39). Ekangavata (only one limb); Sarvangavata (all four limbs).

Avabhahuka — Morbid vayu affects Amsa pradesha (shoulder region) involving siras and snayus at that place resulting in the little bit dragging or contractions of the shoulder joint. Bahu madhye sira vyadhah (Ast. Hrid Nid.15/43; Su.Shareera 8)

Amshashosha — Vitiated vayu drys the shleshaka shleshma at Amsa sandhi region resulting in the emaciation of the muscles of scapula—Amsa shosha (Ast. Hrid Nid.15/43).

Phakka Roga — Vitiated breast milk (stanya dusti). Child shows chestahani and shosha and the child does not walk even after one year (?Rickets). According to origin—Kheerajam (milk vitiated by kapha and the milk is known as Phakka dugda). It obstructs the srotas resulting into malnourished dhatus. Garbhajam—pregnancy during lactation leading to insufficient milk; Vyadhijam—other diseases, jwara, grahani (dysentery), Atisara (diarrhoea) produces weakness of the child.

After careful study of above mentioned diseases, we can say that all Pangu (paraplegia), Khanja, Avabahuka, Amsashosha cases cannot be considered as poliomyelitis (Ashtanga Hridaya Nidana 15/43). In the above mentioned diseases we will not find fever symptom which plays major role to produce poliomyelitis.

The diseases which cause paraplegia (pangu) in child as well as in an adult are:

Infantile paraplegia: 1. Infantile encephalitis (various causes), 2. Cerebral diplegia, 3. Meningitis, 4. Hydrocephalous, 5. Acute anterior poliomyelitis, 6. Infective polyneuritis, 7. Spina bifida (congenital malformation).

Adult paraplegia: 1. Injury to spinal cord, 2. Tumor or abscess in spinal region, 3. Tuberculosis of spine etc.

Khanja can be correlated with monoplegia in lower limb. Monoplegia will be seen in the following diseases:

1. Poliomyelitis, 2. Disseminated sclerosis, 3. Ischaemic paralysis of the leg, 4. Spinal tumor, 5. Hysterical monoplegia.

The back should always be examined in all paralysis cases for differential diagnosis of poliomyelitis. Tuberculosis and infection of spine may cause either a spastic or flaccid paralysis of limbs and usually we will get kyphosis as well as sensory and bladder disturbances. In transverse myelitis, the spastic type of paralysis is usually caused with sensory loss.

Spastic hemiplegia and diplegia usually give the history from birth or in some cases from early childhood. In most cases, either left-side or right-side limbs are involved, but sometimes even all the limbs may be paralysed. To some extent, the child is usually affected mentally but not always. The limbs are always spastic and muscles look normal. Contractures are usually much less than in polio which is not treated.

Avabahuka and Amsa shosha, both the diseases are produced by the compression of localised siras in shoulder joint resulting in contraction as well as emaciation in the shoulder region.

The bulk of a normal muscle is related to the age, nutrition, activities etc. and intact nerve supply. For its maintenance it requires sufficient blood supply and adequate exercise. When one or other of these factors is disturbed, may lead to muscular wasting and even atrophy. We may consider the following diseases in which the muscular wasting and even atrophy may be seen . They are: 1. Paralytic brachial neuritis, 2. Rib compression syndrome, 3. Acute poliomyelitis. Paralytic brachial neuritis, the presence of sensory changes, the absence of fever and a normal CSF are against the diagnosis of acute poliomyelitis.

Rib compression syndromes are produced by compression of the inner cord of the brachial plexus leading to localised muscular wasting.

Paralysis (Pakshaghata) can be differentiated very easily from poliomyelitis, because the causative factors of hemiplegia are different from polio. These include—cerebral thrombosis, cerebral embolism, cerebral haemorrhage, hypertension, cerebral tumor, cerebral abscess, acute encephalitis, acute meningitis, and interspinal neoplasm.

Complications

Urinary tract infections, atelectasis, pneumonia, myocarditis, and pulmonary edema may occur. Complications occur most frequently when there is respriatory muscle involvement and water and electrolyte disturbances (esp. those on continuous artificial respiration). Pulmonary edema and shock are the usual terminal events in fatal cases of poliomyelitis. Myocarditis is seen in 10-20 per cent of cases and may lead to death. Hypertension can occur which may sometimes turn into malignant type. Urinary tract infection is usually due to catheterization. Phlebothrombosis of legs with or without pulmonary embolism may occur in adults. Pneumonia is mostly due to staph, aureus and gram negative bacilli; chronic anxiety and depression, may also occur.

Prognosis

During the febrile period, paralysis may develop or progress. Mild weakness of small muscles is more likely to regress than severe weakness of large muscles. Bulbar poliomyelitis may occur in 5-30 per cent of paralytic cases and carries the highest mortality rate (upto 50 per cent).

Management of Poliomyelitis

During Acute Stage:

The broad principles of management are:

1. Strict bed rest—to minimise the extent and severity of paralysis.
2. Symptomatic relief—of discomfort to muscle tightness and spasm.
3. Suitable body alignment—to avoid excess skeletal deformity in paralytic cases.
4. Maintenance of fluid intake—to maintain adequate fluid and salt balance in the body.
5. Respiratory insufficiency and pooling of secretions in the throat should be watched for to maintain air way.
6. Periodic assessment for the improvement or deterioration in the condition of the patient.

During Convalescence

The accent should be on physiotherapy.

Treatment

Cranial nerve involvement must be detected promptly. Maintain comfortable but changing position in a "polio bed"; firm mattress, foot board, sponge rubber pads or rolls, sandbags, and light splints. Change of position, hot packs for the extremities, and anlagesic drugs usually control muscle spasm and pain. Faecal impaction and urinary retention (especially with paraplegia) must be managed. In cases of respiratory paralysis or weakness, intensive care is needed. Maintain a clear airway, remove secretions, and maintain ventilation if necessary by intubation and mechanical assistance.

To prevent deformity, active exercise is avoided during fever but passive range of motion exercises are carried out, as well as frequent changes in position. As soon as the fever has subsided, early mobilization and active exercise under skilled direction is begun. Early bracing and splinting may be helpful.

In the management of Bulbar poliomyelitis, the main concern is to maintain an airway and avoid risks of inhalation of saliva, food or vomiting. With this in view, the head should be kept low by slightly raising the foot end of the bed and child placed in prone position with face to one side. The mouth, throat, and nose frequently aspirated as necessary. Tracheostomy may be required because of vocal cord paralysis or because of rope sign caused by constriction of the hypopharynx. Mechanical respiratory aid, may be necessary in some cases. If tube or oral feeding incite vomiting, fluids may have to be given parenterally for a few days to maintain fluid and electrolyte balance.

In the management of respiratory failure due to paralysis of diaphragm and/or intercostal muscles, the child is to be placed in a respirator. Antibiotics such as Ampicillin, Cephalosporin may be administered if there is any infection preferably based on culture senstitivity of the organism grown.

Ayurvedic Chikitsa

As soon as the patient comes to the Hospital, careful clinical examination should be carried out systematically in a specially prepared pro forma. After examination the patient should be kept under appropriate treatment according to the condition or stage of the illness. Usually, the patient will be brought in acute or chronic stage.

Acute Stage

Acute stage may be broadly divided into two groups:

I. During Fever Stage
II. During post-Polio Stage

I. *Fever Stage*: First seven days is considered as 'Ama' Stage in Ayurveda. For the convenience of management, we may divided this fever stage into three groups:

1. Pre-paralytic stage
2. Paralytic stage
3. Post-paralytic stage

1. *Pre-paralytic stage*: It is a fact that one cannot diagnose poliomyelitis in pre-paralytic stage from the clinical features alone. However, if proper steps are taken, we can prevent further progression to paralytic stage. Even if all precautions are taken, if paralysis occurs, there will be less severity.

Ayurveda clearly says that during fever, patient is very weak; particularly in varsha ritu, child will have Avarabala due to first stage of visargakala. If child met with Adhighata i.e. injury, trauma etc. it leads to provocation of vata dosha resulting into many vatavyadhis.

If child comes with symptoms, pre-paralytic stage, (see under Diagnostic Features and Clinical Manifestations), the following precautions have been advised:

(i) Complete rest in bed. Patient should be kept warm with the help of woollen clothes.
(ii) To improve indigestion, the following measures are useful:
    (a) Luke warm water should be given whenever the child gets thirst.

(b) Milk boiled with long pepper (Piper longum) should be given.

(c) Previously, if child is consuming solid foods, fresh and hot Lapsi (Yavagu) is given, after seeing the appetite.

(d) Fresh 'Yusha' prepared with green gram should be given.

(e) Khichidi prepared with green gram is to be given in liquid form.

(iii) If there is constipation, it should be relieved by simple laxatives or shodhan basti.

(a) Castor oil 10 to 15 ml. OR

(b) Rasayan Haritaki Churna 250 mg—500 mg at bed time with luke warm water, OR

(c) Shodhan Basti (Triphala quath 100—150 ml mixed with 50 ml of Til oil).

(iv) *Drugs*: Any one of the following drugs should be given for Jwara:

(a) Gulvel satva 125 mg. thrice daily with honey.

(b) Tribhuvana Keerti Ras 125 mg. thrice daily with honey.

(c) Mruthyunjaya Ras 125 mg. thrice daily with honey.

(d) Mahasudarshan Ganvati 125 mg. thrice daily with honey.

(e) If jwara (fever) is associaed with diarrhoea/ dysentery—Sanjeevani vati 125 mg. thrice daily with honey, Kutajarishta/ Jeerakadyarishta, 5 ml. mixed with water should be given.

(v) Intramuscular injections should be avoided as far as possible, particularly during June to September months; and prefer oral medications for risk group children (one to 5 years age group).

2. *Paralytic Stage*: In this stage complete rest should be given and the child should be kept with adequate supports for affected limbs with the help of soft pillows and pads—'Polio bed.' Proper nursing should be given to avoid deformities and

contractures. Anti-jwaraghna (anti-pyretic) therapy should be continued till temperature relieved completely.

As soon as the temperature comes down, the patient will get good appetite and passes stools regularly and restlessness, tiredness, muscle tenderness in limbs will disappear and patient looks cheerful.

3. *Post-Paralytic Stage* : After temperature comes down the management is as follows upto 8 days.

(i) Luke warm medicated oil should be applied gently (Samvahana type) to whole body with Mahanaryana Taila, OR Bala Taila, OR Ksheerabala Taila etc.

(ii) Brahmi oil, OR Ksheerabala oil can be applied on head and keep oil swab over head.

(iii) Fomentation is to be avoided.

(iv) If there is no relapse of fever, the following oral medication is advocated:

  (a) Vata Vidvamsa Ras OR Brihat Vata Vidvamsa Ras 125 mg. thrice daily with honey.

  (b) Brahmi vati OR Brahmi vati with Gold 125 mg. thrice daily with honey.

  (c) Aswagandharishta OR Dashamoolarishta—2 to 5 ml. thrice daily with water.

  (d) Shatavari churna OR Shatavari kalpa OR Shatavari ghrita 2.5 gm. (half-tea spoon) thrice daily with milk.

II. *Post Polio Management:* This can be considered under two headings:

1. Management of Residual symptoms of Paralysis
2. Management of old and chronic patients with contractures and deformities.

1. *Management of Residual Post-Polio Paralysis*: In this stage, the fever completely subsides and the residual symptoms of fever, i.e. muscle paralysis will be seen. After proper assessment of the muscles affected in limbs and the trunk, the following management should be continued till the desired results are obtained.

Apart from the oral medications advocated above, the following Panchakarma measures should be selected according to the condition of the patient:

(i) Oil Massage
(ii) Fomentation
(iii) Murdha Taila
(iv) Basti Therapy

Oil Massage (Abhyanga-Bahya-Snehana): The patient who is fit to undergo Abhyanga must be taken to the Panchakarma Therapy Room, and informed about the procedure to be done to the concerned attendants. The patient is asked to remove the clothes except Kaupeena (loin cloth). The patient should be advised to empty the bladder and bowels (urine and stool) before coming to the massage table. Initially, the child should get gentle massage i.e. Samvahana type and after some days we can advise Unmardhana type of massage to whole body according to the condition of the patient. While doing massage, the child should not cry and special care should be taken to the affected limbs or region. Rotation type of massage with the help of palm should be done to the joints and up and down movements with the help of fingers should be done to the other parts.

Pradhana Karma: The Abhyanga will be done in the following postures:

(i) Seated with both of the legs extended: In this posture the patient will get massage to the head, shoulders, hands and legs.
(ii) Lying on the left side of the body—In this posture, proper massage can be done to the right hand, right leg, right ear etc.
(iii) Lying on the back side of the body—In this posture, the patient will get the massage to the face, chest, abdomen, groin and legs.
(iv) Lying on the front side of the body—In this posture, the child will get the massage to the neck, back, lumbar region, buttocks, thighs, and fore legs.

(v) Lying on the right side of the body—In this posture, the child will get the massage to the left side of the body and to the left ear.

(vi) Lying on the back side of the body—and seated with both the legs extended.

To obtain the desired results 5-10 minutes of massage in each posture should be carried out.

In some patients, they cannot sit due to the paralysis of spinal muscles. For them, the massage can be done in lying posture only.

If the child is fit for fomentation i.e. Swedana therapy, after completion of the massage, he/she should undergo for the next treatment. Otherwise, the child will be given hot water bath after half-an-hour.

Advantages of Massage: One who does Abhyanga once daily will have the following benefits:

(i) It enhances age.
(ii) It relieves weakness of work.
(iii) Enhances eyesight.
(iv) Strengthens the body.
(v) Relieves the vata in the body.
(vi) Induces sleep.
(vii) Gives good colour to the skin.
(viii) It resists the body against exhaustion and exertion.
(ix) Body becomes smooth, flabby, strong and charming.
(x) It tones up the tissues of the body.

Vata predominates in the tactile sensory organs and these organs are lodged in the skin. The massage is found very useful to the skin.

Fomentation (Swedana Therapy): The patient who is fit to undergo fomentation i.e. Swedana Therapy, must first complete Oil Massage, before coming to Swedana therapy. Initially, the fomentation should be given slowly with minimum heat for less duration. Gradually we should increase the period of fomentation. Many varieties of fomentation have been advocated in Ayurveda. For polio patients, one should select the fomentation which is easily implemented and economically cheap, convenient to the physician and the patient because we have to continue for a longer period.

Two steps are very useful:

(i) Nadi Swedana (Steam fomentation) with the help of tube.

(ii) Sankara Swedana i.e. with medicated bolus.

Nadi Swedana: It is process by which the person is made to perspire by using a tube through which medicated steam will be passed on the affected part of the body.

For Nadi Swedana, we require 10 litres of pressure cooker; the lids outlet should be fitted with two metre long rubber tube.

Drugs: 1. Nirgundi patra (leaves of Vitex nigundo); 2. Dashamoola Choorna.

2/3 water should be poured into cooker and add Nirgundi patra and Dashamoola and keep it on stove. When steam starts coming out of the tube, the tolerable steam should be made to pass over the affected parts for 10 to 15 minutes. After completion of the Swedana, the child should be covered with a cloth to protect from cold air. After half an hour the child should get a hot water bath and rest.

Shastika Shali-Pinda Sweda: Shastika shali pinda sweda is one of the important fomentation methods used for the patients who are getting emaciation in their muscles and also useful for deformities in the joints. It checks the emaciation and gives strength to the muscles and ligaments. This treatment needs more persons and requires lot of time for preparation and as well as for performing the treatment. Hence, this treatment should be more useful, whenever the emaciation is seen in the muscles particularly in chronic cases.

Contents of Pinda Sweda:

(a) Balamoola Choorna	100 grams
(b) Dashamoola Choorna	100 grams
(c) Water	4 litres (4000 ml.)
(d) Rice	500 grams
(e) Milk	1/2 litre (500 ml.)
(f) 2 cloth pieces	18" X 18"

Apart from Balamoola choorna, some physicians take Mamsarohini choorna in equal quantities.

Method of Preparation:Take 200 grams of Balamoola and Dashamoola choorna; add 4 litres of water and boil it in a vessel and reduce it upto 1 litre of decoction. From this, 1/2 litre decoction should be taken in a separate vessel and equal quantity of milk, 500 grams of rice and cook like a paste. The cooked paste is kept in two clean cloth pieces measuring 18" X 18" and tied them in the form of a bolus (pinda). The remaining half decoction should be used for dipping the bolus while decoction is sufficiently warmed. 50 grams of Amalaki choorna is kept in water overnight and prepare paste.

Poorva Karma (Pre-operative Procedure): Remove all cloths of the patient and take him on a wooden table and apply Bala taila to the head first. Then the same oil is to be applied to the whole body and do gentle massage for 15 minutes. After massage, apply Amalaki paste over the head and tie with a piece of cloth.

Pradhan Karma (Operative Procedure): One member from either side has to hold the pinda in their right hands, after making it suitably warmed by keeping in decoction. The temperature of the pinda has to be tested by keeping left hand on it—whether the heat suitable to the patient or not. After confirmation of the temperature, give gentle massage with bolus on the body and the bolus will be changed as soon as its temperature becomes less. Every time we must test the temperature of the bolus before massage; in this way the massage should be done slowly for a period of 15 to 30 minutes.

Paaschat Karma (Post-operative Procedure): After completion of Pinda sweda, the contents of the bolus should be mixed with the remaining decoction and make it luke warm and apply this paste to the affected part of the body. After 10 to 15 minutes, the paste should be removed and advised to take hot water bath.

Uses: It makes the body supple, removes the stiffness of the joints, cleans the srotas of the body and brings better circulation. It increases the body weight by correcting the emaciation of the muscles.

Murdha Taila (Application of Oil Over Head): Application of oil to the head is very beneficial. If one applies oil regularly, he/ she does not suffer from headache, baldness, greying of hair, his sense organs work properly, and gets sound sleep. It is useful in several diseases of head and nervous system. Murdha taila is of 4 types:

(i) Shiro Abhyanga (Application of oil over head)
(ii) Shiro Seka (pouring of oil on the head)
(iii) Shiro Pichu (keeping a cloth dipped in oil on head)
(iv) Shirovasti (oil is kept over head)—Ashtanga Hridaya Su. 2/23.

In polio patients, Shiro Abhyanga, Shiro Pichu, and Shiro Seka are very useful and can be advocated. Shiro Abhyanga and Shiro Pichu are advisable regularly as soon as patient's temperature comes down to normal.

Shiro Abhyanga: Application of the oil to the head is known as Shiro Abhyanga. Head is one of the important vital organs (Marmas) and having all the sense organs in it and hence one should protect it from strain and stress by doing Shiroabhyanga daily. If one applies oil to the head daily, they can be free from all diseases pertaining to the head. It has been noted that one who does Shiroabhyanga daily will not suffer from headache, baldness, greying of hair and he will get sound sleep and his sense organs will get good nourishment.

Shiro Pichu : Cotton or gauz dipped in medicated ghee or oil should be kept over Anterior fontanelle and this is known as Shiro Pichu. It gives nourishment to all the sense organs.

Shiro Seka: It is popularly known in the name of '*Shirodhara.*' Pouring of fluid like decoction, medicated oil, medicated milk, medicated butter milk, water etc. over head continuously for a specific period is called Shirodhara. Selection of fluids or oils depends upon the disease and condition of the patient. In polio, medicated oils should be taken for Dhara. They are antivatic in nature, particularly, Ksheerabala Taila, Bala Taila, Tila Taila etc.

Technique of Shira-Seka (Shiro-dhara)

Apparatus required for Dhara

(i) Table containing the extra projection from the table to keep head over it and it should be round and concave having a hole in the centre—acts as an outlet for the oil which is pured over head.

(ii) *Automatic Dhara Instrument*: Specially prepared for Dhara Treatment.

Dhara Paatra: It is a shallow, about 5-6" in depth wide mouthed and curved bottomed, half litre capacity vessel having a hole in the centre of the bottom. In the hole cotton should be kept to allow oil continuously in the form of stream.

Procedure for Dhara: First apply oil to the head and do little massage and then to whole body. Ask the patient to lie on back on the table and keep head on extra projection of the table. He should be in the comfortable position. The Dhara-Paatra should be hanged 4 fingers above the patient forehead. Start the automatic Dhara instrument and allow the oil to flow down on forehead. It will be adjusted to required thickness of the stream. The oil which is coming over the head should be collected in a separate vessel and the temperatue should be maintained constantly. The flow should not stop till the required time is over. Normally, 20-30 minutes is the duration for Dhara and it can be continued for 15 to 21 days. After completion of Dhara, we should clean and dry the head and advice complete rest.

Basti: It is a procedure in which medicated oils or fluids introduced through the anus by an instrument (Basti Yantra) is known as 'Basti Therapy.' Basti is one of the important therapies advocated to treat the various vata vyadhies.

Many varieties of Basti have been described in Ayurveda. But, Matra Basti is one of the safest and uncomplicated amongst all bastis and easy to administer even to the child.

Instrument: 100 ml. metal syringe can be used to give Matra Basti.

Procedure: Massage should be done to whole body after passing natural urges. Special massage should be done to the buttocks. Ask the patient to lie down on the table on his left side with left leg straight and keep the right leg on it by flexing hip and knee. Take 30 to 50 ml of medicated warm oil mixed with one gram of Saindhava lavana in a metal syringe and introduced into the anus with low pressure without giving any jerk. Then light massage should be done on buttocks so that medicated oil should not come out from the anus.

This basti should not be done on empty stomach. The child should have some food before he is ready to undertake Basti therapy. After Basti, the child should allow to lie down upto one hour. Care should be taken to pass stool after 2 hours; if he gets hungry, luke warm milk or khichdi must be given. This Matra basti treatment should be continued upto 8 days continuously without interruption.

Management of Old and Chronic Patients

In old and chronic patients, if they do not get oil massage, fomentation, and Basti, they are prone to get emaciation, contractures and deformities in the affected limbs. According to the condition of the patient, we have to plan the management and rehabilitation to make him independent.

Emaciation of Muscles

If there is emaciation without any contractures and deformities, the patient should be advised the following measures:

1. Oil massage with Mahamashadi taila or Mahanarayana taila, to be continued regularly.
2. Fomentation with Nadi Sweda initially and then Shastika shali pinda sweda should be advised 15 to 21 days course with suitable intervals.
3. Orally, anti-vatik drugs mentioned above should be continued.
4. Specially the Brimhana (anabolic drugs should be continued for longer duration.
   (i) Aswagandha leha 1 spoon twice daily with milk OR
   (ii) Shatavari ghrita 1 spoon twice daily with milk.
5. Matra basti with Bala taila OR Ksheerabala taila OR

Mahamashadi taila should be given 8 days along with oil massage and Nadi Sweda regularly.

6. If patient is walking with maximum limping due to emaciation of the muscles, we must give some simple wooden splints. By doing this we can avoid deformities in healthy limb.

Contractures and Deformities

If there are contractures with or without bony deformities, the following measures should be advised:

The management which is advised for emaciation of the muscles should be implemented:

1. Oil massage, fomentation, oral antivatik and Brimhana drugs, Matra Basti etc.
2. Simple exercises, splints.
3. If there is no relief, we should refer the case to an Orthopaedic Surgeon to remove contractures and deformities. Later on, we should continue the above management.
4. In the management of contractures and deformities, we should take the help of simple splints, walkers and calipers to achieve maximum results whenever necessary.

Repeat the same treatments with suitable intervals according to the condition of the patient for about 3-5 years period.

Prognosis of Poliomyelitis (Untreated)

During the febrile period, paralysis may develop or progress. Mild weakness of small muscles is more likely to regress than severe weakness of large muscles. Bulbar poliomyelitis may occur in 5-30 per cent of paralytic cases and carries the highest mortality rate (upto 50 per cent); in these cases, it is greatly influenced by the age, and the presence of shock, pulmonary edema, superimposed infection, or other medical complications.

Many persons with paralytic poliomyelitis recover completely, and in most of them muscle function returning to some degree. Only a few remain totally paralysed. The more life threatening the disease in the acute stage, the more frequent is complete functional recovery, if patient survives; paralysis of the respiratory centre disappears completely. Similarly, dysfunction of the 9th and 10th cranial nerves is followed by total recovery in most instances although, mild palato-pharyngeal weakness may occasionally persist for life. Paralysis of muscles of respiration often disappears completely, and in most instances, the final vital capacity is adequate to maintain ventilation. In a very few instances, chronic respiratory care is necessary. In weak extremities about 60 per cent of the total strength that they will ever recover in 3 months, 80 per cent within 6 months, but improvement may continue as long as 2 years.

Clinical Research Reports on the Management of Poliomyelitis

In modern medicine, except Physiotherapy and Orthopaedic surgery (in contractures and deformities), there is no any oral or parenteral therapy available to treat an already affected individual with poliomyelitis.

Ayurveda appears to offer some hope in the management of poliomyelitis cases, especially in the paralytic stage and in the post-polio management. Some of the available reports are mentioned below for guidance during the management of poliomyelitis.

1. Intensive research work has been done under C.C.R.A.S. (1975-79) on a "study of Kkhanja and Pangu (Poliomyelitis)" under the guidance of Vd. H.S. Kasture Deshpande et al at Ahmedabad. Out of 100 cases which were studied in this series, 26 patients were affected in left lower extremity, 32 were affected with Right lower extremity whereas 42 cases have been affected in both lower extremities. From this study, it has been seen that 27 cases were of acute poliomyelitis and 73 patients were of chronic duration. Regarding the results obtained—11 patients were cured, 87 relieved, whereas 2 patients were unchanged.
2. In 1980 Ramachandran P. et al have studied 50 polio cases and reported encouraging results with Rasa taila.

3. In chronic polio cases, Snehana and Pinda Sweda along with Matra basti with Mahanarayana Taila have shown encouraging results as observed by Sarma et al (1983).
4. Yadaiah, P. studied 92 patients with polio with different treatment groups during the period 1981-85 as part of thesis work. The following conclusions have been drawn:
   (i) The prevalence of Balapakshaghata is more in male children (63.7 per cent) than females.
   (ii) It is observed that even after vaccination, many children were seen suffering from this disease, mainly due to improper administration of the polio vaccine as per the standard recommendations, e.g. improper storage, transportation, dosage etc. It is, therefore, suggested that proper care should be taken for immunization.
   (iii) From the results, it has been revealed that the incidence of Bala Pakshaghata is comparatively more in varsha ritu (rainy season) than other ritus. In varsha ritu, physiologically, the body gets weakness due to first part of visarga kala and poor appetite leads to suitable atmosphere for multiplication of any virus (Skandagraha). Normally, in varsha ritu, vata gets provocated, and in weak body if any trauma occurs, further derangement of vata takes place resulting into vata-vyadhi in that particular organ. Therefore, it is recommended that to avoid injections and trauma (abhighata) especially in varsha ritu for below 2 years of age.
   (iv) In the present study it has been observed that in preparalytic stage, many cases (77.45 per cent) reported the history of injection. From this, it can be strongly recommended that in varsha ritu, if the child gets fever, unless absolutely necessary (e.g. Intravenous fluid therapy), treat with simple drugs such as antipyretics and avoid intramuscular injections.

(v) It has been observed that lower extremities are more affected (91.3 per cent) than the upper extremities.

(vi) The study has established that continuous Bala taila Matra basti is superior to other treatments practically in almost all the aspects for acute patients (The other treatment group had Tila taila matra basti). The statistical and even clinical results indicated that in this treatment, recovery is faster than the other treatments. In view of this, it is strongly advocated to administer continuous Bala Taila Matra Basti for acute cases to obtain desirable results. This treatment is simple in nature and can be administered even without admitting the patient including children below one year.

(vii) In chronic cases the treatment of continuous Tila taila Matra basti is recommended for obtaining the faster relief. (The other treatment procedures tested were—Bala taila Matra basti 15 days in the doses of 30 ml.; Pinda sweda for 15 days; Bala Taila Abhyanga and Nirgundi Patra Nadi Sweda for 2 months.)

(viii) The study has indicated that the muscles of left knee extensors have gained significant muscle power with continuous Bala taila Matra Basti in acute cases. Hence, it can be suggested that this treatment is advocated for the muscles of left knee extensors.

(ix) The study has revealed that the continuous Bala taila Matra Basti in acute cases is superior to the other treatments, particularly in the improvement of Hip extensors of left side affected cases. In view of this it is advocated to administer in improvement of Hip extensors of left side affected cases.

(x) All the treatments considered in this study have shown statistically significant 5 per cent increase in bodyweight in all the cases in the course of treatment (15 days course). From this it emerges that increase in the body weight implies the reduction in vatavyadhies which is a desirable sign.

(xi) The present study revealed that the reduction of chesta in vrutti and increase in muscle power in all cases have turned out to be statistically significant at 5 per cent level in the course of the treatment. It suggests that almost all cases have gained the muscle power in each treatment.

(xii) In this study Matra basti treatment has not shown any complications and side effects during and after the treatment. From this, it can be recommended that the Matra basti can be administered for children even in out-patient department level.

5. 125 polio cases were studied in Ayurveda Hospital, Kayachikitsa Department Akola during the period 1985-90. The conclusions were as follows:

Table 2.31

S. No.	*Results*	*No. of Pts.*	*(in %)*
1.	Complete relief	1	4.0
2.	Marked Improvement	11	8.8
3.	Moderate improvement	33	26.4
4.	Mild improvement	76	60.8

(i) From this study it has been observed that right and left leg affections have shown good improvement. Those cases with both legs affected have not shown encouraging results. However, in these patients, one limb (either right or left leg) has shown improvement in their muscle power upto 3-4 grade whereas the muscle power of the another limb improved 1 to 2 grade. Hence, these children cannot walk without splints. With the help of simple splints, they are walking.

(ii) The children who are affected with upper extremities have not shown encouraging results.

(iii) Matra Basti has shown comparatively encouraging results than other treatments adopted. This therapy is very easy to administer the patient. Matra basti patients have not shown any side effects or complications.

(iv) Though Pinda Sweda has shown encouraging results in some patients, but it consumes much time and needs more man-power. Also, it cannot be given in summer season (Greeshma ritu).

(v) It has been observed that few patients have got good improvement after Sneha and Swedana treatments.

6. Dr. Tarun Kumar L. Swamy, Head, Department of Panchakarma, Government Akhandanand Ayurvedic Hospital, Bhadra, Ahmedabad-380001, reports the method adopted at Mashoor Hospital, Government Manibhahan Hospital and Government Akhandanad Hospital, Ahmedabad, in an article "Baal Vata Vyadhi—Polio and Panchakarma Chikitsa—Baal Rog Nidan Chikitsa, Special Issue, Harish Pharma, Vijaygarh, Aligarh, as follows:

Treatment is carried out in two groups of patients:

I. Recently acquired Polio case—When polio affected child comes within 30 days from the onset of attack.

II. Those polio children who come after 30 days of the attack.

I. *Recently Acquired Polio (Khanja, Pangu Treatment)*

Children with fever, rooja and paralysis of a limb:

1. | | |
|---|---|
| Sitophaladi Choorna | 500 mg |
| Tribhuvana Kirtiras | 125 mg |
| Shaabar Shring Bhasma | 125 mg |
| Pravaal Bhasma | 125 mg |
| Guduchi Satva | 125 mg |

Three times daily with warm water.

2. Samshamanivati, one pill thrice daily with water OR Sudarshan Ghanvati, one pill thrice daily with water.
3. Amritarishta 10 ml and Dashamoolarishta 10 ml—equal parts with water, thrice daily.

4. Dashaang lep OR Lep gutika, mixed with Shuddh Guggulu—to be applied externally, twice daily; along with Baaluka Sweda.
5. Basti—Til Taila Matra Basti 40 ml OR Narayana Taila.
6. Kati-Snan (Hip-bath)—Dashamoola Quath and hot water to be used.
7. Avagaah Sweda to be done till complete relief.

II. *Uncomplicated Polio-Paralytic Treatment*

This procedure is adopted for those patients who come after one month of polio attack.

1. Abhyang: Bala taila, Chandanabala Lakshadi taila, Narayana taila, Panchguna taila—any one of these can be used. While performing Abhyang, special attention is to be paid to the part affected.
2. Swedana: In Swedana, Shastikshali Pinda Sweda is advised. Of all the Swedana procedures, Pinda swedana appears to be best for polio patients.
   (i) Shastikshali Pinda Sweda procedure—see above.
   (ii) Avagaah Sweda—water mixed with Dashamoola Quath is used.
3. Basti Therapy: Matra Basti—Tila taila OR Narayana taila 40 ml (using glycerine syringe for the technique), at a time.
   Rajyapan Basti—at a time.
   Course: One day Matra Basti and one day Rajyapan Basti can be done. A course of 8 days, 16 days, or 30 days can be adopted.
   Preparation of Rajyapan Basti

Mustadi Quath	100 ml
Mamsa Ras	60 ml
Milk	50 ml
Ghee	20 ml
Honey	10 ml
Saindhav lavana	2 gram
Prakshepa Dravya	3 gram

All ingredients are prepared as done in Nirooh Basti and

administered at warm temperature using syringe and depending on the strength of the individual.

Aushadh Upachar (Drug Treatment)

1. Aswagandha Churna 2 grams (gm)
   Ajasthith Bhasma 250 mgram (mg)
   Shuddh Karaskar Churna 125 mgram(mg)
   Suvarna Makshik Bhasma 125 mgram(mg)
   Praval Panchamrit 125 mgram(mg)
   To be used three times daily with milk.
2. Navjeevan Ras, one pill thrice daily OR
   Vishtinguk Bati, one pill thrice daily with milk.
3. Khanjan Kaari Ras, one pill twice daily OR
   Brihat Vatchintamani Ras, one pill twice daily
4. Yogaraj Guggulu, one pill twice daily OR
   Panchamrit Loh Guggulu, one pill twice daily with milk
5. Dashamoolarishta 10 ml
   Aswagandharishta 10 ml—thrice daily with water.

Fascial Paralysis (Due to Polio)

Jyotishmati Taila—5 drops, twice daily with milk; along with application of Shiro Dhara using Bala taila OR Narayana Taila.

Physiotherapy: Along with the above treatment, appropriate muscular exercises are recommended for every polio affected child.

Prevention

The current widespread practice of active immunization with either oral polio or injectable polio vaccine has greatly helped in the prevention of the disease. There are no contraindications for the administration of the vaccine except that it should not be given to children who are acutely ill or are having diarrhoea. Passive immunisation with human normal immunoglobulin in a dose of 0.25-0.3 ml per Kg. body wt. has been found to be protective but is not required when active immunization is done. If passive immunization is done, the subject should be actively immunised against polio after few weeks.

Occurrence of more than one case in a household is not usual and in the house, isolation is not necessary because by the time the child is diagnosed to be suffering from poliomyelitis, other children in the family have already been infected, most often with silent infections, and most of the adults are immune.

During epidemics, contacts should be confined to bed at the first sign of illness. Tonsillectomy during an epidemic is best postponed. There is no evidence that closing of schools or camps influence the course of the epidemic. However, children may be advised to avoid moving in crowded places and swimming pools during such time. Since the polio virus is destroyed by chlorine and potassium permanganate, suitable treatment of water supplies and swimming pools ensures safety.

Prevention of Poliomyelitis in Ayurveda

The following preventive measures may be applied to all children to prevent poliomyelitis (Yadaiah):

1. Child should not be exposed to cold in rainy season.
2. Wear woollen or warm clothes to the child.
3. Apply Tila oil to whole body and do light massage every day before bathing.
4. Keep Til oil swab on Brahmarandhra (Anterior Fontanelle) for 24 hours upto the age of 2 years.
5. Drop Til oil in both the ears.
6. For bathing apply turmeric and besan instead of soap.
7. Give fumigation or Sharshapa or Hingu or Vacha every day after bath upto one year.
8. If child gets fever, avoid injections as far as possible during June to September months, and prefer oral medications and complete rest.
9. Try to give boiled water to avoid digestive troubles.
10. Proper care should be taken to avoid constipation.
11. Fever, diarrhoea, indigestion, common cold, cough etc. can be treated with simple medicines.
12. Avoid fear psychosis.

13. Diet—Breast milk should be given priority and should be continued at least upto six months.
14. In between 6th and 8th month, child's ear should be nitted with needle specially in winter season.

Along with the above principles, expectant mothers must be educated about the importance of balanced diets, role of physical exercises and proper medical care. Package of treatments normally practiced for post-natal care in rural areas like oil massage, Fomentation, Brimhana (anabolic diets), complete rest etc. must be advocated.

Ayurvedic References for the Above Guidelines in the Prevention of Maternal and Childhood Diseases

1. Proper antenatal check-up on Ayurvedic lines for the pregnant ladies.
2. Diet during pregnancy—month wise as advised in Ayurvedic classics.
3. Proper post-natal care—oil massage, fomentation, Brimhana (anabolic) diet, complete rest.
4. Health education
5. Prevention of neo-natal and childhood diseases:
   (i) Honey, Ghee and paste of the Gold mixed together should be given three times daily to the child on the first day after delivery (Sushruta Samhita Shareer 6/9) to develop immunity.
   (ii) Everyday oil should be dropped into both the ears and apply oil on Shrungataka region (Sushruta Samhita Shareer 10/23)—Ears are the seat of vata dosha and oil keeps not to provocate it. Shrungataka is one of the Sadhya Pranahara marmas. Application of oil and gently pressing on this vital areas may give current stimulation as well as nutrition to the brain every day.
   (iii) Keep oil swab on head and apply oil on Brahmarandhra continuously for children (Ashtanga Sangraha Uttara p.13).—Keeping continuously oil swab on Brahmarandhra (anterior fontanelle) on

the head of children suggests that the brain will get nourishment and soothing effect to the central nervous system. Sushruta has mentioned Pichu Dhara treatment for Pakshaghata patients. From this we can say that all the sense organs will get nourishment from this Pichu. Acupuncture and Acupressure have given prime importance to this point, because it is said to control all the organs and flow of energy in the body (Vinaya Kumar).

(iv) Oil massage should be done everyday with Vatashamaka and Brimhana oils before bath (Sushruta Samhita Shareer 10/23).—It enhances age, strengthens the body, induces sleep, gives good colour and smoothness to the skin, enhancés eyesight, the body will not be susceptible to the diseases duet to vata, resists the body against exhaustion, and exertion, and tones up the tissues of the body. So, the oil massage helps in many skin disorders and vatavyadhies and everyday application enhances the immunity and resists the diseases.

(v) Fumigation should be given to the child everyday (Charaka Samhita Shareer 8/4).—After bath everyday fumigation with Sharshapa, Guggulu, Vacha etc. should be given. Acharya Sushruta says that the Raksha Karma should be given to the children. By doing this fumigation, all the germs can be killed in that area including viruses and bacteria.

(vi) All clothes should be fumigated with Guggulu, Sharshapa etc. after washing properly (Ashtanga Sangraha Uttara p.10)—see above for reasoning.

(vii) In between 6th and 8th month the child's ear should be knitted with needle specially in winter season (Ashtanga Sangraha Uttara p.12).

(viii) The child should be protected from all sorts of injuries (Ashtanga Hridaya Uttara 1/15)—The idea may be that the child will get injury as test dose. This is more explicitly shown in Acupuncture Therapy where ears are thought to control all the organs of the body both anatomically and physiologically (Vinaya Kumar), and thus increase the acquired immunity of the body to various diseases like Poliomyelitis and Tetanus which are more provoked through injury.

(ix) Prolonged breast feeding to the child (Sushruta Samhita Sutra 35/29)—It has been scientifically established that (Sabin, 1955) the placentally transmitted antibodies are known to diminish at a regular rate and the persistence is influenced by the original titre. The majority of infants between five and six months are devoid of placentally transmitted antibodies. Therefore, Sabin points out that as soon as the maternally transmitted antibodies disappear from the circulation, the breast feeding plays further role. If the milk contains anti-poliomyelitis substances it effects the alimentary canal where the virus establishes.

It is well-known fact that in rural areas, after delivery, Indian ladies get vigorous anti-vatik treatment such as oil massage to whole body, fumigation, hot water bath, complete rest, Brimhana (anabolic) diet for a period of one to one and half months. These treatments may produce antibodies against all the diseases in the body of mother which may get transfer through breast milk to the child.

REFERENCES

1. Vinaya Kumar, A., Infectious Diseases: Diagnosis and Management in Clinical Practice, CBS Publishers and Distributors, Delhi (1994 Ed.)
2. Yadaiah, P., Management of Poliomyelitis, Jaya Publications, Akola (1991 Ed.)—A Monograph.
3. Tarun Kumar L. Swamy, Baal Vata Vyadhi—Polio and Panchakarma Chikitsa, Baal Rog Nidaan Chikitsa, Special Issue, Harish Pharma, Vijayagarh (Aligarh).

4. Ghosh. D., Baal Rog Ki Katin Samasya—Pakshaghat, ibid.
5. Purohit, Baal Angaaghat, ibid.
6. Tripathi,B., Baal Pakshaghat, Vaat-Vyadhi Chikitsa, Nirmal Ayurved Samsthan, Aligarh.
7. Vinaya Kumar, A., Principles of Ayurvedic Therapeutics, Indian Books Centre, Satguru Publications, Delhi (1995), Ist Ed. (Sources for Ayurvedic Practitioners and Students Series, Volume One).
8. Vinaya Kumar, A., Recent Trends in the Epidemeology of Poliomyelitis, Continuing Medical Education—2, The Journal of General Medicine, Oct-Dec. 1993, Vol. 6, No. 1.
9. Ramachandran Nair P., et al, Effect of Bhadradarvadi Taila and Sahacaradi Taila in Khanja and Pangu, Jl. of Res.Ayu.Siddha, Vol. X, No.1 & 2, 1989.
10. Charaka Samhita
11. Sushruta Samhita
12. Ashtangra Hridaya
13. Ashtanga Sangraha

Clinical Report

Treatment of Chronic Cases of Sasaveeya Vata (Poliomyelitis)—P. Ramachandran Nair, et al. (*JRAS*:1:3:1980).

Twelve patients were included in the trial, dividing them into two groups at random. Indukanta Ghrita with mastu 3 to 5 gm, was given to all patients for first 14 days as Srothorodhahara measure followed by Virecha on fifteenth day with castor oil in either group. Second phase of treatment for 41 days beginning from the sixteenth day was meant for vatahara and brumhana measures. Indukanta Ghrita along with mamsa rasa was given internally and tila taila externally in Block II. Rasa taila with Bala kvatha 30 ml was administered in Block I along with Rasa taila for external application. Block I showed more improvement leading to 46 per cent relief in comparison to 35 per cent in Block II. As the mamsa rasa is common in both the medicines it was assumed that Rasa taila used externally in Block I was responsible for good result.

In the light of the results of the pilot study, trial was continued with the necessary changes to assess and ascertain the medicine which was responsible for better results in Block

I. 50 cases of Saisaveeyavata were selected from the Outpatient Department and they were grouped at random for the trial. Criteria for selection of cases, duration of the illness, duration of the trial, parameters for assessment etc. was identical as in the above pilot study. The pattern of treatment, medicines etc. were also maintained as given in the pilot study with the only change in external application of Rasa taila in both the groups.

Results

41 per cent and 36 per cent relief was observed in Block I and Block II respectively. Out of 25 cases in Block I, complete relief in one, marked relief in eight, moderate relief in fifteen, and no relief in one case was noticed as against complete relief in two, marked relief in two, moderate relief in 16 cases and mild relief in five cases in Block II.

Reduction in polymorphs (21 cases) and lymphocytes (9 cases) and increase in 4 cases and 16 cases respectively was observed in Block I—it may be due to the influence of the drugs rather than the chronicity as it is not found in Block II. Increase of haemoglobin is significant in both the blocks. The reduction of eosinophil count in Block II from initial high count is encouraging. Onset of the disease does not seem to influence the result and is independent of duration of illness. The cases with maximum duration (2 years) showed 39 per cent relief as against 42 per cent in minimum duration (3 months). The response was poor in both blocks where deformity had set in. Improvement was pronounced in cases having lesser involvement.

Conclusion

Result is highly significant in both the blocks. The better response in Block I was maintained throughout the trial as seen in the pilot study. The first phase of 15 days treatment, including the external application of Rasa taila and Mamsarasa was common in both the blocks. The higher result in Block I may be attributed to the action of Bala (Sida retusa), the main constituent of Rasa Taila and Bala Kvatha given internally. The result can be improved further by treating them subsequent to correction of the severe deformities and providing them with suitable walking aids.

Effect of Bhadradarvadi Taila and Sahacharadi Taila in Poliomyelitis—Short Research Communication, *JRAS*: IX:3-4:1988).

Bhadradarvadi and Sahacharadi taila were tried in Poliomyelitis on forty children of both the sexes aged one to twelve years. The patients were divided into two groups at random. To group one 10 ml Bhadradarvadi Taila was given orally two times a day and 15 ml Taila as Matra Basti. In group two, 10 ml of Sahacharadi Taila was given orally two times and 15 ml Taila as Matra Basti. Massage with 30 ml of the same Tailas respectively was done for 30 minutes. The results were statistically significant in both the groups and found better in the former group.

Forty children of both the sexes suffering from poliomyelitis, affecting paralysis of lower limbs (lower motor neurone type) with maximum duration of two years was kept as selection criteria and duration of treatment was kept as three months. They were aged 1-12 years and were grouped at random, into two batches.

Result

Children treated with Bhadravati Taila (Gr. I) showed complete relief in two cases, marked relief in two cases, moderate relief in three cases and mild relief in ten cases, whereas Gr. II treated with Sahacharadi Taila showed one case with complete relief, marked relief in two cases, moderate relief in four case and mild relief in seven cases. Two cases in Gr.I and six cases in Gr.II did not show any improvement and condition of one cases in Gr. I was slightly deteriorated due to frequent intercurrent illness like fever, dysentery etc. Results in both the groups were statistically significant (P. less than 0.01). Changes noted in routine blood, stool and urine investigations were within the normal range, except the reduction of eosinophil count in 3-4 years age group in Gr. II (P. less than 0.05). Improvement was better in fresh cases especially in Gr. I.

Recurrence of poliomyelitis after vaccination has been noted in both the groups before they were subject to treatment.

Tailas—Bhadravadi (Vagbhata) and Sahacharadi (Charaka) are well-known for their vatahara properties. Taila is prescribed as an agryoushadha (most effective) for vatarogas (Vagbhata) and the internal and external application of Taila is expected to give good response in vatarogas (Vagbhata). The efficacy of Taila is fortified with Bhadradarvadigana and Sahacharadiyoga. As pakvashaya is the vatashtana, basti is expected to give good relief in vatarogas, especially of lower limbs. Hence the better results are to be attributed to the combined effect of oral, basti and external application of Bhadradarvadi and Sahacharadi Tailas.

PAKSHAGATA AND ITS PRINCIPLE OF TREATMENT IN AYURVEDA

The term Pakshagata literally means paralysis of one half of the body where paksha denotes the right or the left and Aghata or Paralysis denotes the loss of motor function resembling with the concept of karmendriyas. There are two sets of indriyas—1. There are two sets of gyanendriyas that is Chakahu, Shrota, Ghrana, Rasand, and Sparsana and 2. Karmendriyas that is Hasta, Pada, Payu, Pastha, and Vakendriya and Third is mana which is supposed to control and guide them. It is said to have component of both. It is obvious that gyanendrayas are part of the sensory system and the Karmendriyas are that of the motor system. Thus in paralysis there may be loss of all the voluntary function with or without impairment of sensory and psychic functions, depending upon the sight and extent of lesion.

Principle and Management of Pakshaghata

All kinds of vatavyadhi have predominance of Vata. So in general anti-vata treatment is good for all of them including pakshagata. The word anti-vata treatment (vataghana/vatahar) refers to the use of all kinds—drugs, food and life style which will help to subside vata. All the classics have unanimously emphasized that best treatment for pure vata diseases is Snehan both external as well as internal. But if it is associated with Kapha and Ama, Snehana is contraindicated. If one examines at the occurrance of pakshagata all thrombotic lesions have involvement of Kapha. The incidence of cerebovascular thrombotic lesions have involvement of Kapha. The incidence of cerebovascular thrombosis is also reported to be maximum among the C.V.A. About half of the cases of strokes have been identified to have thrombotic lesions. Among the embolic one also, in many cases the source of embolus is broken piece of athreoma which is the part of the general atherosclerosis of arteries. This concept is parallel to the concept of *Dhamanai Pratichya* which is described to be a Nanatmaja vyadhi of Kapha. Other common source of embolus is vegetation of Rheumatic Heart which is an example of 'ama.' Haemorrhage cases are usually serious and are less likely to survive for more than 48 hours. In these cases the management is merely symptomatic. Thus in majority of cases Snehan treatment is contraindicated.

Thus treatment of Pakshagata can be dealt under 3 headings.

1. Preventive treatment.
2. Curative treatment.
3. Residual treatment.

Preventive Treatment

It consists of the identification of the modifiable risk factors and manage them properly e.g. hypertension, hyperlipidemia, hypercholesterolemia, diabetes, over weight etc. In addition, seasonal regimen and daily routine described in Ayurveda must be followed strictly. Asatmendriyarthe samoya and Prangyaparadha have been found to play the important roles in causation of vatavyadi in general and Pakshagata in particular; so to avoid the same, the principle and practise of sadvritta/Achar Rasayana should be followed strictly, as

Astmendriyarthe samyoga and pragyaparadha have been found to play the important roles in causation of vatavyadhi.

Those having family history of hypertension, cardiovascular diseases or paralysis having hypercholesterol and hyperlipidemia should avoid to take fatty diet as far as possible. Intake of bengal gram, garlic and onion is specially recommended for them as they help in keeping the cholesterol within normal range. Similarly practice of yoga and regular exercise may be also be helpful. However, if hypertension is already established strenuous exercise/yoga not be taken up. Shavasan/meditation and Bhakti Yoga are very good for them.

Curative Treatment

Curative treatment can be further divided into two parts—(a) during the attack (b) after the attack.

The management during the attack is primarily different because of the loss of consciousness, which is because of odema, Neuronal shock or compression in the increasing haematoma; so a larger area of the brain is involved during this period which may be gradually reduced if the patient survives with the return of the consciousness and some of the vital functions.

To control the lesion Ayurveda has proposed two active measures (1) Raktamokshana (2) Virechana. Nowadays with the advent of effective hypotensive drugs and diuretics the role of Raktamokshana and Virechana is being limited. Blood letting was being used till few decades back in modern medical system also to control the sudden rise of B.P. But we feel that Raktamokshana may have some additional advantages than only controlling the B.P.

Sodhana therapy has to be resumed as early as possible. Anuvasana and Niruha vasti has to be given to clean the bowel and to control the vata at the root (moolasthans). Irrespective of type of lesion, haemorrhage thrombosis or embolism, it has to be administered. Vasti chikitsa should be resumed in all cases of Pakshaghata.

Virechana therapy should be started as the patient develops consciousness (Ch. Chi 28/83). Virechana is also supposed to help in excreting pitta and also kapha to some extent thus it is likely to have decompressing effect around the pathological lesion reducing the cerebral oedema and pressure symptoms. With the virechana, mutra virechana can be also adopted as it is less cumbersome. The most popular method of today, to promotes diuresis is the rapid infusion of manital. It is usually administered for 2-3 days in the big inning of attack.

Though the B.P. needs control in all cases of stroke, but it should not be permitted to fall down below normal because it has its own disadvantages. It favours thrombosis and ischaemia to brain cells. So the preparation like Makaradhwaja, Yogendra Rasa, Brihatvatchintamani, Vatkulantak are frequently recommended in Ayurveda.

Anticoagulant therapy is being recommended nowadays specially in thrombotic lesions. Ayurveda has so many drugs which have similar effect; most popular in the field of Pakshagata are—arsenic preparations that is, Mallasindur, Navagrahisrorja-bhasma, Sameera-Pannaga Rasa etc. Recently Guggulu has been reported that have anti-coagulant/Anti-thromboic properties. Prothrombin time is increased, firbrinolytic effect has been also demonstrated. Apart from that potent hypocholesterolemic and hypolipidemic action of Guggulu is well established.

Regarding physiotherapy it is proposed that snehana and swedana particularly of the parts affected be gradually adopted as early as possible. Of course in the beginning, only passive movement has to be given.

After Attack

Once the patient has recovered from the initial shock and has regained the consciousness a fairly long standing management has to be done for a period of 3-4 months as described by Shusruta to regain the normal locomotive function. Again the treatment is twofold.

1. Aetiological treatment.
2. Physiotherapy.

As mentioned earlier the preventive treatment has to be continued so that patient does not develop a fresh attack which is known as secondary prevention. The best treatment is Sudha Guggulu which has to be given in doses of 2 gm three times a day for 3 to 9 months. In addition Sushruta has emphasised to prescribe—"Mashitiokya" drugs for Pakshagata what has been called as Medhya drugs by Charaka. Shankhapuspi, Bhrami, Guduci, Manhyuastihi has been said as Medhya Rasayana drugs. Each of them can be used as decoction 2-3 times a day in the dose of 5 gm. each at a time. Further the drugs used for Akshepaka has been also recommended; best of them are Vacha, Aswagandha, Jatamamsi, Mandukparni, Jyotishmati etc.

Both the medhya and anti-akshepaka drugs are likely to improve the psychic, sensory and motor function of brain these are proved to have anti-hypertensive and tranquillising action also. Along the minerals Swarna, Rajat, Shilajeta, Abhrak, Mukhta, Praval etc. have been extensively used. Its mode of action is not known.

Physiotherapy

Under this heading Ayurveda has special contribution to apply 'Shirovasti' and 'Shirodhara.' Local massage, fomentation of differend kinds have been said by Charaka to be the best treatment for stiffness or contractures (Ch. Chi. 28/19). Fomentation also relieves different kinds of pain and inflammation and makes the part soft. Systemic and local use of Snehana provides nourishment and the atrophied part quickly nourished and it also tone up the whole body.

Sushruta has specially prescribed Anu Taila for massage, Sowlwana Taila for Upanaha, Bala Taila for Anuvasana basti.

Residual Treatment

Once the Vata vyadhi occurs, in spite of recovery, residual symptoms /persist; minimum is the lightness of the affected parts (Ch. Chi 28/19). Further it has been said that Pakshaghata having a deep seated lesion may improve or may not. However one should make serious attempt to manage only those cases who are of recent origin, have not developed complications and whose general health is not deteriorated.

The idea of management of the late cases with residual symptoms is only to achieve the maximum functional position of prevention of further attacks and complications. To achieve the same, along with preventive treatment, general treatment of health and local treatment such as physiotherapy (Snehana, Swedana etc.) have to be continued; sometimes surgical treatment is also indicated.

Compound Drugs Mostly Used in Pakshaghata

1. Yogaraj Guggulu.
2. Trayodashanga Guggulu.
3. Brihatvatchintamani Ras.
4. Vrihatvatgajankush.
5. Chintamani Ras
6. Chatyrmukh ras.
7. Yogendra Ras.
8. Tarakeshwar Ras.
9. Himahavat Brindhwansa Ras
10. Vatanasam Rasa.

Medicated

1. Narayan Taila.
2. Bala Taila.
3. Mamasa Taila.

Decoction:

1. Rasana Saptak Kashaya.
2. Medhya Rasayana.
3. Rosona Pinda.

Single Drugs

1. Guggulu.
2. Kupilu.
3. Bhallataka.

4. Aranda.
5. Shunti.
6. Sarpagandha.
7. Rasna.
8. Manduk Parni.
9. Shamkha Puspi.
10. Vacha.
11. Bala.
12. Atibala.
13. Nagabala
14. Aswagandha.
15. Satavari.
16. Kapikachu.

In modern system, management depends on stage and severity of the disease. Mild early cases require only bed rest, splinting and salicylates. In more advanced cases with established deformities, the following must be considered.

1. Rest in bed.
2. Splinting,
3. Salicylates,
4. Analgesics,
5. Non-steroidal Anti-inflammatory drugs (NSAIDS)
6. Specific Antirheumatoid drugs,
7. Immunosuppressive drugs,
8. Systemic corticosteroids and corticotrophin (ACTH)
9. *Physiotherapy*

   The purpose of physiotherapy in rheumatology are:
   (i) Relief of pain.
   (ii) Relief of stiffness.
   (iii) Increase of muscle strength.
   (iv) Restoration of movement.
   (v) Restoration of function.
10. *Orthopaedic Appliances*

    The following are used for correction of the deformities:
    (i) Polythene splints for wrists and hands.
    (ii) Polythene gaiter splints for knees,

(iii) Short calliper with ankle-stop, toe-spring and T-strap for foot drop or instability of ankle, arch, supports, lumbar, correct of spinal brace.

11. Intra-articular corticosteroid injections,
12. Intra-articular radiscolloids,
13. *Surgical Treatment*
    Orthopaedic surgical treatment may be advised at any stage of the disease, whether or not disease activity is fully controlled.

Types of Operation

(i) Tendon repair,
(ii) Nerve decompression,
(iii) Removal of subcutaneous nodules,
(iv) Arthrodesis,
(v) Metacarpal or metatarsal hard resection,
(vi) Synovectomy,
(vii) Osteotomy,
(viii) Prosthetic operations.

14. Treatment of extra-articular manifestations.
15. *Occupational Therapy and Rehabilitation*
    Following the stage of immobilisation occupational therapy should be instituted as required, and therapist can educate patients in the use of functional splints and gadgets needed as aids to daily living.

Nearly all rheumatoid patients require some social help which is best arranged in an early stage by the medical social worker.

Clinical Reports

Effect of Panchakarma Treatment with Masadiyoga on Paksha-vadha—S.Madhvan Pillai et al (*JRAS*:1:2:1980).

The paralysis patients were divided into two groups (56 controlled and 56 treated). The pro formae specially prepared for this disease includes history of patients, signs and symptoms of the disease, duration of treatment and clinical investigations. The basis of diagnosis was according to the description of signs and symptoms on paralysis (Pakshaghata) as described in Charaka Samhita.

Under the treatment, process of Panchakarma chikitsa i.e. Sneha, Sveda, Mriduvirechaka and Vasti were included and this proved useful therapy for the disease; Masha, Atmagupta, Eranda, Bala compound was not found very useful. At the outset of the disease, the treatment appeared beneficial and was found effective on right sided paralysis.

The treatment of Pakshaghata as described by Charaka is mainly based on the use of sneha, sveda and mrdu virechaka karmas. Sushruta, in addition to these suggested vasti. The object of the present trial is to establish the effect of the karmas of sneha, sweda, virechaka and vasti on Pakshaghata. An yoga comprising of Masa, Atmagupta, Eranda and Bala (Masadi) was selected for the preparation of taila and kasaya for the trial. This compound has been prescribed for Pakshavadha in Yogaratnakara. Kasaya and taila for snehapana and vasti were prepared with these drugs. Baspasweda was employed for svedakarma. Eranda taila was given for vireka. A control group was also included for which taila and kasaya were prepared adding small quantity of Manjistha to provide a coloured appearance.

The taila for snehapana was prepared as per the principles of snehapana. 480 ml kasaya, 240 ml honey, 240 ml taila, 30 gm satahva and 15 gm saindhava were used for kasaya vasti. For snehavasti 180 ml of prepared taila was used. Number of vastis were given as per the rules of Yogavasti i.e. three kasayavastis and five snehavastis.

Drugs

Group I

1. Snehapana with Masadi taila—from initial 40 ml on the 1st day with gradual increase of 40 ml per day upto 7 days (280 ml), or till the lakshanas of samyak snigdha were noticed. Snehapana was continued.

2. Sweda—3 days baspa sweda was done after snehapana.
3. Vireka—After sweda, on the following morning 20 or 30 ml Eranda taila was given for vireka.
   After vireka, Masadi kasaya 60 ml was given twice a day for three days. Then the same kasaya with addition of 10 ml Masadi taila was repeated for four days.
4. Vasti—Vasti was prepared and applied for 8 days as mentioned earlier, followed by Masadi kasaya 60 ml + Masadi taila 10 ml twice a day upto 60 days. After 60 days final assessment was done.
5. *Ahara*: During the karmas, peya and vegetables were permitted. In the remaining period morning milk and uppamavu, followed by rice and vegetables in the noon and at night with milk in the evening.
6. *Vihara*: Masadi taila was used for abhyanga; Vyayama was suspended during the period of karmas. In remaining days it was permitted.

Group II

Coloured taila and kasaya as mentioned earlier were prepared for application in all the karmas. Sveda and vireka were carried out as for Group I. Ahara and vihara were also same in both groups.

Results and Discussion

It can be observed that this disease usually affects the people after the age of 40 (84 per cent). The maximum incidence observed was in the series in the age group between 50 and 60 (44.6 per cent). The total number of male cases constitute (66.96 per cent). Of the patients who came for treatment are manual workers. 92.8 per cent of the patients are non-vegetarians. 79.47 per cent of the patients have smoking or drinking or both the habits. Vata, pitta and vatakapha prakrities (86.60 per cent) are more prone to the attack of this disease. Rukshana chinta and ativyayama are the predominant causes of the disease.

Haemoglobin is increased after the treatment almost in all cases and rate of increase in Group I is greater than Group II. Total count and differential count are found normal in both groups. ESR is reduced in both groups with treatment. In Group I rate of reduction is greater. Blood urea and serum proteins stand without notable change by the treatment.

Epithelial cells and pus cells were found less in urine. Bile salts and albumin were also absent. The treatment has slight effect on hookworm. Blood sugar was increased in Group I and the same was reduced in Group II after snehapana. There is no commendable change in serum cholesterol.

There is only slight variation in the results of the clinical features in comparison in both the groups. According to age, the effect of treatment is more in the age between 30-50. The response was comparatively better in females than in males. Treatment is more effective in the right sided paralysis patients. Recent origin cases showed better response than chronic cases. On the basis of Doshanubandha, it was observed that kaphanubhandha showed more relief than the Kevalavataja and Pittanubandhaja cases. 28 per cent of the patients showed blood pressure before treatment. No notable change was seen in blood pressure after the treatment.

Out of six reported to have had complete relief, four cases (66.66 per cent) are in Group I and two (33.33 per cent) in Group II. Out of 24 cases showing marked relief, 11 cases (45.83 per cent) are in Group I and 13 (54.16 per cent) in Group II. Out of 47 moderate relief cases, 26 (55.30 per cent) are in Group I and 21 (44.6 per cent) are in Group II. Out of 33 mild relief cases, 15 (45.45 per cent) are in Group I and 18 (54.55 per cent) are in Group II. There are two cases under no relief in the Group II.

Conclusion

Present trial has shown that chinta (mental worries), ativyayama (over exercise or over activities), non-vegetarian food, smoking and drinking habits are the leading predisposing factors in the consideration of Pakshavadha. It is considered that the person over the age of 50 and who are manual workers are to avoid these particularly if they are of vatapitta, vatakapha prakrities.

Regarding treatment sneha, sveda, mrudu vireka and vasti are effective but compound of Masa, Atmagupta, Eranda and Bala has only slight effect on this disease. Early treatment gives better results and right sided paralysis is more responsive to the treatment.

Management of Pakshavadha—A Clinical Study of 109 Cases— P.K.N. Namboodiri et al (*JRAS*:1:4:1980)

The paper presents the therapeutic measures adopted in the treatment of Pakshavata with a view to ascertain an effective line of treatment for this disease. Emphasis has been given to Panchakarma therapy. 109 cases were selected for this clinical study in three groups. The first two groups were given selective Panchakarma therapy in the form of snehapana, sweda, vireka and a course of vasti. A medicated oil was used in the first group and coloured gingely oil in the second group for panchakarma. Bhadradarvadi kashaya with Dhanwantara gutika and Sahacharadi Taila for Abhyanga, Matra vasti, Pichu and Pratimarsahannasya were administered as preliminary treatment for the first two weeks. A third group of patients were also maintained with this line of treatment (preliminary) through out the course.

The results were discussed in terms of clinical recovery and functional improvement. The observations show that the above treatment provided statistically significant improvement. Better results were noted in Group I and Group III. Response was good in fresh cases.

This treatment was also found effective in hypertension. There was apparent reduction of blood pressure after the treatment and it was statistically significant—diastolic in Group I and systolic in Group II. Thus the above study shows Snehapana and Vireka have a definite role in the therapeutic management of Pakshavadha.

Discussion

Pakshavadha is primarily a disease engendered by vata. The vitiation of vata leads to sira and snayu shoshana and causes the disease (Vagbhata). From the available description we may have to interpret these two words sira and snayu in the context of functions of circulatory and central nervous systems. Snayus are developed from Medodhatu (Charaka), Snehana (Oleation) is the main function of Medodhatu (Vagbhata). The obstruction in the circulation of Rasadhatu deprives the snayus of their nutritive substances and causes shoshana. This occurs when there is a decrease in snehana and increase in Ruksha (dry) quality of vata. Therefore, stress has been given to snehana prayoga in the line of treatment of Pakshavadha. Snehana and swedana followed by vireka (Charaka) as given by Charaka and Vasti (Sushruta and Vriddh Vagbhata) as indicated by Sushruta and Sangrahakara were adopted in this trial. These processes remove the obstruction to the channels (srotorodha), eliminate wastes and help to increase the dhatu.

The decoction of Bhadradarvadi gana (Vagbhata) (Sutra 15:5) consisting of Bhadradaru, Nata, Kushta, Bala, Atibala, and Dashamoola with Dhanvantari gutika (Sahasrayoga) was administered initially for 1-2 weeks. Patients admitted immediately after the stroke without taking any other treatment were responding well to this. Dizziness, mental confusion, restlessness and other symptoms of the stroke and high blood pressure were reduced and they showed general improvement. Cerebral edema is developed after cerebral infarction and ischaemia and neurological deficit are increased due to this edema. Therefore, the main aim of treatment of all cerebrovascular accidents in modern medicine is to reduce the cerebral edema and the intracranial pressure using the drugs like Mannitol or Maniline (Glycerol) by intravenous infusion. Like Mannitol, the above decoction containing Dashamoola etc. has got diuretic effect and this may be the reason for the improvement seen. Dhanvantara gutika is also reported to be possessing sedative action.

Sahacharadi taila is a simple preparation containing three drugs namely—Sahachara, Devadaru and Nagara (Vagbhata, Chikitsa, 21.56). The oil was prepared according to the pakavidhi. Nasal inhalation of this oil (Nasya) stimulates the cortex and fortifies the dosha. It was given along with Murdha Taila (Pichu) and are useful in reducing the residual deficits. Most of the patients had constipation. Sahacharadi Taila was also used for Matra vasti which ensures the regular bowel and bladder movements and removes constipation. It has nutritive and snehana effect too. Other treatments like Abhyanga with gentle massage and physical exercise were also employed in this trial programme which lessen the development of contractures and excite the motor units.

The above treatment was given continuously for 60 days for the patients included in the third group. For others in 1st and 2nd groups this treatment was tried for 1-2 weeks, after which snehapana was started with Mashadiyoga I and Mashadiyoga II respectively. Mashadiyoga is described in Yogaratnakara under the treatment Pakshavata. Mashadiyoga II is a placebo using Tila taila coloured with little quantity of Manjishta. For snehapana 40 ml oil was given on the 1st day and the quantity was increased on subsequent days noting the time taken for digestion of sneha. Samyaksnigdha lakshanas were seen from the 4th to 7th day. Then these patients were subjected to steam bath for 3 consecutive days before giving vireka with Eranda taila. Vasti was started from the 8th day after vireka. All these patients received kashaya with taila of the respective group along with Abhyanga after the vasti till the 60th day and the assessment was done thereafter.

Out of 109 cases studied 90 were males (82.57 per cent), 18 females (16.51 per cent) and one (0.92 per cent) was a child. The highest number of cases (40.37 per cent) reported was in the sixth decade of life. 50 cases had right sided hemiplegia and 59 cases left sided hemiplegia. It was observed that manual workers (65.05 per cent) and vatakapha prakritis (70.64 per cent) were prone to an attack of this disease more commonly.

The classification according to modern medical diagnosis: Internal capsular artery thrombosis ranked first (86.24 per cent) among the causes of hemiplegia followed by haemorrhage (6.42 per cent) and embolism (3.67 per cent). Other cerebral lesion like tumor was suspected in remaining number of patients. This diagnosis was on the basis of history and clinical signs and symptoms.

The extent of paralysis varied from patient to patient. 8.26 per cent cases were having severe stroke, 62.39 per cent cases showed moderate attack and remaining 29.35 per cent cases had mild attack.

Biochemical investigations conducted before and after snehapana and vireka and after vasti reveals that blood sugar and cholesterol levels tend to fall after snehapana and vireka. The level is, however elevated after vasti. Except this no other major improvement was noted with snehapana and vireka. Some patients became generally weak after vasti.

Significant change in diastolic blood pressure was noted in Group.I (P. less than 0.05 greater than 0.02) after the treatment compared to the initial reading. In Group II and Group III, though there was apparent reduction of blood pressure after treatment the values were not significant statistically. But systolic blood pressure was lowered significantly (P. less than 0.01) in Group II. In some cases, where the blood pressure was high, it did not come to the normal range after treatment. Yet the patients got relieved from symptoms of dizziness, headache and mental confusion.

In group wise results, comparatively better results were obtained in Group I and Group III. The percentage of marked improvement was more in Group I and moderate improvement was higher in Group III. The value of X^2 test applied in analysing the result of treatment with the three groups showed that the P is less than 0.05 per cent; the result is statistically significant. The above method of treatment is, therefore, considered to be an effective treatment for Pakshavata. The chance of recovery is good when the duration of illness is less.

However, in cases with disturbed consciousness, this line of treatment did not show any marked improvement.

Conclusion

Use of Bhadradarvadi kashaya with Dhanvantara gutika and Sahacharadi taila shortens the first shock phase and hastens the restoration of movements of the paralysed limbs. It prevents the development of stiffness and spasticity and also regulated the bowel. This line of treatment is found to be effective especially in ingravescent stroke. Snehapana and Vireka are found to be useful for lowering blood pressure in hypertensive patients.

Course of Treatment

1st group

A. 1. Bhadradarvadi kashaya—60 ml
(1-2 weeks before starting Snehapana with Mashadi taila No.1 Madi).
Dhanyantari gutika—1 No.
Thrice a day—7 a.m., 1 p.m., and 5 p.m.

2. Sahacharadi taila — 40 ml for Abhyanga in the forenoon
- do - — 60 ml Matra vasti at 2 p.m.
- do - — 5 ml for Pichu at 4 p.m.
- do - — 5 ml for Nasya at 4 p.m.

B. Snehapana, Virechaka and Vasti (after completion of regimen A)

1. Snehapana — 1-7 days
2. Baspasweda — 8-10 days
3. Vireka — 11th day with Eranda taila 30 ml + hot water at 7 a.m.
4. Samsarjana — 12th and 13th days
Madi No.1 Kashaya 60 ml two times—7 a.m. and 5 p.m.
5. Samana — 14th to 18th days
(i) Mashadi taila No.1 kashaya with Mashadi taila No.1 taila 10 ml—2 times at 7 a.m. and 5 p.m.

(ii) Abhyanga in the forenoon with Mashadi taila No.1 taila—40 ml.

6. Yogavasti 19th to 26th days—8 days

(i) Snehavasti—5—with 180 ml of Mashadi taila No.1 taila on 19th, 21st, 23rd, 25th and 26th days.

(ii) Kashayavasti—3—with kashaya of Mashadi taila No.1 480 ml. Gingely oil 240 ml, Honey 240 ml, Satahwa—30 gm, Saindhava 15 gm, on 20th, 22nd and 24th days.

7. Samana Upto 60th days.

(i) Mashadi taila No.1 kashaya—60 ml + Mashadi taila No.1, taila—10 ml—two times at 7 a.m. and 5 p.m.

(ii) Abhyanga with Mashadi taila No.1, taila 40 ml in the forenoon.

8. Physiotherapy during the samana period.

II Group

A. As in Group I 1-2 weeks.

B. Snehapana, Vasti and Abhyanga with taila and kashaya prepared with of Manjistha. Vireka with Eranda taila and Baspasweda. The course of treatment remains the same as in Group I.

Diet: Light diet with peya and vegetables were given till vireka and full diet during the remaining period with rice and vegetables at noon and night and milk and uppumavu in the morning and milk in the evening.

III Group

A. As in Group I + Physiotherapy up to 60 days. (Snehapana, Baspasweda, Vireka and Vasti were not given)

Full diet—till the completion of the course.

Role of Hingutriguna Taila in the Treatment of Pakshaghata—Hemiplega: Prem Kishore and M.N. Padhi (*JRAS*:IX:1-2:1988)

The clinical study to assess the effect of Hingutriguna Taila along with Abhayanga have been conducted on 35 patients of Paksaghata. The Medical Research Council criteria for gradation of muscle weakness has been adopted in addition to other subjective and objective parameters for the diagnosis of the disease and assessment of the results. The observations indicate that the disease is more common in males in the age range of 61 years and above and the paralysis of grade I is most commonly observed. The effect of the treatment has been obvious within a short period of 2 weeks and definite relief has been observed after 4-6 weeks of treatment.

The treatment of the disease in Ayurveda has been based on a set of principles involving sodhana as well as Samanacikitsa. The preparations of Guggulu and Abhayanga have been very commonly administered.

In recent years a series of studies have been conducted to study the effect of Guggulu (Tripathy et at 1971-75), Vastisnehamasamana, and only Samana treatment (Rao et al 1976), Amivasana Vasti and Niruha Vasti (Prasad et al 1976) have been reported to bring improvement. The Panchakarma therapy consisting of Vireka, Vasti, etc. (Pillai et al 1980, Namboodiri et al 1980), Sirovasti with Prasarini Taila (Ananda et al 1976) and compound preparations like Astavarga Kvatha and Dhanwatara Yoga (Rajagopalan et al 1975) have also been reported efficacious. However, the efficacy of these treatments has been a limited one. Some of these treatments are quite costly and cumbersome to the patients. As such, the search is continuing to evolve a simple, cheap and easily available treatment for this disease.

In this quest, the preparation, Hingutriguna Taila has been selected for trial along with Abhayanga of the affected portions. This taila has been prepared with Rasona and Eranda as its main ingredients (Vagbhata). These ingredients have been individually recommended or tried for the treatment of Vatavyadhi. A preliminary study of this preparation has demonstrated its efficacy in the treatment of different Vatavyadhi including Paksaghata and Gridhrasi (Padhi et al 1981). The studies, therefore, have been further continued to assess the definite role of this preparation in the treatment of Paksaghata.

Materials and Methods

Selection of Patients

The patients for trial have been selected on the basis of the following criteria.

1. Loss of function of one side of the body (the muscle weakness of grade 0, 1, 2, and 3 only).
2. Numbers of the affected side.

The patients were subjected to detailed clinical examinations and the revelations of the history and physcial examination have been recorded in a prescribed pro forma. In addition, the pathological investigations of stool, urine and blood as well as serum cholesterol of routine nature were conducted.

Treatment

The treatment consisting of the following internal and external medication had been prescribed to the patients for a period of 4-5 weeks.

1. Hingutriguna Taila—5 ml. 2-3 times a day with warm water.
2. Abhayanga with Tila Taila etc., and Pinda Sweda twice a day.

In addition the patients had also been prescribed certain medicines such as Visatinduka Vati for relief of pain and Sarpagandha preparations for hypertension etc.

The diet consisting of Upuma in break-fast, rice, dal and curry for lunch and chapati, dal, curry and milk for dinner had been provided throughout the course of treatment.

Results

The effect of the treatment had been obvious within two weeks of the treatment and improvement in muscle power had been noted in most of the patients who continued treatment for two weeks (Table 2.32).

Table 2.32: *Showing Degree of Paralysis Involving Separate Portions Parts/Muscle Group*

S. No.	Limb	Part/Muscle-Group	Total No.	Grade and No. of Parts			
				0	*1*	*2*	*3*
1.	Upper	Arm—Forearm (Big-muscles group)	27	10	2	9	6
2.	Upper	Palm—fingers (Small-muscles group)	27	11	6	5	5
3.	Lower	Thigh—leg—foot (Big-muscles group)	27	3	5	13	6
4.	Lower	Toes (Small-muscles group)	27	14	3	4	6

Table 2.33: *Showing the Gradewise Improvement of Muscle Power Who Continued the Treatment for 2 Weeks—24 Cases.*

S. No.	Grade Before	No. or Parts/ Muscles Group	Grade After Treatment & No. of Patients					
			0	*1*	*2*	*3*	*4*	*5*
1.	0	29	12	14	2	1	–	–
2.	1	15	–	7	7	1	–	–
3.	2	29	–	–	11	16	2	–
4.	3	23	–	–	–	17	6	–
Total		96	12	21	20	35	8	–

Further treatment showed more improvement in the functional capacities of the affected parts and improvement in the degree of relief from paralysis after 4-5 weeks of treatment had been quite significant. The treatment induced complete recovery (Grade V) of the paralysis of or nearly complete recovery i.e. only mild weakness of the affected parts (Grade IV) in about 3/4th of the cases (Table 2.33) The effect of the treatment on other associated afflictions has also been quite significant. Complete recovery had been observed in most of the other clinical manifestations, but the improvement in speech defect and Bell's palsy has not been much significant (Table 2.34).

Table 2.34: *Showing Gradewise Improvement in Muscle Power After 4-6 Weeks of Treatment on 15 cases*

S. No.	*Grade Before Treat.*	*No. or parts/ Muscles Group*	*Grade After Treatment & No. of Patients*					
			0	*1*	*2*	*3*	*4*	*5*
1.	0	14	3	–	3	5	2	1
2.	1	12	–	1	–	2	9	–
3.	2	14	–	–	–	3	11	–
4.	3	20	–	–	–	–	7	13
Total		60	3	1	3	10	29	14

The observations on the effect of the drug on serum cholesterol level showed significant reduction ranging between 8 to 78 mg per cent in 5 patients out of 7 patients on which this observation was feasible.

The classification of the results according to the criteria for assessment indicated definite efficacy of the drug since almost all the patients who completed the treatment for at least 4-5 weeks duration showed definite improvement, although complete recovery has been observed in only 4 such cases.

The age, chronicity or the side involved does not show any significant relationship with the effect of treatment. The effect of the treatment on male patients is more pronounced than the one on females since all the patient got complete relief were males. In some cases occasionally, mild loose motions have been reported which could be controlled by adjustment of the dose or taking slightly warm water or some anti-diarrheal medicines.

Discussion

The trial of Hingutriguna Taila in the patients of Pakshagata had been taken up to evolve alternative methods of treatment for this disease condition, which may be more effective than the other available methods of treatment. The available Ayurvedic treatment of this disease is either based on the preparations of Guggulu or other approaches of treatment such as Panchakarma and Rasa Chikitsa which may be relatively more costly and cumbersome. This simple formulation may prove to be quite significant in the treatment of Pakshagata and other Vatavyadhies as well as in certain other disease conditions. It has been observed that most of the patients have been males and the incidence is relatively more in the age group of 61 years and above. The patient under observation have been suffering from the disease for a short period in most of the cases. In addition to the paralysis of limbs of either side which is the cardinal clinical manifestation of the disease, pain in the body, speech defect, Bell's palsy had been other common associated signs/symptoms. The observations on the degree of paralysis, though started later and could be completed only on 27 patients, indicate varying degree of paralysis among which Grade -0 paralysis was most commonly observed while other grades i.e. Grade-1, 2 and 3 have also been frequently noted in different parts of the limbs. The observations on serum cholesterol indicate its level on higher side in most of the patients. It may be mentioned that the serum cholesterol level of 200 mg per cent and more has been considered higher in the patients of obesity, paralysis and coronary heart disease (Tewari et al 1980, Tripathi 1975).

The efficacy of the treatment is very well in conformity with preliminary observations (Padhi et al 1981). The assessment of muscle power according to the M.R.C. scale/criteria showed gradual improvement in the condition of the patients. The effect of the treatment on lowering the serum cholesterol level though observed in small number of patients yet it offers significant areas for further study.

As already mentioned the efficacy of the formulation may be attributed to the Rasa, Guna, Virya and Vipaka of the ingredients of this formulation, especially Rasona and Eranda which are in contrast to the factors responsible for this disease. The hypocholesterolaemic, regenerative effect of the drug could also be responsible for the relief of pathological conditions such as atherosclerosis. The impact of Abhyanga on physiotherapy and its nerve nourishing effect may also be helpful in inducing the recovery.

These observations / study conclusively establish the role of this preparation in the treatment of Pakshagata.

Effect of Bhadradarvadi Taila and Sahacharadi Taila in Khanja and Pangu (Monoplegia and Paraplegia)—P. Ramachandran Nair et al (*JRAS*:X:1-2:1989)

Summary

Walking disability due to the drawing up (contractions) of the kandaras (muscle-tendons) of one leg by deranged vayu situated at kati region is called as Khanja; when both legs are similarly affected, the disease is called Pangu. Since the disease originates at Kati Katyasritavata-Apanavaya is involved. The main complaints—disturbed visceral reflux (micturition and defaecation), loss of sensation, inability to walk are due to Apana vaigunya. Dhatukshaya and Margavarana due to an aghata on Kunkundare marma or a lesion due to any reason to spinal cord are the two basic factors for this disease. The institute has taken up intensive research trials to evolve an effective therapy against this disease. A research trial was conducted to assess the efficacy of Bhadradarvadi Taila and Sahacharadi Taila on Khanja and Pangu.

Forty patients were selected and divided into two groups at random. Bhadradarvadi Taila (Group I) and Sahacharadi Taila (Group II) were administered 20 ml at 7 a.m. and 5 p.m. orally; matrabasti with 60 ml. and abhyanga with 50 ml. On assessment after 30 days treatment, a course of snehapana and yogavasti was prescribed in those cases where improvement was less than 30 per cent.The results of the study was analysed at the end of the trial i.e. after 90 days. The result in both groups were found statistically significant. Routine blood, stool, urine, and radiological investigations did not show any significant changes as a result of treatment. Sahacharadi Taila was found more effective in the diseases of viral origin and degenerative cases. But both preparations showed good response in intervertebral disc prolapse cases.

Introduction

The Institute at Cheruthuruthy has taken up intensive research studies with a view to evolve an effective therapy for this disease. The studies so far conducted revealed that the Ayurvedic line of treatment gives good relief to Khanja and Pangu patients. Internal and external application of medicated oils help in restoration of muscle strength and power. A research trial conducted with Sahacharadi (Sahacara 3 parts, Devadaru 2 parts and Shunti 1 part) Taila showed that it has good effect in Khanja and Pangu patients, conducted by Nair et al in 1984. This prompted us to initiate studies to compare the efficacy of Sahacharadi preparation vis a vis other well-known preparations. Results of the comparative study with Nirgundi has already been reported by Nair in 1984. In this study efficacy of Sahacara oil has been compared with that of Bhadradarvadi. Internal and external application of these oils also gave good response. Bhadradarvadi gana (Vagbhata) is considered to be an effective medicine for vata diseases in general. Hrasuapanchamoola and Brahatpanchamoola are well-known for Vatanulomana and hence were expected to give good response in urinary and excretory organs—systems.

Bạla and Atibala are considered good for Brumhana and Devadaru, Tagara and Kustha for vatahara properties.

Materials and Methods

40 patients of either sex were selected from the Outpatient Department of the Institute for the trial. Patients were between the age group of 15 to 70 years and grouped into two at random as Group I and II. Bhadradarvadi Taila Sahacharadi Taila (Charaka Sam. Chi. 28) were selected for the study. Tila Taila (Sesamum oil) was medicated with respective yogas for preparing Bhadradarvadi Taila and Sahacharadi Taila. Routine tests were done including X-ray of the lumbosacral and thoracic regions before and after therapy. Clinical symptoms were taken as main criteria for selection. Signs and symptoms were graded and marks allotted (numerical values as per criteria of assessment). The following were taken into consideration for grading: control over urinary bladder, control over rectum, sensory changes, muscle power, fasciculations (muscle twitching), chorea, pain, clonus (ankle) patella, muscle tone, Deep tendon reflexes, abdominal reflexes, pressing power and walking speed. Assessment was done initially, periodically, and at the end of the trial and recorded. Trial period was fixed as 90 days and was divided into 3 stages of 30 days each. Bhadradarvadi Taila and Sachacharadi Taila were administered in Group I and Group II respectively. Taila was administered orally in small doses of 20 ml at 7 a.m. and 5 p.m. as Samana sneha in both the groups for 30 days in the first stage. Abhyanga was given with respective oils in both the groups for 30 minutes. Complete assessment was made on completion of the first stage. The cases in which more than 30 per cent of improvement was noted, the same line of treatment was continued till the end of the trial—i.e. for 90 days. The cases in which improvement was less than 30 per cent were changed over to the second stage of the trial. A course of snehapana with respective oil was given in the second stage. If the improvement was more than 15 per cent on completion of snehapana, sweda and vireca, a second course of snehapana was administered.

Remaining cases were transferred to the third stage of the trial. A course of yoga basti (Vagbhata) (5 anuvasanas and 3 niroohas) was given in the third stage. On assessment after a course of basti, if the improvement was more than 20 per cent, a second course of basti treatment was given, while others were discontinued, from the trial. Usual hospital diet was prescribed to all patients.

Clinical improvement was graded as (i) complete relief (disappearance of all signs and symptoms), (ii) marked relief (61-99 per cent relief), (iii) moderate relief (31-60 per cent), (iv) mild relief (10-30 per cent) and (v) no relief (upto 10 per cent).

Table 2.35: *Diet*

Morning	*Noon*	*Evening*	*Night*
I. at 7 a.m. Milk 200ml +10 g. sugar	at 12.30 p.m. rice 250 g+ vegetables 200 g	at 4 p.m. milk 150 ml+ 10 g sugar	at 7.30 p.m. rice gruel 150 g + green gram 25 gm

II. Rice gruel at 8.30 p.m.

On Snehapana period, little rice gruel was prescribed after complete digestion of sneha consumed.

Result

Marked relief and moderate relief were noted in 7 cases in each and mild relief in 3 cases in Group I (Bhadradarvadi), marked relief in eight cases, moderate relief and mild relief in five cases each was reported in Group II (Sachacharadi). Three cases in Group I and two cases in Group II did not respond to the treatment. On statistical analysis, the results in both the groups were significant. On assessment of the improvement after 30 days of treatment, 30 per cent and more relief was noted in 7 and 12 cases respectively in Group I and Group II. Only in two cases out of thirteen, and in four cases out of eight, snehapana could be given due to the indigestion/complication.

In remaining cases same samana treatment was continued for both the groups. The result in snehapana patients was less than 15 per cent improvement, hence a course of basti was prescribed for both the groups. Better result was observed in fresh cases than in the chronic cases. According to modern diagnosis, aetiology due to intervertebral disc prolapse and of viral origin showed better response in Bhadradarvadi group as well as Sahacharadi group. Radiological investigations revealed fracture/disc prolapse/dislocation of vertebra in seven cases and five cases in Gr I and II respectively. Arthritis of spine was found in four cases in Gr II. However, no radiological change was observed on final assessment after completion of the trial. The changes in blood investigations reports were negligible and within normal limits. The results of stool and urine tests was also not significant.

Table 2.36: *Modern Diagnosis and Result*

	Diagnosis	*Group I*	*Result*	*Group II*	*Result*
		Frequency	*%*	*Frequency*	*%*
I.	Inflammatory				
(i)	Bacterial	1	27.28	–	–
(ii)	Viral	5	45.72	3	66.50
(iii)	Degenerative	7	38.81	6	51.48
II.	Traumatic				
(i)	Fracture and Dislocation	3	23.21	5	42.28
(ii)	Osteoarthritis	–	–	4	49.28
(iii)	Intervertebral Disc prolapse	3	75.23	1	59.05
III.	Congenital	1	36.54	1	21.5
	Total	20		20	

Discussion

Tila taila is considered to be an effective remedy for vataroga especially where Apana vayu is involved. It's efficacy considerably increases by the samskarana (processing) with Vatahara dravyas. The ingredients of Bhadradarvadi Taila, Bala and Atibala possess guru and snigdha gunas, Balya, Rasayana and vatahara properties and are good remedy for healing up of internal and external injuries (Bhavamisra-Bhavaprakasa); and hence they may be responsible for healing of lesions in the spinal cord which results in this disease. Tagara is recommended in diseases connected with brain like Apasmara and Unmada. In addition it is also an effective drug against Bhoothagraha, hence it is expected to give good response in neurological afflictions of viral/bacterial origin (Bhavamisra). Kushta is considered to be an agryaoushadha for vatarogas and massage with a mixture of kustha choorna, honey and ghee is recommended to increase the muscle power (Bhavamishra). Devadaru is well-known for its vatahara properties (Bhavamisra) and Dashamoola for sophahara, soolahara, anulomana and Tridosha samana properties (Vagbhata). All these properties of the ingredients of Bhadradarvadi Taila may be responsible for the improvement seen. Sahachara is an effective drug for vatarogas in general. Pharmacological studies on rats has shown that it possess significant anti-inflammatory activity. The Katutiktarasas and sophohara and soolahara properties of Dahacara in combination of taila may be responsible for the improvement in Khanja and Pangu patients, especially in the cases of inflammatory origin and it is also effective in the disease of viral origin.

Conclusion

Bhadradarvadi Taila and Sahacharadi Taila were found effective in Khanja and Pangu. Results in both groups were statistically significant. Sahacharadi Taila was found more effective in viral origin and degenerative cases and in both the groups, good results were shown in intervertebral disc prolapse cases.

MUSCULAR DYSTROPHY
PSEUDOHYPERTROPHIC MUSCULAR DYSTROPHY

Muscular Dystrophies

These inherited myopathic disorders are characterized by progressive muscular weakness and wasting. They are subdivided by mode of inheritance, age of onset, and clinical features as shown in the (Table 2.37).

In the Duchenne type, pseudohypertrophy of muscles frequently occurs at some stage; intellectual retardation is common; and there may be skeletal deformities, muscle contractures, and cardiac involvement. The serum creatine phosphokinase level is increased, specially in the Duchenne and Becker varieties, and mildly also increased in limb-girdle dystrophy. Electromyography may help to confirm that weakness in myopathic rather than neurogenic. Similarly, histopathologic examination of muscle biopsy may help to confirm that weakness is due to a primary disorder of muscle and to distinguish between various muscle diseases.

There is no specific treatment, but it is important to encourage patients to lead as normal lives as possible. Prolonged bed rest must be avoided, as inactivity often leads to worsening of the underlying muscle disease. Physical therapy and orthopaedic procedures may help to counteract deformities or contractures.

Ayurvedic Concept of Muscular Dystrophies

It may be mentioned here that hypertrophy consists of a uniform enlargement of all constituent parts of an organ and the functional capacity of the organ increasing at the same time. False hypertrophy of an organ which is characterised by an enlargement of the organ which is not due to an increase in the pareonchym, but in some other constituents (intercellular tissue or adipose tissue) while the parenchyma remains normal or even atrophied and the function of the organ is diminished. As said above the pseudomuscular dystrophy is genetically determined sex-linked recessive type of myopathy.

Table 2.37: *The Muscular Dystrophies*

Disorder	*Inheritance*	*Age at Onset (years)*	*Distribution*	*Prognosis*
Duchenne type	X-linked recessive	1-5	Pelvic, then shoulder girdle; later limb and resp. muscles	Rapid progression. Death within about 15 years.
Becker's	X-linked recessive	5-25	Pelvic, then shoulder girdle	Slow progression. May have normal life span.
Limb-girdle (Erb's)	Autosomal recessive (may be sporadic or dominant)	10-30	Pelvic or shoulder girdle initially, with later spread to the other	Variable severity and rate of progression. Possible severe disability in middle life.
Facioscapulo humoral	Autosomal dominant	Any age	Face and shoulder girdle initially, later pelvic girdle and legs	Slow progression. Minor disability. Usually normal life span.

Distal	Autosomal dominant	40-60	Onset distally in extremities; proximal involvement later.	Slow progression.
Ocular	Autosomal dominant	Any age	External ocular muscles. May also be mild weakness of face, neck and arms.	
Oculopharyngeal	Autosomal dominant	Any age	As the ocular form, but with dysphagia	

Though in the broad classification of diseases, a category known as Adibala Pravritta diseases have been included, there appears to be no reference to a disease identifiable to pseudohypertrophic muscular dystrophy in the Ayurvedic classics (Sushruta Samhita Sutrasthana XXIV.) But a line of treatment for any disease known or otherwise can be thought of if the Samprapti of the disease is understood.

According to Ayurveda, Mamsakashaya may be present under the following conditions:

(i) Where there is Raktakshaya (Susrutha Samhita: Sutrasthana XV:7).

(ii) Mamasa vaha sroto dusthi including Rakta vaha dhamani dusthi (Sushruta Samhita: Sareera IX:12).

(iii) Asthi gata kupita vata (Charaka Samhita: Chikitsasthana:XXVIII:33).

(iv) Majja gata kupita vata (Charaka Samhita:Sutrasthana:XXVIII:14).

Mamsavriddhi or Mamsavriddhi like states are mentioned in Samamamsaja—diseases like Adhimamsa and Mamsasanghata (Sushruta Sa: Sutrasthana XXIV:12). Since in this disease vriddhi and kshaya both are seen side by side, the general dictum that all vridhis are due to nourishing factor and hence it is followed by kapha and all kshayas are due to non-nourishing component and hence it is followed by vata can be inferred (Vagbhata: Ashtaga Sangraha Sutra-XIX). If kapha and its samanaguna ama causes srotorodha thereby causing vridhi in a particular part, the same srotorodha can cause vata prakopa which in turn cause wasting or sosha of the region affected by it.

Ayurveda visualises 13 agnis which are responsible for digestion and metabolism. Each dhatu has corresponding agni which is responsible for the metabolism of the respective, dhatu. The increase or decrease of particular dhatu depends on the sada or deepti (decrease or increase) of the respective dhatvagni (Vagbhata, Ashtanga Hridaya. Sutra XI: 34):

From the above it can be inferred that whenever the Rakta vaha dhamani is impaired, Mamsagni is in deepta and Medogni is in sada-vastha, the condition similar to pseudohypertrophic muscular dystrophy may be produced. Therefore, the line of treatment according to Ayurveda for the above condition must comprise of not only Brimhana measures but also srotorodhahara, raktaprasadana and dhatvagni deepana measures.

Clinical Report

Pseudohypertrophic, Muscular Dystrophy—An Ayurvedic Approach— P. Ramachandran Nair et al (*JRAS*:1:3:1980).

Materials and Methods

Eight cases of pseudohypertrophic muscular dystrophy of either sex in age group of 9 to 19 years were selected from the Out-patient Department of Indian Institute of Panchakarma, Cheruthuruthy. All the cases were earlier diagnosed to be pseudohypertrophic muscular dystrophy in the Medical College Hospitals after thorough examination.

Treatment

Taking various Ayurvedic principles into account, the course of treatment at in-patient level was fixed at 10 weeks. It comprised of three phases. First phase is exclusively meant for Srotorodhahara and Dhatvagnideepana; second phase being Raktaprasadana and Raktavahadhamani sodhana and Medohara followed by, third phase exclusively constituted by Mamsasoshahara measures. The following medicines were administered at different phases of the treatment:

First Phase (14 days)

Shatdharana ghrita 5 to 10 gm—morning and evening.
Sahacharadi kashaya 30 to 60 ml—morning and evening.
Kottamchukkadi Taila for gentle external application.
Sathahwa Kalka for udwartana.

Second Phase (28 days)

Gugguluthiktaka Kashaya 30 to 40 ml—morning and evening.

Lohasava + Balarishta—15 ml—twice after food.

Third Phase (28 days)

Indukanta Ghrita 5 to 10 gms with Rasa Taila 3 to 5 ml—morning and evening.

Balarishta—15 ml to 30 ml twice after food.

Narasimha Choorna—1 gm twice a day.

Rasa Taila for external application.

All the above medicines were prepared according to the recipes in Sahasrayoga and Arogyakalpa druma. Shatdharana ghrita was prepared taking the drugs mentioned in Sushruta Samhita under Shatdharana Choorna Yoga as per the general ghritapaka vidhi.

Discussion and Conlusion

Presence of considerable amount of creatine in urine indicates of muscular dystrophies. There was no indication of decrease in these high values after completion of trial. Serum creatine in most of the cases either remained normal or increased a little within the normal range. In all the cases the ESR decreased, five cases of high ESR came to normal while in one case even though it showed decrease it did not come within normal. The reduction after trial suggests some change in the chronicity and it may be due to use of Guggulu thiktaka Ghrita and Gugguluthiktaka Kashaya in the middle phase of the trial. The values of total count and differential count and Haemoglobin were within the normal range before and after the trial and VDRL was negative in all the cases.

All the patients showed increase in grip strength indicating improvement in palmar and forearm muscles. The strength gained by upper limbs and lower limbs in terms of ability to lift weight and pressing power respectively even though minimal, the tendency was always on the improving side. Considering the fact that the period between the initial and final weight taken was only 10 weeks, the medicines certainly exerted positive influence towards gaining weight in almost all the cases, except one.

The changes in deep tendon reflexes noted were appearance of biceps reflex in one case and ankle reflex in two cases. Two cases of initially exaggerated ankle jerk were restored to normal after trial.

The condition of lower limbs, trunk and upper limbs before and after trial were assessed for muscle power. In all the cases the results were encouraging and these findings have been employed in arriving at the results. Out of eight cases studied, three (37.5 per cent) showed marked relief, two cases moderate relief (25 per cent) and three cases (37.5 per cent) mild relief.

3

ENDOCRINOLOGY

OBESITY (STHAULYA)

Obesity is a complex disorder that may be defined as an increase in weight of over 10 per cent above "normal," due to generalized deposition of fat in the body.

"Normal" or "desirable" weight, however, is difficult to determine; the standard age, height, and weight tables ordinarily used for practical clinical purposes are not always acceptable to everyone. It is important to differentiate weight increase due to depot fat from the increase due to body water or lean body mass. Weight gain due to obesity should be distinguished from that due strictly to fluid retention in edematous states (e.g. ascites, heart failure).

From a metabolic point of view, all obesity has a common cause: intake of more calories than are required for energy metabolism. The reason for differences in the food intake energy utilizations of various individuals, which make it possible for one person to utilize calories more "efficiently" than another, are not always known. Many clinicians feel that the metabolic changes in obesity are a result of obesity rather than a cause of it.

Some studies suggest that there are 2 major types of obesity based upon the number of as well as the size of the fat cells. Patients with so-called hypertrophic or adult-onset obesity usually have a normal fixed number of fat cells and gain weight by fatty deposition or hypertrophy of the normal number of cells. The patient with hypertrophic obesity is reasonably amenable to weight reduction. In the hyperplastic-hypertrophic type of obesity, where both the number and size of fat cells increase during childhood, weight reduction is difficult to achieve and to maintain. A high rate of weight reduction failure must be accepted, and particular effort must be made to minimize the metabolic consequences (e.g. hyperglycaemia) without inducing secondary physical disability and psychologic depression.

Aetiology

Although most cases of obesity are due to simple over-eating resulting from emotional, familial, metabolic and genetic factors, a few endocrine and metabolic disorders lead to specific types of obesity (e.g. Cushing's syndrome and hypothalamic lesions). It is particularly difficult to explain the phenomena of fluid retention and fat mobilisation and storage in obesity. Hypothyroidism is rarely a cause of obesity.

Complications

The association of obesity with increased morbidity, and mortality rates is well-known. Hypertension, diabetes mellitus, gall bladder disease, gout and possibly coronary atherosclerosis are frequently associated with obesity. There is an unexplained increase in the incidence of certain types of cancer (breast, endometrium, gall bladder, colon) in the obese in individuals. Obesity presents special hazards in pregnancy and in surgical patients. The psychologic and cosmetic implications of obesity are also significant factors. An obesity hypovetilation syndrome has been described in extremely obese individuals who show little or no evidence of primary disease of the heart or lungs.

Prognosis and Treatment

Specific weight reducing chemical agents and hormones (e.g. thyroid, chorionic gonadotropin), singly or in combination are either ineffective or hazardous and have no place in the treatment of obesity. Juvenile onset obesity is often very difficult to ıreat, possibly because of some ill-defined metabolic disorder, and it is important to institute a therapeutic programme as early as possible.

The Concept of Obesity in Ayurveda

Ayurvedic classics have recognized the drawbacks of obese (sthula) persons and described eight defects in corpulent (Medaswi) persons.

Asta-Dosha of Obesity

1. Those who are of too corpulent category are deficient in longevity.
2. They are slow in movement.
3. They find it difficult to indulge in sexual intercourse.
4. They are weak.
5. They emit bad-smell.
6. They have much of sweating.
7. They have much of hunger.
8. They have much of thirst.—(C. 54. Chapter 21/4 Niranaya Sagar, 116/117)

Etiology of Medaswita (Obesity)

Excessive corpulence is caused by over intake of heavy, sweet, cooling, and unctuous food, want of physical exercise, abstinence from sexual intercourse, day-sleep, uninterrupted cheerfulness, lack of mental exercise and heredity.

As a result, in fatty persons initially only the fat is excessively deposited. Other dhatus do not grow and nourished as required.

Samprapti (Pathogenesis)

The evolution of the disease is as follows:

1. The excessive use of Santarpaniya ahar having Guru, Madhura, Snigdha drava qualities, causes kaphavriddhi. The kapha is a dominant dosha vitiated by initiating factors.
2. Amashaya is a prominent place of the increased kapha. It is accumulated here. Thus Sthaulya is Amashya Samuttha Roga.
3. The impaired digestion due to Agnimandya—the lack of Agni function is responsible for the formation of Ama and Kapha Dosha. This is a basic vitiation phenomenon.

4. The Ahar Rasa along with the Ama circulates through the Srotas (channels) and settles in Medovaha srotas. This is the place for starting further vitiation.
5. The Medodhara Kala is vitiated. Hence the abdomen gains the weight and size. It increases the girth due to accumulation of Meda (fat).
6. Later on, the Meda is spread in other parts of the body and the tissues gain thickness due to accumulated fat (Meda).

Rupa or Manifestations

On completion of the Dosa—Dushya Sammurchhana (Samprapti), the symptoms are manifested. They are called Rupa or Lakshanas. Ayurvedic classics have mentioned following rupas: In addition to Asta-Dosha:

1. Shortening of life
2. Dyspnea on exertion
3. Delusion (Moha)
4. Kasa; swasa
5. Increased unctuousness in the body
6. Distension of the body
7. Flabby and pendulous mass move in the body

Management

The principles of treatment of all diseases cited in nut-shell by Ayurvedic physician, Acharya Charaka describes the measures to be adopted as under:

Elimination therapy, alleviation therapy and avoidance of causative factors—these three principles along with three proper procedure should be adopted for the treatment of disease in general and medoroga in particular. Of all these, avoidance of etiological factors forms the back-bone of the treatment.

Hence a wise physician should plan for the treatment by administering drugs, prescribing diet and encouraging useful regimen to correct the condition, without doing adverse or harmful effect on the patient's life.

The fat reducing diet, habits, and life style are advocated as Pathya or wholesome; conversely, the Apathya or unwholesome diet, habit and addictions causing deteriorating effect, obstructing the progress in improvement and aggravating the medo-vriddhi are to be avoided with care and patience. For a long period medical check-up and follow-up are desirable.

The regular life, diet control, moderate and regular exercise and medicine all together have efficacy in reducing the bodyweight, abdominal girth and restoring the health.

Drugs

1. Dasang Guggulu, 3 pills thrice a day for 30 days (Bhavaprakasha).
2. Trushanadaya Lauha, 500 mg twice a day for 30 days (Yogratnakara).

Both these recipes are effective to reduce the body weight. Among these two, the Dasang Guggulu is superior for the management of Medoroga.

To sum up, the Medoroga is not cured but controlled by the awareness of patients, faithfulness to the physicians instructions and drug-therapy. All these together bring encouraging results.

Clinical Report

Patients having clinical picture of medoswita in the age group of 20 to 60 years are selected. The subjective and objective criteria were taken into consideration for selecting the patients.(Total No. 30 patients)

A. Subjective criteria—Snighdagatrata, Swedadhikya, Khudhadhikya, Nidra, and Trishnadhikya having been present.
B. Objective criteria—body weight, girth, subcutaneous fat measurement of thickness by callipers.
C. Estimation of serum cholesterol and serum lipid in blood.

Observation and Discussion

It was observed that out of 30 patients selected for study, Nidradhikya was reported by 70 per cent, snigdhagatrata in

66.66 per cent, kshudra-swasa in 66.66 per cent, swedadhikya and tandradhikya in 66.63 per cent as a common complaint.

Along with this, gad-gadvanit gatrasaad, moha and Daurbalya developed later on as a result of Medodusti janya srotodusthi.

14 patients treated with Dasang Guggulu had shown a considerable relief in Medodusti janyalakshanas. The cardinal symptom of obesity was found relieved in many and wide range of cases. There was apparent reduction of bodyweight in all cases during treatment. The effect on serum cholesterol level and lipid was also found significant. The effect of the drug was strenghened by restricted diet and exercise too.

Conclusion

The present study revealed that medicine has shown satisfactory result in the management of obesity. It was effective in reducing body weight and symptoms of Medodusti. (A.B. Nirmal and B.M. Nirmal).

HYPERLIPIDEMIA AND OBESITY

The principal circulating lipids (fats) in humans are of 4 types. (i) triglycerides, (ii) free cholesterol, (iii) cholesteryl esters, and (iv) phospholipids. These are transported as spherical macromolecular complexes termed *lipoproteins*, wherein an inner core of hydrophobic lipids (triglycerides and cholesteryl esters) is encased by a membrane of unimolecular thickness consisting of various proteins (apolipoproteins, or simply apoproteins) in association with hydrophilic lipids (free cholesterol and phospholipids).

An excess or deficiency of certain lipoproteins can result from primary genetic disorders or may be secondary to acquired metabolic dysfunctions. In all cases of hyperlipoproteinemia, secondary forms should be ruled out before a diagnosis of primary genetic hyperlipoproteinemia is made. The secondary form of hyperlipoproteinemia are commonly due to: uncontrolled diabetes mellitus, hypopituitarism, lipodystrophy, renal failure with azotemia, severe hypothyroidism, hypergammaglobulin disorders, or advanced nephrotic syndrome (with serum albumin below 2g/dl). These lipemic manifestations are seen in genetically predisposed persons with mild diabetes mellitus or hyperestrogenemia (as in pregnancy or with oral contraceptive therapy) or in those who use alcohol excessively.

Treatment

Treatment of the secondary hyperlipoproteinemias consists, where possible, of treatment of the primary disorder, e.g., hypothyroidism, nephrotic syndrome, obstructive jaundice, or estrogen excess due to use of oral contraceptives. In primary hyperlipoproteinemia, no one diet is effective in all the lipid transport disorders. Similarly, none of the pharmacologic agents are universally effective. An understanding of lipid transport mechanisms and drug actions has improved the therapeutic approach to the hyperlipidemic patient.

Ayurvedic Management

Concept

Hypercholesteraemia is a condition common in these days due to the emotional stress, nicotine from the cigarette smoking, coffee drinking and partaking of a few large meals frequently and due to other factors that lead to higher or fluctuating levels of the free fatty acids. Cholesterol elevation is a metabolic derangement and may be associated with various disorders of different aetiology like diabetes mellitus, nephrosis, obesity, myxoedema, xanthomatosis, obstructive jaundice, hypotituitarism, idiopathic hypercholesterolaemia etc. Atheroscelososis and coronary heart disease are the major complications of hypercholesterolaemia.

Lipids are identical to Snehas described in Ayurveda. Medas, one of the seven Dhatus has been comprehended under the heading of Snehas. A few scholars of Ayurveda (Kasture and Dwarakanath) opined that muscle fat—Vasa is identical to Medas so far it relates to the properties; Vasa is an Upa-Dhatu of Mamsa-Dhatu from which Medo-Dhatu is derived by the action of concerned Dhatwagni. Bhava Misra has not considered them as synonymous terms. Considering this it is perhaps logical not to keep the derived lipid cholesterol beyond the periphery of Meda and Vasa. They are akin to each other. Elevation in cholesterol is likely to elevate the Medo-dhatu. This might be the reason for Acharya Sushruta's observation that increased Sneha contents of the body leads to excessive accumulation of Meda causing Sthaulya (corpulence/obesity). Co-existence of the higher levels of the cholesterol and the obesity has been further confirmed by many workers, although Satyavati (1966) reported 0 per cent relationship between cholesterol and Meda being a part as well as whole. So a drug affecting Meda is likely to affect the cholesterol too.

The Materia Medica of Ayurveda mentions of a few drugs that can be used in the disturbances of Meda. Gum Guggulu, turmeric, onion, garlic, holy-basil, Indian-berbery, black-butamin, bengal-gram, mango, ginger etc. are a few that have been taken up for study in this field; compound preparations like Arogyavardhini, Navaka Guggulu, Amritadhya Guggulu, Vidangadi Loha, Loharasayana etc. have been prescribed for obesity in Ayurvedic texts (Bhaishajaratnavali).

Clinical Reports

A Clinical Evaluation of Arogyavardhini as a Hypocholesteramic Agent with Special Reference to Obesity/Corpulence—Tewari N.S. and Jain P.C. *JRAS*:1:1:1980).

Arogyavardhini, a formulation, from Rasa-Ratna-Samuchaya which is said as Deepani-pachani-pathya-hrudya-medovinashini—was taken up for clinical trial. It is widely used for the skin disorders Kusht-Adhkar in the field of Ayurveda. It is a herbo-mineral preparation having 12 ingredients—containing five bhasmas i.e. of mercury, sulphur, iron, mica and copper—each one part with double the quantity of the three myrobalans, three parts of black butamin, four parts of pure gum Guggulu, four parts of root of Plumbago zeylanica and four parts of Picrorrhiza kurroa.

101 patients having cholesterol levels of above 200 mg per cent were chosen by total extraction method (by Zlatkis et al 1953). In addition to routine tests including blood sugar, coagulation time in 25 patients with Lee and White method were carried out. The trial drug Arogyavardhini was prepared in the pharmacy department of the State Ayurvedic College, Lucknow. It was administered in dose of 6 tablets (about 720 mg) of Arogyavardhini daily in three equally divided doses with water. The follow-up continued for two weeks. The subjects were allowed routine diet without non-vegetarian and heavy fat diet. A record of associated diseases and other complications is also noted.

The patients were also divided into three groups based on cholesterol level as: A (200-250mg per cent); B (251-300 mg per cent) and C (above 300 mg per cent).

Table 3.1: *Showing the Distribution of Associated Diseases in the Study*

Associated Diseases	*No. of cases*	*Percentage*
1. Obesity	48	47.6%
2. Diabetes mellitus	12	11.9%
3. Hypertension	6	5.9%
4. Arthritis	4	3.9%
5. Angina pectoris	4	3.9%
6. Ischaemic heart disease	3	3.0%
7. Nephritis	3	3.0%
8. Obstructive jaundice	2	2.0%
9. Hemiplegia	2	2.0%
10. Primary sterility	2	2.0%
11. Idiopathic hypercholestero-laemia	15	14.8%
Total	101	100.0%

Table 3.2: *Showing the Common Clinical Features Found in 48 Cases of Obesity Having Hypercholesterolemia*

Signs & Symptoms	*No. of Cases*	*Percentage*
1. Body ache and joint pains (Krathan and Angavasad)	36	75.0%
2. Dyspnea (Kshudra-shwas)	22	45.8%
3. Feeling of heaviness in the body (Angashaithilya)	16	33.3%
4. General weakness (Ashakti)	12	25.0%
5. Numbness, tingling and burning sensation (Kara pada dah)	10	20.8%
6. Polyuria and intense thirst (Trishna)	9	18.8%
7. Vertigo (Moha)	5	10.4%
8. Profuse sweating with bad odour (Kshutsweda-daur-gandhya)	4	8.3%
9. Increased appetite	3	6.3%

Observations and Results

Females (69) outnumbered the males (32) in all the three groups. Serum cholesterol elevations has relation with the advancement of age with its peak reaching in fourth decade of age with absence in first and after seventh decade. The associated diseases and clinical features observed in the 48 cases of obesity are shown in the tables.

Subjective improvement was observed in the body ache and joint pains, dyspnea, feeling of heaviness, general weakness, and numbness, tingling and burning sensation by the treatment. There was complete recovery in cases where there are mild symptoms.

The time taken for the action of the drug in reducing the excessive cholesterol is well in the range of 7-21 days noted by many workers with different drugs. Significant fall was observed in all the three groups A, B, and C by 5 per cent, 8 per cent and 14 per cent respectively by the end of the two weeks of treatment.

Table 3.3: *Cholesterol levels in three differnt groups*

Groups	*Mean S. cholesterol in mgms %* Initial	After 2 Weeks	After 12 Weeks	*Total Fall in mg%*	*Total Fall in mg%*
1. Group A (200-250 mg%)	225	214	173.0	52	23.0
2. Group B (250-300 mg%)	276	254	206.5	69.5	25.4
3. Group C (301 mg% and above)	330	283.8	209.8	120.2	36.4

About 80 per cent of cases under trial showed the hypocholesteraemic action of the drug expressing the fall varying from 10.5 per cent to 60 per cent in comparison to their pretherapy value after 12 weeks of treatment. 20 per cent of the cases which showed either no response or fluctuating levels of the cholesterol were associated with other diseases like diabetes mellitus and nephritis. The fall in serum cholesterol was directly proportional to pretherapy value. Fall of 23 per cent, 25.4 per cent and 36.4 per cent respectively in the three groups at the end of 12 weeks of the treatment in three different groups is in favour of this.

In group B and C, the fall in the level of the cholesterol became stationary for a fortnight after six to eight weeks of the trial; although the drug was taken and the fall was continued afterwards. This suggests that escape phenomenon might be a cause to an increased endogenous synthesis of cholesterol as a result of feed response of the drug in reducing the cholesterol; it showed highly significant P value of less than 0.011 in group A and B and less than 0.001 in Group C.

Effect on Blood Coagulation Time

This was carried out only in 25 cases which were initially found below the lowest limit of normal range i.e. 4 minutes in 74 per cent of cases. At the end of 12 weeks of treatment with the trial drug, the coagulation time was increased by a mean of about 40.5 per cent in all the cases. It was further confirmed that there is co-existence between the hypercholesteraemia and decreased blood coagulation time. Higher the level of cholesterol, lower was the coagulation time as observed in several cases.

Effect on Body Weight

The drug did not show reduction in body weight where it was in excessive in cases of obesity. There was slight reduction in a few cases ranging from 0.5 kg to 2.6 kg; but that was not found stationary and statistically significant.

Toxicity of the Drug

The drug did not show any side effects even with higher doses. Initially there was the stationary block in the fall of cholesterol at the end of 6 to 8 weeks of trial due to escape phenomenon. Maximum dose given was 1.5 gm. per day which was gradually tapered down to original one afterwards. Moreover, the drug did not show any toxicity even after the use beyond three months. Hence, it may be recorded that the drug is quite safe and free of any toxicity.

Possible Mode of Action of the Drug

It is not possible to make any specific comment on the mode of action of the drug regarding the cholesterol reduction. It may be presumed as due to combined action of the ingredients of the drug that act on the different stages of cholesterol metabolism.

Sitosterol present in Plumbago zeylanica inhibits cholesterol absorption from the intestines, although it is of less importance, as normally only 0.3 gm of the cholesterol is absorbed from the intestines unless the individual ingests large amount of cholesterol rich diet.

Other ingredients of the drug like Picrorhiza kurrora, black butamen, Phyllanthus embelica, mercury, sulphur and iron bhasmas act as a cholagogues and hence the secretion of the bile acids and salts that help in metabolic pathways of the cholesterol. Picrorhiza kurroa (Kutaki) draws much more attention in this reference as it covers half the amount of the total drug and is an established cholagogue increasing the hepatic insufficiency.

Resins present in Gum-Guggulu, black butamen and Terminalia belerica inhibit the reabsorption of bile salts and acids subjecting them to be excreted out with the faeces by the laxative action of P. kurroa, black-butamen, Gum-Guggulu, P. embelica, T. chebula, mercury and sulphur. Thus the drug reduces the excessive cholesterol by increasing the catabolism to the cholesterol.

Conclusion and Discussion

101 cases having hypercholesteraemia of three different groups (mild, moderate and severe) have been tried with the composite drug Arogyavardhini. At the end of three months of the trial, the reduction in serum cholesterol was 23 per cent, 25.4 per cent, and 36.4 per cent in three different groups respectively having a mean fall of 29.1per cent, which is comparable with other hypocholesteromic agents. The drug showed uniformity in action on the reduced blood coagulation time also which has been recorded as a co-existence with hypercholesteria. It has been calculated that a reduction of serum cholesterol by 15 per cent would result in a decreased risk of coronary heart disease by 35 per cent.

Thus the drug can be of use in cases of ischaemic heart diseases as the drug has a significant hypocholesteraemic effect along with a tendency to elevate the blood coagulation time. The drug may be further beneficial in preventing the premature atherosclerosis as it is amply proved that atherosclerosis can be cured, if not calcified. Tissue cholesterol may be drained if the serum cholesterol is lowered down because the tissue cholesterol and serum cholesterol are exchangeable.

The drug can be of use in case of the early lesion of atherosclerosis and prevents complications when used for long time. The drug is free of toxicity even after prolonged use. Moreover the drug is easily available in the market and can be easily prepared in the pharmacy.

Endogenous synthesis is solely responsible for about 80 per cent of the total day to day formation of the cholesterol, irrespective of the oral feeding of cholesterol. The accumulation of the cholesterol in the blood depends upon the formation of the cholesterol and its excretion in the liver. Moreover, most of the lipids are metabolised in the central pool of the metabolism i.e. liver.

Hence, there is every possibility that the hypocholesteraemic action of the Arogyavardhini might be only due to the presence of Kutaki (Picrorhiza kurroa) which is a proved cholagogue. Therefore, there is a very useful need to have a comparative trial of the single drug Kutaki for reducing the cholesterol and body weight where medoroga prevails. Further more, Kutaki has been recommended in the Ayurvedic texts to be used in Medoroga in high doses. At the same time, it has also been comprehended amongst the Lekhaniya gana in Charaka Samhita, which further confirms the actions of Kutaki in cases of Medoroga (corpulency/obesity).

A Double Blind Clinical Trial with Ayush-55—An Ayurvedic Compound Preparation in Obese Cases—K. Kuppurajan et al (*JRAS*: 1:2:1980)

Summary

The results of a double blind clinical trial with Ayush-55 an indigenous compound preparation in obese patients are reported. Ayush-55 caused a significant decreases in Erythrocyte sedimentation rate and lowered both the systolic and diastolic blood pressure in obese patients. There was no change in the body weight or in the levels of blood lipids. There was also no toxicity or side effect during the course of the treatment. Though this did not prove to be an ideal anti-obesity drug, but it has shown good therapeutic utility in the treatment of conditions like arthritis with high ESR and BP to which obese are commonly prone.

The compound preparation Arogyavardhini has been clinically studied in obesity and was found to exert beneficial effect in obese cases (N.S. Tewari and Jain (1979, Abstracts of drug potentials in Indian Medicinal Plants). Recently a double blind clinical trial with this preparation has shown that the drug improved the liver function appreciably in acute viral hepatitis. (A.B. Vaidya, 1980:I: J.M.R). Ayush-55 is a modified formulation of Arogyavardhini and contains Triphala, Shilajatu, Guggulu, Chitrakmula, and Tikta apart from mercury, sulphur and oxides of iron and mica. Ayush-55 was supplied by Regional Research Institute, Calcutta in the form of tablet of 500 mg each. The report presents the results of the effect of a double blind clinical trial with Ayush-55 in cases of obesity.

Composition of Ayush-55 Drug

Purified mercury 1 part; Purified Sulphur 1 part; Lauha Bhasma 1 part; Abrak Bhasma 1 part; Triphala 6 parts (each 2 parts); Shilajatu 3 parts; Guggulu 5 parts; Chitrakmula 4 parts; Katuki-22 parts; Processed in Nimba swarasa.

The patients were randomised and Ayush-55 was administered in doses of 3 gm/day (2 capsules thrice daily). Similar colour capsules containing starch powder served as the control for this Study. Total of 15 patients were included initially in the study of which 13 patients completed the trial. After the inital treatment for 3 months with either the placebo or the drug, the patients were put on crossover treatment respectively for another three months with an interval of 15 days in between. They were advised to take normal food and were followed up every fortnight for the entire period of treatment.

Results and Discussion

It is clear from the studies that Ayush-55 caused a significant decrease in systolic and diastolic blood pressure. There was no change in the body weight or in any of the body measurements.

It also caused a significant decrease in ESR. There was a slight reduction in SGPT and total lipids during the drug treatment. The other biochemical parametres (Bl. sugar, Bl. urea, SGOT, Thymol turbidity, Alkaline phosphatase, Total proteins, Haemoglobin), did not show any variation during the drug treatment.

The results indicated that the drug Ayush-55 was free from any toxicity or side effects at the dose tries in this study. Though there was a slight reduction in the level of total lipids, the drug did not produce appreciable reduction in body weight. As such this could not be considered as an ideal anti-obesity drug. However, the significant reduction in ESR as well as systolic and diastolic blood pressure observed in the patients during drug treatment in contrast with placebo treatment indicated its utility as anti-inflammatory and hypotensive drug. This can be attributed to either the properties of the constituents of the preparation or of the combined action of all the drugs of this compound. The oleoresin and steroidal fraction of Guggulu as well as the crude Guggulu which is one of the constituents of Ayush-55 are knwon to exhibit marked anti-inflammatory and anti-arthritic properties. They are also known to prolong coagulation time and prothrobin time. The observed reduction in ESR may be attributed to this property of Guggulu.

The standard line of treatment of hypertension includes Arogyavardhini compound whose modification is Ayush-55. Here the mode of action of it may be through vasodilation thereby facilitating greater peripheral circulation. V.K. Sharma et al have observed that Arogyavardhini when administered at a dose of 720 mg/day for 2 to 3 weeks reduced cholesterol and ESR levels in obese cases. The drug also increased the blood clotting time.

The drug Ayush-55 is Arogyavardhini compound slightly modified by substituting Tamrabhasma with Guggulu. Tamrabhasma itself is recognised as lekhna drug. Since much light has been thrown in the recent years about the role of trace elements in the blood on general metabolism, it was considered worthwhile to study of the effect of Arogyavardhini with the addition of Guggulu.

The obese cases who were included in this study did not have abnormal lipid values. In hyperlipidaemic and hypercholesterolaemic patients the effect of Ayush-55 is to be studied separately. Since in such cases, also the Tamrabhasma can play a useful role it is proposed to study the effect of Ayush-55 with the addition of Tamrabhasma in obesity as well as in lipid disorders. As far as the present study is concerned only it be said that it is a good drug in the treatment of conditions like arthritis and hypertension in general and in particular obese patients.

REFERENCES

1. Tewari, N.S., Jain P.C., A Clinical Evaluation of Arogyavardhini as a Hypocholesteraemic Agent with Special Reference to Obesity/Corpulence, *JRAS*:1:1:1980.
2. Kuppurajan K, et al; A Double Blind Clinical Trial with Ayush-55—An Ayurvedic Compound Preparation in Obese Cases., *JRAS*:1:2:1980.
3. Kotiyal J.P., Singh D.S., Bisht D.B., Study of Hypolipidaemic Effect of Commiphora Mukul (Gum Guggulu) Fraction 'A' in Obesity: *JRAS*:1:3:1980.
4. Mrs. S. Ghai.; C.M. Ghai, Obesity and Its Management in Ayurveda, *JNIMA*: XXXV : 8 : 1993.
5. Salutgi S.B., Phadanik B.S., Effect of an Indigenous Drug "Lipidsol" on the Haematology and Metabolic Profile in Goats: *Ayurveda Samachar*: 15:11:1993.
6. Nirmal B.M., Nirmal A.B., Etiopathogenesis and Principles of Management of Medoroga (Obesity)—An Ayurvedic Approach: *Ayurveda Samachar*: 15:7:1993.
7. Nirmal A.B., Nirmal B.M., Triple Management Measures in Obesity (Medaswita), *Ayurveda Samachar*: 15:12:1993.

MADHUMEHA (DIABETES MELLITUS)
(Prameha with Special Reference to Madhumeha vis-a-vis Diabetes Mellitus)

Relationship

'Prameha' is related to Mootravaha srotas. Thus obstinate urinary disorders with increased urinary flow are grouped together as Pramehas. Those with decreased quantity of urine are included separately under Mootrakricchara, Mootraghata and Ashmari.

Definition

The word 'Prameha' is derived from the root Miha-Sechane, which means excessive watering. Pra stands for excessive quantity or increased frequency (Va. Ni. 10/7).

General Considerations

Charaka has given entire description of Diabetes under one heading, 'Prameha,' whereas Sushruta has given a detailed description in 3 chapters:

1. Prameha (Diabetes in general)—20 types
2. Prameha Pidicas (Complications)—7 types
3. Madhumeha (Diabetes Mellitus)—One type.

Analysing Ayurvedic classics, we come across different typology for Prameha —

1. (a) Sahaj (Genetic)
   (b) Uttarkalaj (Acquired)
2. (a) Sthoola Pramehi (Obese diabetics)
   (b) Krisha Pramehi (Asthenic diabetics)
3. (a) Aavrittavatajanya (Due to channel obstruction)
   (b) Shuddhavatajanya (Due to aggravation of Shuddh vata)
4. (a) Swatantara (Primary or independent)
   (b) Pratantara (Secondary, as a result of other urinary disorders)

Pathogenesis (Samprapti)

Samprapti comprises of five components i.e., (Ghatakas):

Dosha, Dooshya, Adhisthana, Ama and Agni.

1. *Dosha:* Tridosha i.e. Vata, Pitta, and Kapha; vata being most predominant.
2. *Dooshya*: Generally all the dhatus are vitiated. These are:
   - (i) Bahu Abaddh Medas—Surplus and unutilized fat or adipose tissue.
   - (ii) Mamsa (Muscular tissue)
   - (iii) Kleda (intracellular and extracellular fluids of the body)
   - (iv) Shukra (semen)
   - (v) Shonita: Blood
   - (vi) Vasa (Muscle fat)
   - (vii) Majja (Marrow tissue)
   - (viii) Lasika (Fluids and Plasma)
   - (ix) Rasa (Blood Plasma)
   - (x) Ojus (Vital substances in the body, meant for resistance)

   It implies that the disease does not affect a particular organ or system of the body. It rather affects the whole body.
3. *Adhishtana*: The main Srotas involved in the disease are:
   - (i) Mootra vaha srotas
   - (ii) Medo vaha srotas

   The type of Vikriti is Atipravritti (i.e. excessive flow) and Vimargagamana (i.e. improper flow)
4. *Agni*: The main cause of Medodhatu dusthi and Medovriddhi is Mandyata of Medodhatwagni.
5. *Ama*: Dhatwagni mandyata results into the production of Ama (Ama Anna Rasa, Mala Samchaya, Dosha Dusthi).

Diagnostic Features (Nidana Mukhya Lakshana)

Common symptoms for all the pramehas is that urine is increased in quantity (polyuria) and is altered in consistency (Avil mootrata).

Clinical Manifestations

Prameha can be divided into three major categories—vataja, pittaja, and kaphaja. The varieties of kaphaja meha have the following characteristic features:

1. The urine resembling water (Udak meha).
2. The urine resembling sugarcane juice (Ikshu valika)
3. The urine having density (Sandra meha)
4. The urine having density below and transparency in the upper layer (Sandraprasad meha)
5. The urine having white colour (Shukla meha)
6. The urine containing seminal fluid (Shukra meha)
7. The urine having cold touch (Sheeta meha)
8. The urine passing out slowly (Shanair meha)
9. The urine containing slimy material like saliva (Laala meha)
10. The urine containing sand like substances (Sikta meha)

Six varieties of pittaja meha have the following characteristics as per Charaka:

1. The urine resembling the solution of alkalies (Kshara meha)
2. Urine having black colour (Kaala meha)
3. Urine having yellow colour like turmeric (Haridra meha)
4. Urine having indigo colour (Neela meha)
5. Urine having yellow colour like Manjishta (Manjishta meha) and
6. Urine having blood in it (Rakta meha).

Charaka describes four types of Vataja meha with the following characteristics:

1. Urine mixed with majja or bone-marrowlike looking (Majja meha)
2. Urine mixed with Ojas (Oja meha or Madhumeha)
3. Urine mixed with Vasa or muscle fat (Vasa meha)
4. Urine mixed with lasika or lymph (Lasika meha) or Hasti meha.

These four varieties are caused by the Apakarshana (diminution) of dhatus (C. Chi. 6/9-11).

Note: Vagbhata uses the term Sura meha for Sandra prasad meha and Pishta meha for Shukla meha and Alala meha. He has rather described Lavana meha and Fena meha.

Course of the Disease

Shleshma dosha and Medas dhatu (formed by Medoagni Mandya), possess similar nature. Thus, they combine with each other interacting with mamsa and kleda to result into the disease prameha. The disease progresses with involvement of further more doshas and more dhatus. The complications arise in the form of Prameha pidicas, with the disease progression. Vata aggravation predominated and Madhumeha result which is difficult to cure. (A.H. Ni. 10/20). In modern parlance, it may be explained as the potential diabetics or stress diabetic change to frank or uncontrolled diabetes, if uncared for. It has also been noticed that N.I.D.D.M. (Noninsulin Dependent Diabetes Mellitus) sometimes changes to I.D.D.M. (Insulin Dependent Diabetes Mellitus) with progression of the disease.

Diagnosis

Turbid urine in excessive quantity has been considered as a chief diagnostic feature of Prameha. Hyperglycemia and glycosuria are important evidences to suggest diabetes mellitus with modern viewpoint, although, a glucose tolerance test is done for confirmation. Clinical features as illustrated earlier conform different types of pramehas. Sushruta considers sweetish taste of urine as prodromal symptom of prameha. Charaka describes the same by attraction of ants to the urine. Although it seems that these should be the diagnostic features instead of prodromal symptoms for the disease (C. Chi. 6/14).

Differential Diagnosis

Prameha and Madhumeha are to be differentiated from each other. Prameha is a collection of polyuric states of the body. It is of 20 different types. Madhumeha is its specific type, caused by vatika predominance. Madhumeha has poor prognosis. Urinary alteration in some types of pramehas may be similar to the urinary changes in Raktapitta. Differentiation is done with the help of premonitory symptoms (C.Chi. 6/54).

Complications (Upadravas)

Diabetes mellitus is known to give rise to complications like—early cataract, neuropathy, angiopathy, retinopathy, foot ulcer, and recurrent infections. However, complications of prameha as enumerated by Charaka are thirst, diarrhoea, fever, burning sensation, weakness, anorexia, and indigestion (C. Ni. 4/48). For Vataja, Pittaja, and Kaphaja mehas, Sushruta and Vaghbhata describe the complications like Aruci, vomiting, cough, peenas, fever, thirst, acidity, diarrhoea, insomnia, numbness, shivering, colic pain, and constipation (A.H.Ni. 1/22-24). In some chronic stages carbuncles which putrify the muscle tissues like Alaji and Vidradhi appear. A brief description of Prameha pidicas (Diabetic carbuncles) follows:

Prameha Pidicas (Diabetic Carbuncles)

Charaka has described 7 types of Pidicas—Alaji, Sharavika, Kacchhapika, Jalani, Sarshapi, Vinata, and Vidradhi (C.Su. 17/83-89). Apart from these seven, Vagbhata describes 3 more varieties—Masoorika, Putrini, and Vidarika (A.H.Ni. 10/25, 26). Vidradhi is of two types—Bahya and Abhyantara. Similar to Vagbhata, Sushruta also describes ten pidicas. Sharavika, Kacchapika, and Jalani have poor prognosis as per Charaka. The pidicas thus described may in turn give rise to complications like—thirst, hiccough, unconsciousness (may be due to toxaemia), fever (due to infection and inflammation) etc. (C.Ch. Su. 17/111).

Pidica Without Prameha ?—A question arises here, whether, Pidica may occur without prameha or not. Charaka clarifies this by stating that Pidica may occur due to vitiation of Medas, even without existence of Prameha (C. Su. 17/104).

Management (Chikitsa)

Charaka advocates Samshodhana therapy for obese and strong diabetics. It aims at reducing the kapha aggravating diet (i.e. carbohydrate diet) apart from decreasing the total quantity of diet (i.e. cutting calorie overload). Weak and emaciated patients should be given Bramghana therapy (to improve nourishment). Yavagu (Barley) is considered an important diet for prameha. Some effective antidiabetic formulations have been mentioned in the name of Pramehaghna yogas in Ayurvedic classics, though they have mild to moderate effect clinically. Some of them are:

A decoction constituted of Daruhaldi, Devadaru, Amla, Harad, Baheda and Nagarmotha in equal quantities helps treating prameha.

Similarly, fresh Amla juice taken with honey and haldi gives good result. Some specific formulations mentioned by Charaka for Kaphaja Pramehas are:

- Harad, Kayafar, Nagarmotha, and Pathani lodhra (Decoction)
- Haldi, Daruhaldi, Tagar and Vidanga (decoction)
- Lodhrasava/Madhawasava
- Dantyasava
- Bhallatakasava etc.

For Pittaja Pramehas

- Khasa, Lodhra, Arjuna, Lala chandana (decoction)
- Khasa, Nagarmotha, Amla, Bahera (decoction)
- Neema, Arjuna, Amla, Haldi, Neelkamal (decoction) etc.

For Vataja pramehas

- Trikantakadi Sneha
- Fala Trikadi Kwatha etc.

Some drugs and food products have been researched for their hypoglycemic and antidiabetic activities with favourable results. Few of them are enlisted here:

Legumes, blackgrams (Phaseolus mungo), Melia azadirachta, Allium cepa, Allium sativum, Acacia catechu, Albizzia lebbeck, Cassia auriculata, Cyamopsis tetragonoloba, Dietary fibres, Dolichos biflorus, Eugenia jambolana, Glycine soja, Jasad Bhasma, Mucuna pruriens, Ocimum sanctum, Tinosporia cordifolia, Tribhang shila, Trichosanthes dioica, Vinca rosea, Vitamin C etc.

Prognosis (Sadhya-Asadhyata)

Prameha is included under the eight Maharogas and is thus difficult to be treated in general. Doshik specification reveals that kaphaj pramehas are less typical; Paittika pramehas are more typical and Vataja pramehas are most typical with treatment point of view, i.e. Vataja pramehas are Asadhya. Even, modern medicine has no permanent remedy for the disease diabetes. Drugs may be used to decrease glucose absorption, to increase serum insulin levels or to enhance peripheral utilisation of glucose; thus, the relief so obtained is temporary.

Clinical Reports (Anubhoot Prayoga)

Experimental Studies

Many preliminary experimental studies have been conducted on albino rats, rabbits, and dogs to find out the hypoglycaemic antidiabetic activities of certain drugs. Animals are injected with Alloxan or Streptozotocin to produce diabetes experimentally. Few examples are cited here:

Swerchirin (50mg/kg/bodyweight/per oral) isolated from hexane fraction of Swertia chirayata lowered blood sugar levels in streptozotocin treated hyperglycaemic rats, only in milder diabetics (Saxena et al 1991).

Powedered whole seed of Leucaena leucocephala when fed to hyperglycaemic (alloxanised) albino rats, lowered blood sugar levels (Singhal et al 1982).

Leguminous seeds of Acacia catechu, Acacia suma and Albizzia adoratissima were found to lower blood sugar levels in normoglycemic albino rats (Singh et al 1976).

Studies on the effect of a hypoglycaemic principle from Allium cepa Linn were made. It was found effective in alloxan induced diabetics (Augusti 1973).

Clinical Experiences

Clinically, Jambu (Eugenia jambolana) seed powder was found effective in mild to moderate diabetics. The clinical trials were conducted on patients in S.S. Hospital, Banaras Hindu University. In other works, Pterocarpus marsupium

(Vijay sara) was found effective in diabetes (mild to moderate). Nimb oil reduces blood sugar levels in diabetic patients clinically (Nimbola-key Pharma). Leguminous diet and a diet containing Vitamin C helps lowering blood sugar levels. The author found Bilwa (Aegle marmelos) effective in 50 patients of N.I.D.D.M. in a preliminary research carried out at S.S. Hospital Varanasi. The effect is mild to moderate. These drugs may be used in the inital stages of N.I.D.D.M. with dietary precautions. In later stages, they may be used as an adjuvant to therapy to decrease the dose of modern medicine and to give a better sense of well-being.

REFERENCES

1. Augusti K.T. Studies on the Effect of a Hypoglycaemic Principle from Allium Cepa Linn., IJMR.J.61,7, July 1973.
2. Bharti A. Clinical Study on Madhumeha vis-a-vis Diabetes Mellitus and Its Treatment with Bilwa (Aegle marmelos), M.D., Thesis, 1991.
3. Singh K.N., Mittal R.K., and Barthwal K.C., Hypoglycaemic Activity of Acacia catechu, Acacia suma and Albizzia odoratissima Seed Diet in Normal Albion Rats. X, IJMR. 1976.
4. Saxena A.M., Bajpai M.B., and Mukherjee S.K., Swerchirin Induced Blood Sugar Lowering of Streptozotocin—Treated Hyperglycaemic Rats., Ind. Jl.Exp. Biology. July, 1991.
5. Singhal P.C., Gupta R.K., Singh J.B., and Joshi L.D., Preliminary Studies on Hypoglycaemic and Hypocholesterolaemic Activities of Leucaena leucocephala (Lam) de wit.-Ind. Jl. MEd. Res.76. December 1982.

Sanskrit References

1. Samanyam lakshanam tesham prabhootavila mootrata ... Va.Ni.10/7.
2. Kalenupekshita sarva yadyanti madhumehatam...A.H.Ni. 10/20.
3. Mootre abhidhavanti pipalikashcha ... C. Ci. 6/14.
4. Haridra varna rudhiram ca mootram ...
   ... raktasya pittasya hi sa prakopah ..... C. Ci. 6/54.
5. Upadravastu khalu pramchinam ......
   .... tat prasangat bhavanti .... C. Ni.4/48.
6. Sharavika kachhapika jalini .... vinatmata. ... C. Su. 17/83-89.
7. Trita shwasa mamsa sankatha.....
   ....pidicanamupadravah. .....C .Su. 17/111.
8. Vina prameha ayeta jayante dushta medasah ....C. Su. 17/104
9. Sapoorvaroopa .... yadi na pradushtam .... C. Ci. 6/56.

Terminology

Prameha—Urinary disorders with increased quantity or turbidity.
Madhumeha—Diabetes mellitus
Mootrakricchara—Dysuria
Mootraghata—Oliguria/Anuria.
Ashmari—Stone (lithiasis) of urinary tract.
Prameha pidica—Diabetic carbuncle.
Sahaja—Genetic
Uttarakalaj—Acquired
Sthoola—Obese
Krisha—Asthenic.

MADHUMEHA

Historically speaking Madhumeha or Diabetes mellitus is known from Vedic times. Even in Puranas and Kavyas the description of Madhumeha and its treatment are given. In *Raghuvansa,* which is considered to be one of the best epic (Mahakavya), an indirect narration of Madhumeha is found. It seems to be metaphor (Rupak). The cause and treatment of sterility of king Dilip, the great grandfather of Lord Rama, is suggestive of the treatment of Diabetes mellitus. The story runs like this. "The king Dilip had no issue. So he consulted his preceptor Vasistha Maharshi. Maharshi said that you have forgotten to bow down and serve the cow Kamadhenu and due to the curse of Kamadhenu you have got no issue. So he advised to start the Seva (service) of the cow. Thereupon king Dilip whole-heartedly serves the cow and in the end due to the blessings of the cow Kamadhenu, king Dilip gets a son through Queen Sudeshna." Here also a description of Devdaru is given. According to the above description the following facts can be inferred:

(i) In old times, everybody was required to serve cows. That is why a cow is called Kamadhenu i.e. cow is the source of health, wealth and prosperity. (ii) The whole-hearted service of the cow is the preventive and curative treatment of certain metabolic disorders like Madhumeha. (iii) The treatment of Madhumeha is possible with Devdaru i.e. Sedarus Deodara.

Compare this treatment with Sushruta's treatment of Madhumeha. Sushruta says—

महाधनो वा श्यामकनीवार वृत्तिरामलककपित्थतिन्दुकाश्मत्तक फलाहारो मृगै: सह वसेत्, तन्मूत्रशकृभक्ष: सततमनुव्रजेद्गा:। (सु. चि. ११-१२)

A religious ceremony viz. 'Gotrivit' or 'Gotrat' is being performed in the beginning of monsoon i.e. in the month of Ashadha. The lady, who wants Saubhagya i.e. long life of her husband, performs this ceremony. She feeds a cow about 1 kg. of Yava (barley) and the barleys which comes out with the faeces of the cow are collected. They are then thoroughly washed. These barleys are to be eaten by the lady for 3 days. This religious ceremony resembles the treatment of 'Prameha' according to Charaka. Charaka says—

खराश्वगोहंसपृवद्भृतानां तथा यवानां विविधाश्च भक्ष्या:। (च. चि. ६-२४)

Yava are to be given for eating to animals like donkey, horse, cow, bear etc., and are to be collected from their faecal matter. They are to be consumed in the form of different types of food.

From the above, it may very easily be inferred that our Acharyas have combined religion with Ayurveda and our religious ceremonies are meant for curative and preventive treatment of certain diseases.

Classification of Madhumeha (Diabetes Mellitus)

Madhumeha is classified by the Acharyas in different ways as under:

I. सहज (Congenital or Juvenile)

II. स्थूलप्रमेही (Obese Diabetic), कृशप्रमेही (Asthenic type)

III. आवृतवातजन्य (Due to obstruction of channels), शुद्धवातजन्य (Due to Shuddha Vata)

IV. स्वतंत्र (Independent), परतंत्र (As a result of other urinary disorders)

The above classification is based on the classification done by Maharshi Charaka. If required, other classifications can also be made. But in my opinion the above classification is a complete one in all respects.

The Samprapti of Madhumeha

The *Samprapti* comprises of five components i.e. घटक. They are—Dosha, Dushya, Srotas, Ama and Agni. In Madhumeha the components of pathogenesis are as under:

(i) Dosha-Tridosha i.e. Vata, Pitta, Kapha, Vata being most predominant. Vata may be provoked by obstruction (आवृतवात) or may be independently provoked (शुद्धवात).

(ii) Dushya i.e. Dhatus (Tissues). Generally all the Dhatus are vitiated in Madhumeha. Main Dhatus are (a) बहुअबदूधमेदस् (Surplus and unutilised fat or adipose tissue), (b) मांस (Muscular tissue), (c) क्लेद (Fluids of the body i.e. intracellular and extra-cellular fluids), (d) शुक्र (Semen), (e) शोणित (Blood), (f) वसा (Muscle fat), (g) मज्जा (Marrow tissue), (h) लसिका (Fluids & Plasma), (i) रस (Blood Plasma), (j) ओजस (Vital substance or the Biochemical substances in the body meant for resistance or immunity).

In the above, it is clear that all the body tissues are vitiated in Madhumeha i.e. Diabetes mellitus. This is a disease in which any of the tissues or organs may be damaged. The disease is not localized in any one organ of the body but may vitiate any of the important organs.

Another important thing to be marked in the above description is that Ayurveda gives maximum importance to the derangement of fat metabolism (बहु अबदूधमेदस्, वसा, मज्जा etc.) while the modern science considers this disease to be mainly due to the derangement of carbohydrate metabolism.

In diabetes mellitus not only the fat metabolism is disturbed but the fluid balance is also disturbed as suggested by the derangement of क्लेद-लसिका-रस etc.

The muscles and blood are also damaged as can be seen from the production of dermatitis, boils, carbuncles i.e. (प्रमेह पिड़का). Thus Prameha manifests its effects in any part or tissue of the body.

Srotas

The main Srotas i.e. system involved is मूत्रवहस्रोतस and मेदोवहस्रोतस, though other Srotas are not exempt. The type of pathological changes (विकृति) of the Srotas may be Atipravriti (excessive flow) and विमार्गगमन (extravasation or improper flow).

Agni

The main Agni involved in this disease is Dhatvagnimandya i.e. less functioning of hormones mainly मेदोधात्वग्नि. Here a short description regarding Agni and Ama is necessary. Agnis though many in the body, are classified as (1) Jatharagni, (2) Dhatwagnies, and (3) Bhutagnies. Thus totally there are 13 Agnies in the body. They are useful for digestion, transformation, assimilation and utilisation of the nutrient material. By this description of Agnis, it may very well be said that all the enzymes, hormones are to be put under the heading of Agni. These Agnies are vitiated in 3 ways i.e. excessive functioning (तीक्ष्णाग्नि), under functioning (मन्दाग्नि) or erratic functioning (विषमाग्नि). In hyperfunctioning of Agni (तीक्ष्णाग्नि) the body tissues are burnt off, and in hypo-functioning the nutrient material is not utilized or transformed properly, resulting thereby in accumulation (दोषसंचय or आम).

In Prameha मन्दाग्नि at the level of Dhatwagni takes place.

Ama

As narrated above Dhatwagni Mandya results in the production of Ama. Ama is mainly of 3 types (1) आम अन्न रस i.e. Chyle, (2) मलसंचय i.e. accumulation of undigested nutrient material, and (3) प्रथमदोष दुष्टि i.e the sudden and insidious beginning of vitiated Dosha. In diabetes mellitus the result of आम is accumulation of waste matter in the body, that is why Acharyas have mentioned दन्तादीनां मलाढ्यत्वं (collection of sordes on tongue and on other parts of the body like ear, teeth, tongue, etc.) and विक्कणता (stickiness on the skin and mucous membrane) as the Poorvarupas (prodromals) of Praméha.

Thus *Prameha* is a disease produced due to आम resulting in the vitiation of any of the *Dhatus* (Tissues) mainly *Medas* (fat). *Kleda* (fluids of the body) and *Mamsa* (muscular tissues). It also vitiates blood and its components and results in decreased immunity of resistance i.e. *Ojas-Kshaya.*

The pathogenesis of *Prameha* is general and Madhumeha runs as under (1) Firstly, *Shlesma-Dusti* is the primary factor in the production of *Prameha. Dusta* (vitiated) Shleshma circulates in the body. The *Dhatus* in the body are loose i.e. not compact i.e. unutilised (2) Secondly, Meda (fat or adipose tissue) may be in excess, unbound and unutilised.

The *Shleshma* combines with this type of *Medas* because both *Meda* and *Shleshma possess* similar properties. The combination of vitiated *Shleshma* with the Medas produces vitiation of *Medas.*

(3) Thirdly both the vitiated *Medas* and *Shleshma* come in contact with *Mamsa Dhatu* (Muscular tissues) and also with *Kleda* (fluids) in the body; and vitiate them. (4) If Mamsa is vitiated, dermatitis and other skin diseases like *Prameha Peedaka* (carbuncles, boils, ringworm etc.) are produced and (5) if Kleda is vitiated, urine quantity is increased and the *Dhatus* also flow out with urine, (6) In the long run the *Mutravaha Srotas* (Nephrons and tubules) are obstructed (स्रोतोरोध) and Diabetic kidney disorder (nephritis) takes place.

From the above pathogenesis it is seen that (1) Prameha is not the disease of only urinary tract. There is derangement of fat metabolism. That fat is surplus and unutilised. So it is necessary to assess at what level of the fat metabolism there is disturbance. Thirdly the *Kleda* i.e. fluid balance in the body is disturbed. Some components in the fluids are either excess or diminished so that they are either accumulated in the body or thrown out of the body with urine e.g. sugar is in excess in the blood and though necessary as fuel during exercise and work, is excreted through urine. Thus the body cannot resist exercise, work or infection. Thus the working capacity is diminished.

The modern science believes that carbohydrate metabolism is primarily deranged in diabetes mellitus, while Ayurveda believes the disease primarily to be due to the disturbance in the fat metabolism. The question is open for further research. Later on, the protein metabolism is also disturbed. Thus it is a chronic metabolic disorder in which all the three metabolisms i.e. carbohydrate, fat and protein metabolism are disturbed. It is possible that other metabolisms like calcium, iron etc. may also be disturbed. So the disease is considered to be Maha-Vyadhi (difficult to cure or incurable). Thus the disease *Madhumeha* is produced due to *Dhatu-Agni-Mandya* i.e. decreased functioning of the Dhatu-Agni i.e. Metabolism.

Prodromal Symptoms

There are many premonitory symptoms as the disease is a chronic one. They are: sweet taste, excessive thirst and appetite, dryness in the mouth and throat, excessive accumulation of waste matter in the channels (स्रोतस) thereby producing stickiness in the skin, hairs are also sticking to feather (केशानां जटीलीभाव:). There is lethargy (आलस्य), drowsiness (तन्द्रा) or excessive sleep: either burning (दाह) or hyposensitiveness (सुप्तता) in the limbs, hands and feet: a typical odour in the urine and the urine becomes sweet so that the ants are attracted to the urine. These symptoms, though considered to be the premonitory symptoms (पूर्वरूप) are symptoms which attract the attention of the patient to consult a doctor, who decides whether the patient is suffering from Diabetes or not. It may be said that in fact, Diabetes mellitus does not manifest any of the symptoms directly related to blood or urine, but it produces symptoms other than the symptoms of the urinary tract. Many a times Diabetes mellitus is diagnosed accidently. The patient, well built in body, consults a physician, with the complaints of debility or dermatitis or progressive myopia and is diagnosed as a patient of diabetes mellitus. The urine colour, consistency are generally normal and show no abnormality by eye observation. Thus the premonitoy symptoms are really the symptoms of *Madhumeha.*

Signs and Symptoms

The urine is kashaya (astringent) and sweet in taste, white in colour resembling *Madhu. Madhu* has 2 meanings (1) Honey (2) Alcohol. Honey is sweet and astringent in taste, yellow or white in colour and has a typical odour. The same is the colour, taste of alcohol. Moreover in alcohol there is fermentation. So also it is possible that the diabetic urine may undergo fermentation on preserving for a night or two.

Complications (उपद्रव)

Diabetes mellitus is a disease of deranged metabolism and the Ojas (resistance power) undergoes Kshaya i.e. it lowers the *vitality.* Thus the patient is susceptible to infection very easily and once there is infection, it is difficult to cure. Sushruta, while describing the curability or otherwise of Vrana (uclers) has said that the Vrana in a diabetic patient is very difficult to cure.

कुष्ठिनां विषजुष्टानां शोषिणां मधुमेहिनाम् ।
व्रणाः कृच्छ्रेण रुह्यन्ति येषां चापि व्रणे व्रणाः॥

Prameha Pidaka are example of secondary infections. They are also *Krichra-Sadhya* or difficult to cure (असाध्य).

Due to the disturbance of metabolism, no organ is exempt from undergoing *Vikriti* (pathological change). Thus arteries undergo atherosclerosis; Heart undergo hypertrophy and enlargement. There is a possibility of damage in nervous system resulting in दाह (neuritis) or पक्षवध (Hemiplegia). The मूत्रवहस्रोतस are also damaged resulting in Diabetic nephritis.

Heart may be enlarged resulting in congestive cardiac failure. Thus any of the body organs may be damaged.

Another grave complication is संन्यास (coma). When accumulation of *Ama Dosha* takes place in blood and disturbs the brain, specially the sensory centres of the brain मूर्च्छा (unconsciousness) and संन्यास (coma) takes place. In fact मद, मूर्च्छा and संन्यास are the three stages of loosing consciousness. The first stage is मद in which the patient gets giddiness, the second stages is मूर्च्छा in which the patient gradually loses consciousness and in the third stage the patient passes into coma i.e. संन्यास. This is due to the accumulation of ketone bodie, a side product of deranged fat and protein metabolism which may be compared with *Ama-Dosha* or *Mala Sanchaya.*

Thus diabeties mellitus is a disease of deranged metabolism and leads to any of the grave complications.

Treatment (चिकित्सासूत्र)

The principles of treatment in a diabetic patient may be classified as under:

1. There are two types of diabetics (1) स्थूलप्रमेही (Obese) (2) कृशप्रमेही (asthetic type). In स्थूल (obese) the treatment must be mainly based on proper utilisation of excess fat i.e. he should be given (i) शोधनं (purificatory process), (ii) अपतर्पण reduction in body weight by way of diet control or drugs). व्यायाम (exercise) etc.

2. In the कृशप्रमेही asthenic type, the treatment should be mainly based on the line of increasing stamina and vitality by way of tonics (बृंहण) diet, drugs etc. The patient should never be given excessive *Langhana* or *Apatarpana* i.e. he should not be starved.

3. The patient, whether obese or Asthenic, suffers from the complications like *Gulma, Kshaya* (Tuberculosis), pain in abdomen etc. if he is given excessive *Apatarpana* (Langhan or starvation etc.) He should always be given some food. A diabetic and an obese person generally suffers from excessive appetite and thirst and so some type of nutrition should always be given to them. I have come across a patient, who is a Juvenile diabetic, he was kept on insulin and other modern hypoglycemic drugs. He suddenly started discomfort in abdomen with gas etc., then severe pain in abdomen. Next day he got vomiting.

The vomit contained the same food which was ingested the previous day i.e. 14 hours before. He was admitted in Irwin Hospital but no diagnosis could be done; then he consulted me. I diagnosed the case as *Gulma* and *Alasaka* i.e. Pyloric spasm due to insulin. Then I stopped all hypoglycemic drugs and kept him only on garlic. The patient then never suffered from pain and his blood sugar had been normal gradually. He is having perfect health now and is free from diabetes.

The following are the articles of food which can be given to the diabetic:

(i) *Cereals:* Yava (Barley) are the best. Different preparations of food, prepared from Barley can be given e.g. *Mantha, Odana, Apupa, Bread, Roti* etc. This is the subject of pharmaceutics and foodstuffs. So the method of preparations of barley is not dealt with here. Wheat can also be given.

Rice: This is controversial. Ayurveda prescribes old rice (पुराणशाली) as one of the cereals, which can be prescribed to the diabetic patients. While according to the modern science Rice due to starch and carbohydrate, are considered to be increasing diabetes and obesity.

I would like to draw here the attention and also ask the scientists working in the field of nutrition, the percentage of diabetics and obese persons staying in the area, where the people are mainly rice eaters e.g. Bengal, Assam, Bihar, Tamil Nadu, Kerala and other South Indian provinces and compare with the provinces where rice is either rarely taken or not taken e.g. Punjab, Rajasthan etc. A survey should be done in this field also. So far as I know, the percentage of obesity is much less in South Indian States and Eastern States as compared with Rajasthan, Punjab and some parts of UP where Rice is rarely taken. This proves that old rice can be prescribed to the diabetics and the modern concept requires to be reassessed.

Pulses: *Mung* (green grams), Chanaka (Bengal grams), *Matha, Adhaki* etc. can be taken.

Vegetables: All types of bitter vegetables (तिक्तशाक) e.g. Karela, Methi etc. should be given.

Adjuvants: Oils—best is Mustard oil (सर्वपतैल). The preparations of food are many and so they are not mentioned here. But according to Ayurveda one should start with light diet (लघु भक्ष्य) or (लघु आहार) and then gradually increase the quantity of food. It is a rule that one should keep complete attention on the conditions of *Agni* i.e. digestion. Diabetes, being a disease of deranged metabolism, special attention should be kept on the condition of digestion and metabolism.

As previously said in the historical aspect, *Yava* (Barley) collected from the faeces of cow are the best as food. They are pre-digested and contain some of the enzymes of the cows and other beasts and might be helping in substituting emzymes or might produce some enzymes which may be necessary for proper metabolic functions. Other preparations of Barley can also be prescribed.

Exercise: Hard exercises are prescribed for diabetics and obese persons. This is meant for proper utilisation of the fat and consumes the glucose and fat in the body. The methods can be changed in the present times according to the habitat (देश) and time (काल). But the exercises are very necessary.

Some of the hard, productive exercises prescribed by Sushruta are as under:

(1) Exercises (व्यायाम) (2) Fighting (नियुद्ध) (3) Games (क्रीडा) (4) To ride an elephant, horse etc. and walking (गजचर्या, तुरगचर्या, रथचर्या, पादचर्या).

Over and above the above mentioned heavy exercises, there are other exercises according to the financial position and also according to the community. There are (i) for poor class, the diabetic should walk about 100 miles, bare footed, not staying more than one night in the same place, should eat only the things available by begging and keeping restraint on his sense organs (मुनिः इव संयतात्मा).

(ii) For rich diabetics—they should eat only *Shyamaka*, Kodrava etc., *Amalaka, Kapitha* etc. and reside with the cattle. The food stuff for them should be *Ruksha* (free from fat) or they may stay with the cows and eat the above with the urine and faeces of the cow. Compare this with the metaphor in Raghuvamsha.

(iii) For others—either farming or digging a well etc.

From the above, it will be seen that the exercises prescribed by the Acharyas are very hard and productive. In short for diabetics exercise serves the purposes of (1) utilising the fat and (2) metabolising sugar, fat and carbohydrates and also proteins.

In the present day civilisation, when these types of exercises are not possible, one should regularly play some out-door games, do some productive labour, or the best is different types of yogic exercises.

Yoga now-a-days has attracted the attention of Western people. The greatest drawback in our country is that we cannot appreciate the Indian things, customs or literature in the beginning but we are ready to accept, when we hear the same from the Western countries. In Yoga also the same thing has happened. When our Acharyas and Yogies propagated Yoga in America and other countries, they were accepted there and they did research work. But our Indian research workers were not only criticising the Yoga but they discarded Yoga to be humbug and propagated Yoga as only for Yogies and did not accept it as a scientific method. But when the same Yoga was scientifically studied in the Western countries, our research scholars now-a-days are working on Yoga even in India.

Yoga improves all sorts of metabolism in the body. So diabetics should perform different types of Yoga. Yoga will definitely help in diabetes mellitus.

Drugs: As regards drugs, there are so many drugs and formulations but the main drugs are either bitter (तिक्त) or astringent (कषाय) in taste. They improve the fat and carbohydrate metabolism. Some of the medicines are given below:

Kwatha (decoction) 1. *Darvi*, Surahwa, Trifala, Musta. 2. Trifala, Daruhaldi, Vishala, Musta.

The above two decoctions are different—only in one drug. The first contains Surahwa (Deodaru) and the second contains Vishala. Vishala is drastic purgative and so can be used in constipated persons.

The author of this paper has assessed the hypoglycemic action of the above two decoctions. The effect is 1. Hypoglycemic and 2. long lasting. About 20 cases of Diabetes mellitus were studied. Their blood sugar was estimated, G.T.T. done and the results were found to be promising. The aricle has been published in 'Ayu' the authentic quarterly of Gujarat Ayurveda University.

As mentioned above, garlic is also worth trying. One of my students, who was accidently diagnosed as severe diabetic suffered from *Gulma* and *Alasaka* (Pyloric spasm) as a result of improper use of Insulin and other modern oral hypoglycemic drugs, was given only garlic paste (लशुनकल्क) with 10 ml. of grount nut oil. All modern antidiabetic drugs were stopped. The blood sugar level gradually decreased and at present he is having normal blood sugar, though he eats everything including rice. The author then tried garlic in other patients also. All of them have got reduction in blood sugar level. This suggests that garlic might be producing insulin and other hormones. According to Ayurveda, garlic is digestive, tonic, bactericidal, wormicide and tonic.

It may be pointed out here that *Lasuna* (garlic) has not been mentioned as a remedy for diabetes mellitus or *prameha*. It is possible that the hypoglycemic action of *Lasuna* might be due to its action on digestion and metabolism. Ayurveda, as already narrated previously believes diabetes mellitus as a disease of *Mandagni* at *Dhatwagni* level i.e. a disease of deranged metabolism. *Lasuna* might have acted on the *Agni*. There is a vast scope for research on this drug also.

The other medicines are all the bitter drugs and diet e.g. Guduchi (Tinospora cordifolia), Methi, Karvellaka etc. The juice of all these drugs can be used as hypoglycemic. It is possible that the action may not be as quick as insulin or other modern hypoglycemic drugs. But they definitely act on diabetes.

Rasayana

Rasayana (Rejuvenators) drugs are very useful in all diseases, specially in chronic diseases. Rasayana means that line of treatment which maintains 1. the flow of Rasa *Dhatu* (nutrient material) properly, 2. maintains good health, 3. delays old age, 4. stops decay and degeneration and 5. prevents and cures diseases. There are so many varieties of Rasayana drugs e.g. some are *Karshana Rasayanas* (for obese persons), some are *Brihana* (for lean and thin persons for increasing weight), some are digestives e.g. Pippali (long pepper) etc., some are acting on maintaining cholesterol at normal level e.g. Guggulu. In short, *Rasayana* therapy is meant for maintaining normal biochemical values and production of hormones necessary for maintenance of good health. Here it is necessary to decide which type of *Rasayana* may be useful for diabetics. The drug of choice is 1. Shilajatu 2. Guggulu and 3. Haritaki (myrobalans) and Amalaki. Shilajatu is useful in this disease. For obese persons Guggulu may also be used as Guggulu has been proved as hypocholesteremic drug.

Thus for the treatment of Diabetes Mellitus, *Ahara* (diet), *Achara* (daily regimen), *Vyayama* (exercise), Drugs (hypoglycemic drugs), *Rasayana* therapy (Rejuvenation therapy) may be properly prescribed for long time. I am sure that by the prolonged use of the above treatment, the patient will not only be free from Diabetes Mellitus but can live a long (दीर्घजीवितीय) life, healthy (सुखायु) and will be useful to the society (हितायु).

Diagnosis of 20 Sub-Types of Prameha Based on Physical and Chemical Examination of Urine in Proved Cases of Diabetes Mellitus

The paper attempts at providing scope for comparing the twenty varieties of Prameha with Diabetes mellitus. The parameters like fasting blood sugar, body weight etc. were utilised in this regard. It is, however, felt that further study on a large population may possibly provide scope and basis to correlate.

Introduction

There has been a view among some scholars that 20 types of Prameha are different forms of urinary/metabolic disorders, for example *Udakameha* diabetes insipidus, *Sandrameha* as Chyluria, Sukrameha as Spermatorrhoea, *Sikatamha*as *Lithuria, Kalameha, Raktameha* and *Manjisthameha* as Haematurea and Haridrameha as Biluria and similarly *Vasameha* as Lipuria and *Majjameha* as Gonorhoea etc. *Ikshumeha, Sheetmeha* and *Madhumeha* have been compared with alimentary glycosuria, renal glycosuria and diabetes respectively. According to such descriptions *Prameha* is a collective name of so many disorders of urinary tract and other systemic diseases of varying etiology and pathology requiring almost different types of treatment for their amelioration. The prognosis of these diseases are also entirely different. The only thing in common to them is presence of urinary symptoms and an enquiry was made to appreciate urinary disorders vis-a-vis *Prameha.* At the outset, if it is considered that Prameha as a hereditary disease there is no binding that all the 20 types of Prameha may not be hereditary. Sushruta described that acquired *Prameha* is a result of excessive eating, rest and so all the 20 types of *Pramehas* may also develop due to these factors. Prodromal symptoms are same for all the 20 types of Pramehas. Pathogenesis for *Paittika* and *Kaphaja Prameha* is very much similar except for the predominance of *Doshas*; of course the Vatik type also follows the same course to certain extent. But there is no difference in pathogenesis of 10 sub-types of *Kaphaja-Pramehas* and , 6 sub-types of *Paittika Pramehas* and 4 sub-types of *Vatika Pramehas* among themselves. Regarding the clinical features of urinary changes, Sushruta clearly mentioned that instead of *Doshas* and *Dushyas* being the same only due to the difference in their proportion (*Samyog-Vishesata*) different manifestations are observed. Same is the case regarding the prognosis and termination of the disease; all the 20 types of *Pramehas* may lead to the stage of *Madhumeha.* Thus starting from the etiology to the prognosis, *Prameha* is a single disease according to Ayurveda with difference only in manifestation depending upon the concentration of *Doshas* and *Dushyas.* Hence it cannot be compared with diseases of varying aetiology and pathology manifesting in urinary disorders. There are other urinary diseases too, where they can find suitable place, for example *Mutrakrichra* and *Mutraghata.* At the same time there is no binding that other systemic diseases do not cause urinary symptoms, for example *Kamala, Raktapitta, Kshtakshina* and such other diseases. Therefore, authors have advanced the view that Diabetes mellitus as a whole is *Prameha* and the sub-types of diabetes mellitus may be sub-types of *Prameha* and the same has been examined critically. The 20 sub-types of the three basic types of Prameha, i.e. Kaphaja, Pittaja, and Vataja are not fundamentally different and they only indicate the stage of the disease.

Thus this study has been done with the premise that all the 20 types of *Prameha* are sub-types of the same disease, which are identified today under the term Diabetes mellitus, contrary to common notion that the 20 types of *Prameha* may be correlated with other diseases than Diabetes mellitus and only *Madhumeha* should be treated as synonymous to Diabetes mellitus. Hence to validate this premise, urine examination has been done in a series of 27 established diabetic patients proved by glucose tolerance test (G.T.T.). It is because the classification of *Prameha* is mainly based on the colour of urine, deposits, consistency, turbidity and a few associated symptoms, urine examination has been carried out according to Ayurveda.

Material and Methods

A series of 27 cases of Diabetes mellitus established by G.T.T. were selected. The patients were advised to bring the total urine voided in the morning. It was kept in a glass jar and was examined physically, chemically and microscopically. The physical examination was carried out particularly to observe the characteristics of sub-types of Prameha described in Ayurveda. The bio-chemical examination was carried out to know the presence of sugar, albumin, phosphate and acetone. The urine was centrifuged and the material settled was examined under microscope for the presence of crystals, and different types of cells and casts, if any. The fasting blood sugar was estimated to find out the existence of any correlation with the urinary changes. Since the emphasis was on the associated symptoms while passing urine, in the diagnosis of different types of *Prameha*, the clinical features were also recorded.

Observations

Findings in individual cases relating to age, sex, bodyweight, fasting blood sugar in mg per cent together with reports of physical, chemical and microscopical examination of the urine and associated symptoms are presented (Table 3.4).

On the basis of the findings of 27 cases, ten have been identified as kaphaja prameha, seven as pittaja prameha and six as vataja prameha and four could not be included into any of the groups. Among *Kaphaja Prameha, Udakameha* (one), *Ikshumeha* (one), *Sandrameha* (two), *Sheetameha* (one) *Shaneirmeha* (four) and *Shuklameha* (one) were noted. The patients of *Pittaja Prameha* were identified to be seven; among them two had *Raktameha* and five had *Haridrameha. Vataja Prameha* were six and among them three had *Vasameha,* two had *Majjameha* and one was having *Sahaja Madhumeha*; this last case was diagnosed as juvenile diabetes.

Comments on (Table 3.4) Udakameha (one case): The patient of Udakameha was passing a colourless urine just like water in physical appearance; sugar was present (+++), no associated symptoms were observed.

Ikshumeha (one case):The urine was turbid and the colour was just like crushed sugar-cane juice and the sugar was present only in traces; microscopic examination revealed presence of epithelial cells.

Sandrameha (two cases): The urine of patients of *Sandrameha* showed phosphate and clacium oxalate in chemical as well as microscopic examination. The deposition of crystals were observed after keeping the urine in the pot for a long time.

Sheetameha (one case):The urine of patient of *Sheetameha* showed presence of sugar in the urine, and there was high frequency of micturition, the patient reported a sensation which was not hot but cold. Hence he was diagnosed as a patient of *Sheetameha.*

Shaniermeha (four cases): The urine of the patients of *Shaniermeha* had strew-coloured and showed presence of sugar only in the urine, and while passing the urine, mild dysuria, burning pain, weakness after micturition, goose skin and shivering sensation. The symptoms indicate mild degree of urethritis.

Shuklameha (one case): The urine was milky white turbid. There was no chyle and the patient complained of shivering while passing urine.

Thus out of 10 types of *Kaphaja Prameha* described, in Ayurveda, 6 types could be identified in this small series of 10 cases of *Kaphaja Prameha.* Seven patients of Diabetes mellitus could be called as of *Pittaja Prameha* in this series.

The urine of the two patients of *Raktameha* was blood red in colour. On chemical examination albumin and sugar were present and on microscopic examination plenty of RBCs were seen (+++) and pus cells were seen; dysuria and burning sensation during micturition were reported.

Of the five cases of *Haridrameha,* one was tumeric yellow and two were lemon yellow urine and two showed pale colour (Ishatapeeta). The patient having turmeric yellow urine showed the presence of RBC+ and epithelial cells on microscopic

Table 3.4: *Ayurvedic Diagnosis of Patients of Diabetes Mellitus Based on Urine Examinations: "Sub-types of Kaphaja Prameha"*

S. No.	*Name*	*Age & Sex*	*Duration of Illness in Years*	*Wt. in Kgs.*	*Fasting Blood Sugar in mg. %*	*Physical Appea-rance of Urine.*	*Chem. Exam.*	*Micro-scopical Exam.*	*Associated Symptoms with Frequency of Micturition*	*Diagnosis*
1.	LMM	4 5F	0.5	75	120	Turbid, Ikshu Ras-like colour	Sugar Traces	Epithelial Cells	Patient cannot retain urine for longer time. Some-time her clothes become wet. Frequen-cy 9 times.	Ikshu meha.
2.	SKR	45 M	0.5	70	175	Straw, mucoid deposits appears after long time.	Sugar + Phosphate present	Calcium oxalates, crystals of triple phosphates	Frequency-8 times.	Sandra-meha.
3.	VNL	76 M	.7	70	128	Straw	Sugar traces, Phosp-hates present	Crystals of triple phosphates.	Frequency-10 times.	Sandra-meha

4.	GMS	47 M	5	59	112	Straw	Sugar traces	—	Cold micturition, Frequency: 50 times.	Sheeta-meha.
5.	RNS	55 M	0.5	55	250	White like water	Sugar +++	—	Frequency: 30 times.	Udaka-meha.
6.	SN	65 M	5	60	110	Straw yellowish deposits at mid Zone	Sugar +	Epithelial cells.	Dysuria, pain, burning, weakness after micturition Frequency: 11 times.	Shanir-meha.
7.	BC	65 M	1	80	105	Straw	Sugar traces	— —	Erection of hairs, dysuria, frequency: 8 times.	Shanir-meha
8.	RSS	52 M	6	65	110	Straw	Sugar traces	—	Hot and difficult micturition, frequency: 18 times.	Shanir-meha.
9.	CNT	70M	4	60	190	Straw	Sugar ++	—	Burning and difficult micturition	Shanir-meha.
10.	HHN	44 M	6	55	184	Milky white	Sugar ++	—	Shivering at the time of micturition	Shukla-meha.
	Mean		3.35	64.9	148.4					

Table 3.5: *Ayurvedic Diagnosis of Patients of Diabetes Mellitus Based on Urine Examinations: "Sub-types of Pittaja Prameha"*

S. No.	*Name*	*Age & Sex*	*Duration of Illness in Years*	*Wt. in Kgs.*	*Fasting Blood Sugar in mg. %*	*Physical Appearance of Urine.*	*Chem. Exam.*	*Microscopical Exam.*	*Associated Symptoms with Frequency of Micturition*	*Diagnosis*
1.	MP	60 M	10	70	190	Red colour-like blood	Albumin, sugar ++	RBC+++ dysuria,	Dribbling of urin, frequency: 15 times.	Rakta-meha
2.	MY	70 M	4	60	137	Reddish colour, whitish deposits appears immediately	Albumin, Sugar +	RBC, pus+ epithelial cells	Pain, dysurea, burning micturition, frequency 15 times.	Rakta-meha
3.	LJC	50 M	5	60	145	Turmeric yellow in colour	Sugar +	RBC + epithelial cells	Shivering and erection of hair frequency. 35 times.	Haridra-meha.
4.	JS	50 M	6	60	300	Lemon yellow in colour	Sugar +++	—	Shivering and erection of hairs, frequency: 17 times.	Haridra-meha.
5.	NNR	52 M	8	70	200	Lemon yellow in colour	Sugar ++	—	Hot micturition, frequency: 7 times	Haridra-meha.
6.	MPC	40 M	7	62	220	Pale (Ishatpeeta)	Sugar ++	—	Frequency: 6 times	Haridra-meha.
7.	VN	35 M	4	40	205	Pale (Ishatpeeta)	Sugar ++	—	Frequency: 5 times	Haridra-meha
	Mean		6.28	60.3	199.57					

Table 3.6: *Ayurvedic Diagnosis of Patients of Diabetes Mellitus Based on Urine Examinations: "Sub-types of Vataja Prameha"*

S. No.	*Name*	*Age & Sex*	*Duration of Illness in Years*	*Wt. in Kgs.*	*Fasting Blood Sugar in mg. %*	*Physical Appearance of Urine.*	*Chem. Exam.*	*Microscopical Exam.*	*Associated symptoms with Frequency of Micturition*	*Diagnosis*
1.	BNS	53 M	8	60	334	Straw mucoid deposits, appeared after keeping longer time, turbidity.	Sugar +++ Albumin traces	—	Frequency: 14 times.	Vasameha
2.	DKP	32 M	8	50	258.8	Straw, colour, turbid.	Albumin, Sugar ++	—	Frequency: 3 times.	Vasameha
3.	SC	52 M	5	62	384.6	Straw and turbid.	Albumin Sugar +++	Yeast bodies	Frequency: 11 times	Vasameha
4.	ARS	90 M	18	40	200	Straw colour, Brownish deposits in lower zone	Albumin, Sugar ++	—	Frequency: 8 times.	Majjameha

S.Name No.	Age & Sex	Duration of Illness in Years	Wt. in Kgs.	Fasting Blood Sugar in mg. %	Physical Appearance of Urine.	Chem. Exam.	Microscopical Exam.	Associated symptoms with Frequency of Micturition	Diagnosis
5. HRM	67 M	20	80	390	Straw colour.	Sugar +++	Epithelial cells, cast.	Frequency: 33 times	Majjameha
6. SK	17 M	1	50	125	Straw colour, turbid mucoid deposits appeared after keeping longer time.	Albumin, Sugar +	Calcium oxalates.	Dysuria, Frequency: 15 times.	Sahaja Madhumeha.
Mean		10	57	282.06					

examination. Care should be taken to ascertain whether the patients was on B-complex therapy.

Of the six types of *Pittaja Prameha* described in Ayurveda, only two were been identified in this small series, and the colour in the urine seems to be related with the presence of RBC.

Of the six patients of *Vataja Prameha,* one was *Sahaja Madhumeha* (Juvenile type) and five were *Apathyanimittaja* (Maturity onset). Urine was mostly straw in colour with little turbidity or brown deposits in a few of the samples. On chemical examination all of them showed the presence of albumin along with sugar, on microscopic examination epithelial cells and yeast bodies have also been demonstrated.

Of the three cases identified as *Vasameha* and two as *Majjameha.* The urine of the patient of *Vasameha* was straw and turbid showing an appearance of *Vasa*; of course albumin was present in all of them. In case of *Majjameha* there were some deposits or floating masses of epithelial cells and casts proving an appearance of *Majja.*

Thus *Dhatukshaya* in urine was observed in all cases of *Vataja Prameha.* Albumin, cells or casts, were seen.

Table 3.7: *Showing the Pattern of Duration of Illness Fasting Blood Sugar and Body Weight in Patients of Different Types of Prameha.*

S. No.	*Types of Prameha*	*No. of Cases*	*Average Duration of Illness in Years*	*Average Fasting Blood Sugar in mg %*	*Average Body Weight in kg.*
1.	Kaphaja Prameha	10	3.55	148.48	64.9
2.	Pittaja Prameha	7	6.38	199.57	60.3
3.	Vataja Prameha	6	10.00	282.06	57.0

It is obvious from the Table 3.7 that duration of illness at the time of registration has an increasing trend in *Kaphaja, Pittaja* and *Vataja Prameha* indicating that these three types of *Prameha* may be the three stages of the disease advancing with the illness. For the first few years, say below 5 years there is proneness of *Kaphaja Prameha* and subsequently the stage of *Pittaja Prameha* was reached. By the end of one decade of illness the patients lands into the stage of *Vataja Prameha.* Uncontrolled and improperly treated diabetes also culminates into this group. A proper management of diabetes has every chance to delay the advancement of illness but at times even reaches that stage of the disease.

The findings like the fasting blood sugar levels and the pattern of body weight confirmed the classification schedule. The fasting blood sugar levels has an increasing trend with the advancement of illness i.e. in different stages of diabetes, *Kaphaja, Pittaja* and *Vataja.* In the stage of *Kaphaja Prameha,* fasting blood sugar level is around 150 mg per cent and in *Pittaja Prameha* it reaches around 200 to 250 mg per cent. Of course in the stage of *Vataja Prameha,* it is above 250 or around 300 mg per cent. Thus a rough clinical correlation between the blood sugar levels and types of *Prameha* can be also established. By implication it means that the diagnosis of *Kaphaja, Pittaja* and *Vitaja Pramehas* are possible even by the estimation of blood sugar levels.

Similarly, the study of the body weight, in patients of different types of Prameha diagnosed on the basis of urine examination mentioned earlier, revealed interesting observations. There is a gradual loss of weight with the advancement of the disease and the minimum weight is recorded in the stage of Vataja Prameha. This is in confirmity with the concept of Ayurveda that in the stage of *Vataja Prameha* there is predominance of Dhatukshaya leading to asthma. Loss of tissue element has also been seen by the urine examination test.

Thus all the three observations i.e. the duration of illness, fasting blood sugar levels and pattern of body weight point to the *Kaphaja, Pittaja* and *Vataja* types of *Prameha* and they may be just only three stages of the same disease.

Discussion

The entire study was planned to study scope of correlation of the concept of *Prameha* and diabetes which is contradictory to the common prevalent view that Diabetes mellitus should be known as *Madhumeha* and rest of the 19 types of *Prameha* be correlated to other metabolic and urinary tract diseases.

Authors have advanced the view that the present concept is a deviation from the spirit and description of *Prameha* in the Ayurvedic texts. Of course, the concept of diabetes mellitus has also much changed during the last three decades in modern medicine as well as in the pathogenesis which was not clearly understood in earlier stages.

In this study a series of 27 patients of Diabetes mellitus having abnormal glucose tolerance test have been selected. Their case histories have been recorded and the urine examination of the morning urine has been done by physical, chemical and microscopic methods. Due emphasis has been given to observe the urinary symptoms and physical characteristics of urine described in Ayurvedic texts in relation to sub-types of Prameha.

In the small series of 27 patients having proven diabetes mellitus, the authors have been able to identify and demonstrate 11 sub-types of Prameha (*Kaphaja-Udaka, Ikshu, Sandra, Sheeta, Shanir* and *Shuklameha; Pittaja-Rakta* and *Haridrameha; Vataja-Vasa, Majja* and *Sahaja Madhumeha*). There is bound to be some controversy in these conclusions but it is sure that apart from signs and symptoms of *Madhumeha* alone, the features of many other sub-types of *Prameha* are surely cognisable in the patients of Diabetes mellitus; the urine examination of *Prameha* patients can be well standardized on a larger series, and that may be helpful in the diagnosis of the metabolic stage of the disease. Thus, it is obvious from the urine examination that *Prameha* as a whole may be treated as synonym to diabetes mellitus.

The other interesting fact that has emerged out of these investigations particularly with reference to duration of illness, body weight and blood sugar levels are worth noting. It has been recorded that with the advancement of illness, blood sugar level goes on increasing and the patient has a trend of decreasing body weight. The clinical features of *Kaphaja Prameha, Pittaja Prameha* and *Vataja Prameha* have been identified to be related with the advancement of the disease in this series. In the patients of early stage i.e. below 5 years of illness, stage of *Kaphaja Prameha* has been observed and within ten years the patient is likely to reach the stage of *Vataja Prameha.* In between five to ten years the predominance of the sign and symptoms of *Paittika Prameha* has been found to be frequent.

This observation is in conformity with the classical description of *Prameha* that the entire disease is one and the manifestation of *Kaphaja, Pittaja* and *Vataja* and is only due to differtation of *Kaphaja, Pittaja* and *Vataja* and is only due to difference in the proportion of *Dosha* and *Dushyas* in the body and further Vaghbhata emphatically described that in the early stage of *Prameha* there is predominance of Kapha and following the Kshaya of the same, there is predominance of *Pitta* and in the later stage there is *Kshaya* of *Kapha* and *Pitta* with predominance of *Vata* alone.

दोषदृष्याविशेषेऽपि तत्संयगोविशेणतः ।
सूत्रभेदेन भेदो सेहेषु कल्पयते ॥
मुत्रवर्णादि भेदेन भेदो मेहेषु कल्पयते ॥

Vaghbhata envisages the concept that in the same patient, *Kaphaja, Pittaja* and *Vataja* stages may be identified at different durations of illness, i.e. different stages of the disease.

It is also in conformity with the observations of Sushruta that if the patients of *Prameha* are not managed properly, they reach the stage of *Madhumeha.* Of course, he conveys something more by this statement than Vaghbhata. According to Vaghbhata, it is a natural history of the disease that in Prameha every patient has to pass from *Kaphaja* to *Pittaja* and then to *Vataja* stage. But Sushruta mentioned that progression of the disease is not only time-oriented but it is also dependent upon the management of disease. If the patients are properly managed, the progression of the disease can be slowed down and if not managed, they may reach the stage of *Madhumeha*, of course quickly.

सर्व एव प्रमेहास्तु कालेनाप्रतिकारिण: ।
मधुमेहत्वमायान्ति तदाऽसाध्या भवन्ति हि ॥
(Sushruta, Nidanasthana, 6/29)

These classical concepts are explainable today in the light of modern investigations. The patients of maturity onset diabetes are insulin-independent in the early stages. The blood insulin level may not be necessarily below than that of normal individuals. But at a later stage the insulin levels fall down and they reach to the stage of insulin-dependent diabetes. The blood sugar level also goes on increasing with the advancement of the disease and the deficiency of the insulin, the body weight may also fall accordingly. In the terminal stage of the disease, patients develop several complications like nephropathy, neuropathy, retinopathy, ketoacidosis etc. which are likely to generate the manifestation of *Vata* as described in Ayurveda. The presence of tissue elements '*Dhatu*' in the urine is also more likely because of nephropathy leading to *Dhatukshaya*.

Thus it is established by these observations that Prameha is one disease and the manifestations of different types of subtypes are duration-oriented. Of course it can be influenced to certain extent by the proper management. Hence the concept of *Prameha* as a whole should be treated on par with the concept of diabetes mellitus and to consider *Madhumeha* alone as diabetes mellitus may be a misnomer. Based on this pilot approach, it is proposed to advance this study on a larger series with inclusion of several other bio-chemical parameters.

REFERENCES

Ashtang Hridaya, 1962: Vidyotini Hindi Commentary by Atridev Gupta, Chowkhamba Sanskrit Series, Varanasi.

Ashtant Sangraha , 1951: By Atridev Gupta, Nirnaya Sagar Press, Bombay.

Charaka Samhita, 1941: With Chakrapani Commentary, Nirnaya Sagar Press, Bombay.

Charak Samhita, 1962: By Kashinath Shastri and G.N. Chaturvedi, Chowkhamba Vidya Bhavan.
Scientific American Journal, 1979: The Causes of Diabetes, by Notkins, A.L. Nov.
Sushruta Samhita, 1968: By Atridev Gupta, Motilal Banarasi Das, Varanasi.
World Health, 1979: Magazine of W.H.O., May.

Clinical and Biochemical Correlation of Different Stages of Diabetes Mellitus with Different Doshic Types of Prameha

Regarding the identity of Prameha confusion is prevailing that Prameha is a urinary syndrome consisting of so many diseases of urinary tract and only 'Madhumeha' should be treated as diabetes mellitus. On the contrary, author has proposed that basically Prameha is one disease associated with an increased frequency and quantity of urine and its turbidity. Madhumeha is only a sub-type of Prameha or the terminal stage of Prameha that's why the rest of the 19 types of Prameha are said to reach the stage of Madhumeha in course of time and early enough if not treated properly. Thus diabetes mellitus should be treated as Prameha. To support this hypothesis at the outset of clinical correlation between diabetes and Prameha has been done on the basis of literature. For this purpose right from definition, classification, pathogenesis, clinical features, concept of treatment all have been taken into account as it is described in the literature of Ayurveda and author finds them well comparable with the concept of diabetes.

Regarding the classification of Prameha, Kaphaja Prameha, Pittaja Prameha and Vataja Prameha, the three main types of this disease, it has been proposed that they resemble very much different stages of diabetes mellitus. It has been observed that with progression of disease there is increase in hyperglycemia and simultaneously fall in plasma insulin. The patients of Kaphaja Prameha have actually hyperinsulinism as compared to normogram and of Pittaja Prameha have moderate insulin and patients of Vataja Prameha have hypo-insulin or ainsulinism. Thus the former two are insulin-independent diabetes of today and the latter one is insulin-dependent diabetes. Plasma cortisol is maximum in Pittaja Prameha. In the literary correlation it has been proposed that in the Kaphaja Prameha there is predominance of growth promoting hormone and in Pittaja Prameha there is predominance of cortisol and catecholamines and in Vataja Prameha there is absolute deficiency of insulin. The same have been found to be true in this study excepting the growth hormone which has not been estimated. But instead of that insulin which has been estimated is also on anabolic hormone has been found to be highest in Kaphaja Prameha. There is always a possibility that insulin-independent type of diabetes leads to the stage of insulin dependent diabetes—Vataja Prameha. It is in confirmity with the categorical statement of Vagbhata that in the initial stage there is predominance of Kapha in every patient of Prameha, but at later stage there is Kapha-Kshaya followed by Pitta-kshaya ultimately leading to Vata-vriddhi-vata-prameha in every case. Thus the concept of different stages of diabetes mellitus is well comparable with the main types of Prameha as described in Ayurveda.

Introduction

By the study of literature on *Prameha* it is evident that *Prameha* as a whole is comparable with the disease known as Diabetes Mellitus in modern medicine and the three clinical types identified as *Kaphaja, Pittaja* and *Vataja Prameha* can be correlated with different stages of diabetes mellitus. Further the 20 sub-types of *Prameha* can be also identified among the same groups and sub-groups (Chandola and Tripathi, under publication).

Previously deficiency of insulin was considered to be the main factor in the pathogenesis of this disease, but lately it has been recognised that there are large number of cases in whom there may not be absolute deficiency of insulin rather there may be hyper-insulinism (Notkins, A.L. 1979). These two types of diabetes are classified as insulin-independent and insulin-dependent types. In the later there is absolute deficiency of insulin and patient cannot be managed without insulin therapy, but in the former the deficiency is relative and these patients can be managed with diet control and oral hypoglycemics.

There are several views regarding the aetiopathology of insulin independent diabetes. Here a hypothesis has been proposed that probably growth promoting hormone may be high in one group (*Kaphaja*) and glucocorticoids in the other group (*Pittaja*) causing hyperglycemia instead of insulin deficiency (Tripathi et al 1972). Diabetes Mellitus is a known progressive disease. The seeds of this disease are already sown in the intrauterine life as it is genetic and it remains for a considerably long time in the latent form. Over eating, excess intake of glucose, sendentary habits, obesity and other factors induce mild diabetes, preferably during the period of stress or infection. This stage is chemical stage of diabetes. It is followed by the stage of acute diabetes with moderate hyperglycemia, glycosuria and typical clinical features, polyuria, polyphagia, polydipsia, requiring appropriate drug treatement. Ultimately the patient passes to stage of chronic diabetes with the severe hyperglycemia. The patient develops complications like nephropathy, neuropathy, retinopathy etc. This is the stage when patient becomes insulin dependent, and now at this stage he cannot be managed without insulin therapy (Medical Clinics of North America, 1965).

Ayurveda has also visualised this type of progression and it has been described that in the initial stage of *Prameha* the *Kapha* is in excess, but there is *Kapha Kshaya* at later stage. Similarly there is excess of *Pitta*, particularly in *Pittaja Prameha* which also lead to Pitta Kshaya at a later stage. So utlimately there is Vata Vriddhi in Kaphaja Prameha as well as in Pittaja Prameha in the terminal stage, when all types of patients of *Prameha* lead to the stage of Madhumeha, subtype of Vataja Prameha *Madhumeha*, sub-type of *Vataja Prameha.*

Thus it is hypothesised that all 20 types of *Pramehas* are different types of diabetes mellitus and *Kaphaja, Pittaja* and *Vataja Prameha* can be correlated with different stages of the same disease. With this hypothesis the present study has been done to investigate if such correlation exists in the patients of *Prameha*/ Diabetes mellitus.

Material and Methods

A small series of 27 patients with the complaints of diabetes mellitus or previously known to be diabetics was selected. The diagnosis was again established and confirmed with the help of glucose tolerance test. These cases were classified as patients of chemical diabetes, acute diabetes and chronic diabetes, depending upon the blood glucose level. The patients upto 130 mg per cent fasting blood sugar as chemical diabetes, 131 to 250 mg per cent fasting blood sugar as acute diabetes and patients having fasting blood sugar level above 250 mg per cent as chronic diabetes.

These patients were subjected to assessment of plasma insulin by radioimmunoassay technique (dextran-coated charcoal immunoassay of insulin described by Herbert, Lau, et al. (I) double antibody method) and plasma cortisol (Matingly, D. Fluorometric method). Unfortunately we did not have facility for the assessment of plasma insulin and cortisol in all cases. Hence it could be done only in 11 cases and growth promoting hormone could not be estimated at all as per proposal of hypothesis.

"Schema showing correlation of different types/stages of diabetes mellitus with types of Prameha"

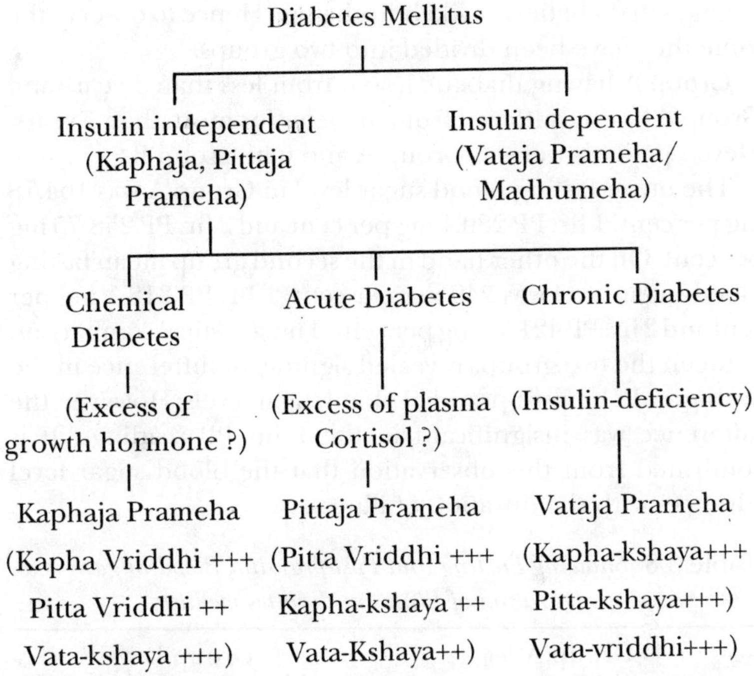

The blood sugar level has been correlated with the plasma insulin and plasma cortisol level and as the diabetes mellitus is a progressing disease, blood glucose, plasma insulin and plasma cortisol have been also correlated with the duration of illness and age of the patients.

In order to compare the derangement in blood glucose, plasma insulin and plasma cortisol in diabetics, in a small series of four normal volunteers these investigations have been also done to serve as normogram.

Observation on Pathogenesis of Diabetes Mellitus

Duration of Illness vis-a-vis Fasting and Post-prandial Blood Sugar

The observations of 17 patients is included herewith who had their fasting and two post-prandial glucose readings and in whom either the plasma cortisol or plasma insulin or both have been estimated. As mentioned earlier with the progression of disease the clinical features and the pathological changes in diabetics are likely to change. Hence to observe the same they have been divided into two groups.

Group A having diabetic lesion from less than 5 years and Group B having suffered from diabetes for more than 5 years. Eleven patients were in Group A and 6 in Group B.

The mean fasting blood sugar level in Group A was 164.78 mg per cent, 1 hr. PP 289.1 mg per cent and 2 hr. PP 258.75 mg per cent. On the other hand in the second group mean fasting blood sugar level was 249 mg per cent, 1 hr. PP 318.1 mg per cent and 2 hr. PP 421.75 mg per cent. The statistical comparison between the two groups revealed significant difference in the fasting and 2 hr. post-prandial blood sugar levels. However, the difference was insignificant in the 1 hr. PP readings. It is confirmed from this observation that the blood sugar level advances with the duration of illness.

Table 3.8: *Showing Fasting and Post-prandial Blood Sugar vis-a-vis Duration of Illness in diabetes mellitus*

	Group A Duration upto five years			Group B Duration above five years		
	Fasting blood sugar mg%	PP Blood sugar mg % 1 hr.	PP Blood sugar mg % 2 hr.	Fasting Blood sugar mg%	PP Blood sugar mg % 1 hr.	PP Blood sugar mg % 2 hr.
Mean	164.78	289.1	258.75	249	318.1	421.75
S.D.	85.74	153.24	89.56	80.44	77.77	118.00
S.E.	25.88	48.49	31.65	32.83	34.72	48.16

Comparison between both Groups–Mean difference:

F = 84.22	PP (1) Hr. = 29	PP (II) Hr. = 163
t = 2.02	t = 0.49	t = 2.83
P = <0.05	P = >0.05	P = <0.10
Significant	Insignificant	Significant

Duration of Illness vis-a-vis Plasma Insulin

Plasma insulin has been estimated in fasting blood sugar of 12 patients of diabetes mellitus; out of that in 8 patients the duration of illness was less than 5 years and in 4 patients it was more than 5 years. The mean plasma insulin was 14.15 μU/ml in Group A and it was only 4.43 μU/ml in Group B. On statistical analysis the mean difference is significant $P < 0.025$. It may be inferred from this observation that with the progression of the disease the insulin deficiency increases and the patients who are insulin-independent in beginning become insulin-dependent at later stage.

Table 3.9: *Showing Plasma Insulin vis-a-vis Duration of Illness in Diabetes Mellitus*

	Group A *Duration of illness upto 5 years* *Plasma insulin μU/ml*	*Group B* *Duration of illness above 5 years* *Plasma insulin μU/ml*
Mean	14.15	4.43
S.D.	10.31	4.80
S.E.	3.64	2.40
Mean difference:	9.72	t = 2.23 P = < 0.025 Significant

Duration of Illness vis-a-vis Plasma Cortisol

Plasma cortisol has been estimated in 14 cases, 9 in Group A and 5 in Group B. The mean plasma cortisol in Group A was 46.82 μg/100 ml and it was 55.03 μg/100 ml in Group B, i.e. patients having duration of illness more than 5 years. It shows that mean plasma cortisol is higher in the chronic cases but the difference is not significant.

Fasting and Post-prandial Blood Sugar vis-a-vis Age in Diabetes Mellitus

The same 17 patients of maturity onset diabetes have been divided into two Groups. Group A between the age of 31-50 years and Group B above 50 years. Seven patients belong to Group A and 10 patients to Group B in this series. Mean fasting blood sugar in mg per cent in Group A was 157.14;1 hour PP 262.28 and 2 hour PP 256. On the other hand in Group B, the mean fasting blood sugar in mg per cent was 220.66 1 hour PP

Table 3.10: *Showing Plasma Cortisol vis-a-vis Duration of Illness in Diabetes Mellitus*

	Group A *Duration of illness upto 5 years* *Plasma cortisol μg/100 ml*	*Group B* *Duration of illness above 5 years* *Plasma cortisol μg/100 ml*
Mean	46.82	55.03
S.D.	19.92	28.19
S.E.	6.64	12.53

330.68 and 2 hour PP 383.06. Thus it is obvious that in the maturity onset patients, the blood sugar is higher in the advance age group. On statistical comparison fasting and 2 hour PP samples have significant difference $P< 0.05$ and < 0.025 respectively. However, the difference is insignificant in 1 hour PP sample. The rise in blood sugar in higher age group is probably due to progression of disease as with the advancing age, the disease is also bound to grow. As it has been observed earlier that with the increase in duration of illness there is decrease in plasma insulin and increase in blood sugar. Hence this factor may be contributory to the present observation also.

Plasma Insulin vis-a-vis Age in Diabetes Mellitus

Plasma insulin has been estimated in 12 patients of diabetes mellitus. Six belong to Group A, having the age group between 31-50 years and 6 in Age Group B, having their age above 50 years. The mean plasma insulin in μU/ml was 11.02 in Group A and 10.8μU/ml in Group B. It shows that with the advancing age there is tendency of fall in plasma insulin in maturity onset diabetes.

Table 3-11: *Showing Fasting and Post-prandial Blood Sugar vis-a-vis Age in Diabetes Mellitus.*

	Group A Age 31 to 50 years			Group B Age above 50 years		
	Fasting Blood Sugar mg%	PP Blood Sugar mg% 1 hr.	2hr.	Fasting Blood Sugar mg%	PP Blood Sugar mg% 1 hr.	2 hr.
Mean	157.14	262.28	256	220.66	330.68	383.06
S.D.	45.44	78.58	85.18	107.7	162.05	133.75
S.E.	17.15	29.65	34.77	34.08	57.26	47.26

Mean Difference:

f=63.52	t=1.66	P < 0.05	Significant
PP 1 hr. 68.4	t=1.06	P > 0.05	Insignificant
PP 2 hr. 127.06	t=2.16	P < 0.025	Significant

It is evident from the Table that in the advance age group the plasma insulin has been recorded even upto 0 μU/ml and as low as 1.2 μU/ml in another case. However, on statistical comparison the difference is insignificant. It shows that in some patients the disease has been started in much later age group. So the duration of illness does not exactly coincide with the age of the patients.

Table 3.12: *Showing Plasma Insulin vis-a-vis Age in Diabetes Mellitus*

	Group A *Plasma insulin μU/ml* *(Age 31-52 years)*	*Group B* *Plasma insulin μU/ml* *(Age above 50 years)*
Mean	11.02	10.8
S.D.	8.52	11.86
S.E.	3.48	4.84

Plasma Cortisol vis-a-vis Age in Diabetes Mellitus

As mentioned earlier plasma cortisol has been estimated in 14 cases; 6 in Group A having their age group between 31-50 years and 8 in Group B in the age group above 50 years. The mean plasma cortisol in μg/100 ml in Group A was 59.003 and in Group B 42.82 μg/100 ml. It reveals that the plasma cortisol has also a tendency to fall down in old age. However this difference is statistically insignificant.

Table 3.13: *Showing Plasma Cortisol vis-a-vis Age in Diabetes Mellitus*

	Group A *Age Group 31-50 years* *Plasma Cortisol μg/100 ml*	*Group B* *Age group above 50 years* *Plasma Cortisol μg/100 ml*
Mean	59.003	42.82
S.D.	30.84	11.15
S.E.	12.58	4.04

Correlation of Different Stages of Diabetes with Plasma Cortisol, Plasma Insulin and Ayurvedic Classification of Prameha

The 17 cases of maturity onset diabetes mellitus investigated in this series have been classified into 3 groups, chemical diabetes, acute diabetes and chronic diabetes on the basis of their fasting blood sugar level as described elsewhere.

Table 3.14: *Showing Pattern of Fasting Blood Sugar in Different Stages of Dibetes Mellitus in a Series of 17 Cases*

S. No.	*Stages of Diabetes*	*Fasting blood Sugar Value in mg%*	*No. of Cases*
1.	Chemical diabetes	110-130	6
2.	Acute diabetes	131-250	8
3.	Chronic diabetes	251 and above	3

The corresponding plasma cortisol and plasma insulin in each group has been classified and given below in the tabular form.

Incidence of different types of Prameha in Patients of Diabetes Mellitus

Table 3.15: *Showing Pattern of Fasting Blood Sugar Plasma Insulin and Plasma Cortisol in Kaphaja Prameha (Chemical Diabetes) (Fasting Blood Sugar Ranging 110-130 mg per cent)*

	Blood Sugar mg%	*Plasma Insulin μU/ml*	*Plasma cortisol μg/100ml*
Mean	115.17	18.4	45.98
S.D.	8.77	14.13	17.59
S.E.	3.58	7.06	7.86

Table 3.16: *Showing Pattern of Fasting Blood Sugar, Plasma Insulin and Plasma Cortisol in Pittaja Prameha (Acute Diabetes) (Fasting Blood Sugar Ranging 131-250 mg per cent)*

	Blood Sugar mg%	*Plasma Insulin μU/ml*	*Plasma Cortisol μg/100ml*
Mean	192.62	7.8	56.37
S.D.	37.30	3.63	27.50
S.E.	13.18	1.48	10.42

Table 3.17: *Showing Pattern of Fasting Blood Sugar, Plasma Insulin and Plasma Cortisol in Vataja Prameha (Chronic Diabetes). (Fasting Blood Sugar Ranging Above 250 mg per cent)*

	Blood Sugar mg%	*Plasma Insulin µU/ml*	*Plasma cortisol µg/100ml*
Mean	358.2	5.25	36.05
S.D.	50.47	7.42	6.36
S.E.	29.17	5.26	4.50

Table 3.18: *Showing the Pattern of Fasting Blood Sugar, Plasma Insulin and Plasma Cortisol in Normal Subjects*

	Fasting Blood sugar mg%	*Plasma Insulin µU/ ml*	*Plasma Cortisol µg/ 100ml*
Mean	81.25	10.85	24.05

Discussion and Conclusion

The interesting observations revealed by the above classification are as follows:

1. As regards the fasting blood sugar is concerned it has got an increasing trend. As the mean fasting blood sugar is 115.17 mg per cent in chemical diabetes, 192.62 mg per cent in acute diabetes and 358.2 mg per cent in chronic diabetes.

2. On the other hand corresponding plasma insulin has a decreasing trend, it is 18.4 µU/ml in chemical diabetes, 7.8 µU/ml in acute diabetes and only 5.25 µU/ml in chronic diabetes.

3. But if we examine the pattern of plasma cortisol, it is 45.98 µg/100ml in chemical diabetes, 56.37 µg/100ml in acute diabetes, and 36.05 µg/100ml in chronic diabetes. Thus the plasma cortisol is at peak in acute diabetes and is lowest in chronic diabetes.

4. The comparative pattern of blood glucose, plasma insulin and plasma cortisol in different stages of diabetes has been studied. It shows that actually there is state of hyperinsulinism and hypercortisonism, in the stage of chemical diabetes as compared to normal. But in the stage of acute diabetes there is the fall in insulin which is just below the normal and we can call it the stage of hypo-insulinism. On the other hand as regards the plasma cortisol, it is at its peak in acute diabetes and as compared to normal it is hypercortisonism. In the stage of chronic diabetes there is further reduction in insulin to the extent that it has reached to the stage of ainsulinism in some cases. But there is simultaneous fall in plasma cortisol level as well.

Correlation

As hypothesised earlier on the basis of literary review, that the stages of diabetes can be correlated with different types of Prameha on the basis of clinical features as follows:

Table 3.19: *Showing the Clinical Correlation*

S. No.	*Stages of Diabetes*	*Types of Prameha*	*Distinguishing Clinical Features*
1.	Chemical diabetes	Kaphaja Prameha	Overweight
2.	Acute diabetes	Pittaja Prameha	Loss of weight, Polyuria, Polydipsia, Polyphagia.
3.	Chronic diabetes	Vataja Prameha	Complications Neuropathy, Nephropathy, Retinopathy.

Apart from the clinical features, insulin and plasma cortisol have been estimated in these patients along with blood glucose estimation. According to Ayurveda all types of Prameha lead to stage of *Madhumeha* by the passage of time and by inadequate management. *Madhumeha* is characterised by severe hyperglycemia and severe glycosuria. Sushruta has mentioned that the entire body becomes excessively sweet in *Madhumeha.* It indicates severe degree of hyperglycemia; as regards urine it has been described to be just like honey that also denotes the presence of sugar in high concentration.

The present observations reveals that there is progressive increase in blood glucose level and patient can be identified as *Kaphaja, Pittaja* and *Vataja Prameha* on the basis of their fasting blood sugar level, as indicated for the different stages of diabetes.

As far as insulin is concerned it possesses anabolic property and is responsible for growth, strength and adiposity in the body. Hence it may be treated to be a substance of *Kaphaja-varga* and has been found to be highest in chemical diabetes. On this basis also it may be identified as *Kaphaja Prameha* and the insulin is lowest in chronic diabetes denoting the relative or complete *Kshaya* of *Kapha.* With the *Kshaya* of *Kapha* in all probabilities, *Vata* is increased. So the stage of very low insulin or ainsulinism leading to severe hyper-glycemia and severe glycosuria associated with several types of complications be compared with *Vataja Prameha.*

On the other hand the adrenal gland as a whole is a symbol of a type of *pitta* or *agni.* Adrenergic activities like rise in blood pressure, expression of anger, flusing of face etc. seems to be *Paittika* activity in the body. It is reported that medullary as well as cortical secretions, synchronise with each other. It has been observedthat plasma cortisol is highest in acute diabetes. Thus high plasma cortisol may be taken as index for the diagnosis of *Pittaja Prameha.* In short the biochemical correlation may be summarised as follows which will facilitate the diagnosis of *Kaphaja, Pittaja* and *Vataja Prameha* by laboratory methods.

Table 3.20: *Showing the Biochemical Correlation with Types of Prameha*

S. No.	*Type of Prameha*	*Plasma Insulin* μ*U/ml*	*Plasma Cortisol* μ*U/100ml*
1.	Kaphaja Prameha	Hyperinsulinism >10.85	Normal or above
2.	Pittaja Prameha	Hypoinsulinism <10.85	Hypercortisonism
3.	Vataja Prameha	Relative ainsulinism 0-5.25	Normal or slightly above.

REFERENCES

1. Aber Louis Notkins, 1979: The Causes of Diabetes, Scientific American, November, 1979.
2. Chandola, H.M. & Tripath, S.N., 1979: Correlation of *Prameha* with Diabetes Mellitus and Evaluation of the Response of C. Tamala on Glucose and Insulin Metabolism, Thesis M.D. (Ay.), I.M.S., B.H.U., Varanasi.
3. Charaka Samhita, 1941: With Chakrapani Commentary, Nirnaya Sagar Press, Bombay.
4. Foa, Picro, P., Bajaj, J.S., Foa, Naomil Glucagon, 1977: Its role in Physiology and Clinical Medicine. Springer Veblag, New York, Heidelberg, Berlin.
5. Herbert, Valau, K.S. Gottheb, C.W., Bieicher, S.J., 1965: coated charcoal immunoassay of insulin J. Clin, Endocr.,, 25, 1365.
6. The Medical Clinics of North America, 1965: Diabetes, Volume 49-Number 4, July.
7. Tripath, S.N. & Singh, V.K., 1972: Concept of *Prameha* (Diabetes-Mellitus) in Indian Medicine, Nagarjuna, Vol. XV., No. 6, 58-67.
8. Chandola, H.M. & Tripathi, S.N.: Diagnosis of 20 sub-types of *Prameha* based on Physical and Chemical Examination of Urine in Proved Cases of Diabetes Mellitus (under publication).

Clinical Reports

Effect of C. tamala (Tej-Patra) on Plasma Insulin vis-a-vis Blood Sugar in Patients of Diabetes Mellitus—H.M. Chandola, S.N. Tripathi and K.N. Udupa (*JRAS*:1:3:1980)

In the previous study attempt has been made to establish the role of C. tamala as an hypoglycaemic agent particularly in the patients of diabetes mellitus and to assess the extent of usefulness, in the management of diabetes. The hypoglycaemic effect of C. tamala was established in long term and short term trials and its immediate effect in a series of 32 diabetic patients indicated that blood glucose level may be effected at different levels. Drug may retard the absorption of glucose, accelerate the transfer of glucose from blood to the tissues or it may actually increase the utilisation of glucose by accelerating the metabolism in different ways. Hence the drug may have hypoglycaemic response but to call it a real antidiabetic, it must be able to influence the release of insulin and accelerate the glucose metabolism and that has not yet been demonstrated. The effect of C. tamala on blood sugar as well as on plasma insulin has also been assessed simultaneously. In this trial radioimmunoassay technique has been adopted to assess the level of insulin in the blood of diabetic patients before and after treatment.

Materials and Methods

In Experiment No.1—five diabetic patients of maturity onset coming to Kayachikitsa OPD of Sir Sunderlal Hospital, BHU, Varanasi were selected and the diagnosis was confirmed by glucose tolerance test in each case. Leaves of C. tamala were procured from the local market commonly available in the name of 'Teja-patra' and used as kitchen spice. The leaves were dried and pulverized and filtered through a fine mesh and packed in 100 gm plastic packets; patients were advised to take orally two heap tea-spoonfuls of the above C. tamala powder four times a day half-an-hour before breakfast, lunch, tea and dinner for 15 days. Diet: the patients were allowed diet that can provide 1800 calories with restriction of sugar, potato and rice. For the assessment of results, fasting blood sugar vis-a-vis plasma insulin has been estimated before and after two weeks treatment with C. tamala powder.

In Experiment No.2—Assessment of immediate response of C.tamala on fasting blood sugar and plasma insulin levels upto two hours after administration of the drug. In this series another set of four patients of diabetes mellitus of maturity onset having abnormal glucose tolerance test were selected for study and all the patients were admitted in Kayachikitsa ward in identical conditions.

Fine powder of C. tamala in the dose of 20 gm was orally administered after the collection of fasting blood sample. For the assessment of results, fasting samples of venous blood were collected before the administration of the drug to estimate fasting blood sugar and plasma insulin levels. It was followed by collection of four blood samples at half an hour intervals upto 2 hours for the estimation of blood sugar and two samples at one hourly interval for the estimation of plasma insulin.

Discussion

By the previous clinical and experimental studies it was demonstrated that the powder of the leaves of C. tamala do have hypoglycaemic property. The reduction of blood glucose is possible in many ways. The action of C. tamala may be either of the two i.e. it may be promoting the insulin secretion or the action may be 'insulin like.' The third possibility is to effect on preventing glycogenolysis. Hence these experiments have been done to see that what is the fate of plasma insulin when C. tamala is administered in the patients of diabetes mellitus. Interestingly enough, improvement in the plasma insulin level has been observed in some cases. The mean plasma insulin before treatment was 14.08 μu/ml and after treatment, it has improved to 23.82 μu/ml. On statistical analysis it is just insignificant; may be due to a smaller series. In the patients in this series along with the fall in glucose, rise in plasma insulin has been observed.

In order to pin-point this of C. tamala on insulin and glucose, immediate effect of the drug has been assessed on plasma insulin and blood glucose in fasting cases for a period of two hours. Gradual fall in the blood glucose has been recorded. Mean fasting blood sugar level was 186 mg per cent with the mean plasma insulin 8 μu/ml but gradually the blood sugar level has fallen to 129.50 mg per cent at the end of two hours with a rise of plasma insulin to 31 μu/ml. Thus the rise of plasma insulin has been demonstrated with the fall of blood sugar in the same sample after the administration of powder of C. tamala for 2 hours.

Conclusion

It may be inferred from these experiments that the drug C. tamala has some definite role to paly with the release of insulin from the beta cells of islets of Langerhans. Of course, further studies in-vitro and in-vivo have to be designed to trace the exact mode of action of the drug. Instead of using the crude drug, different fractions of the drug and active principle may be also used for the purpose of study and trial.

Correlations Between Blood Sugar Levels and Some Biochemical as Well as Ayurvedic Phenomena in the Patients of Madhumeha (Diabetes Mellitus)—S.N. Gupta, S.K. Misra and G. Singh (*JRAS*:II:1:1981).

A study on twenty-four diabetic patients had been performed evaluating Vriddhi and Kshaya of Dhatus and Doshas along with Blood Sugar (fasting), serum cholesterol, SGOT, SGPT, and serum alkaline phosphatase values.

Blood sugar values had been correlated with Vriddhi and Kshaya of Dosha and Dhatu as well as other biochemical factors.

Blood sugar values showed positive correlations with serum cholesterol values (P less than 0.05), Rasa Vriddhi (P less than 0.01) and Kapha Vriddhi (P less than 0.05), while no correlation with other biochemical as well as Dosha-Dhatu factors could be observed.

It means that among the biochemical factors the cholesterol shows high levels as well as positive correlation with blood sugar values (P less than 0.05) and it signifies that the factors responsible for the hyperglycaemia are also responsible for the rise of levels of serum cholesterol. The cholesterol increases according to the severity of the disease.

The established correlations were repeated in order to test their relevance in relation to the Ayurvedic factors and the values of Kshaya and Vriddhi. This may later give us clues to assess Kshaya and Vriddhi only by investigating these values.

Effect of Jambu Fruit Pulp (Eugenia jambolana) on Blood Sugar Levels in Healthy Volunteers and Diabetics—C.V. Nande, P.M. Kale, S.Y. Wagh, D.S. Antarkar, and A.B. Vaidya (*JRAS*:IV:1-4:1983)

Jambu (Eugenia jambolana) is traditionally used for the treatment of Diabetes mellitus. Effect of Jambu fruit pulp was investigated in seven non-diabetics and five diabetic patients. Blood sugar was estimated basically and 1, 2 and 3 hours after administration of Jambu fruit pulp orally (107 to 120 gm) in over night fasting subjects. Blood sugar was estimated on Auto-analyzer using Hoffmans micro-method for this study. In non-diabetics there was small but significant drop in the blood sugar (P less than 0.05) while there was increase in blood sugar in diabetics which was statistically insignificant. Jambu fruit does not seem to have significant role in the management of diabetes.

Siddha Remedy for Diabetes Mellitus—K. Sivaprakasam, Kalavathy K.Rao, R.Yasodha, and G. Veluchamy (*JRAS*:V:1-4:1984).

A clinical trial on diabetes mellitus is carried out on twenty-five patients. The clinical diagnosis was done as per modern and Siddha parameters. Once they are selected for this study, they are advised to cut off all allopathic anti-diabetic medicines. The patients are treated only with Siddha medicines namely Kadal Azhinjil and Triphala tablets. Detailed study was made using modern investigations.

The two drugs chosen for clinical trial are purely of herbal origin and are recommended as anti-diabetic drugs in indigenous system of medicine. (Wealth of India) Kadal Azhinjil botanically identified as Salacia chinensis (Syn. Saptarangi, Cherukorandi) belongs to the family of Hippocrateae. The roots, fruits and barks are of medicinal value and our preparation contains mainly the roots and barks. Triphala has three components mixed in equal proportions. They are Terminalia chebula (Syn. Chebulic myrobalan), Terminalia bellerica (Syn. Belleric myrobalan) and Phyllanthus embelica of Euphorbialceae family and the other two are of Combrataceae family. All these three ingredients have multi-dimensional medicinal value such as laxative, carminative, nervine tonic, and anti-inflammatory and anti-diabetic. These drugs are proved to be non-toxic with clinically dose administered. The selected 25 patients were treated only with these trial drugs: 1. Kadal Azhinjil Choornam 500mg twice a day with water. 2. Triphala tablets 2.5 gm thrice a day with water. All the patients were treated for six months.

Discussion

Encouraging results were obtained. More than 50 per cent reduction in blood sugar was seen in four cases (highly significant). 40 per cent—50 per cent reduction was seen in eleven cases (significant), less than 40 per cent reduction was seen in six cases. No significant reduction was seen in four cases. Highest blood sugar recorded during the trial was 460 mg. It was reduced to 230 mgm after four months of treatment. The lowest high blood sugar recorded before treatment was 190mg. After treatment it came down to 115 mg. Total reduction was about 40 per cent.

Another peculiar finding observed is that these drugs have some unknown specific action on renal tubules by which the renal threshold is increased very much. The urine sugar is brought to normal much earlier to corresponding blood sugar. Even after the blood sugar touched normal the patients are requested to continue the drugs to have a long lasting control.

Clinical Studies of Abraga (Mica) Chendooram in the Management of Diabetes Mellitus (Neerazhivu)—V. Ravi Shanker and M.P. Aggarwal—*JRAS*:IX:1-2:1988).

Abraga Chendooram, a Siddha drug was clinically tried on the ambulatory patients of Diabetes mellitus attending the diabetic clinic at Safdarjung Hospital, New Delhi. During preliminary screen those cases in which reduction in calorie intake controlled the disease effectively or indicated serious complications like Ketoacidosis, nephropathy, or neuropathy, or retinopathy etc. were excluded. The cases taken up for study were mild and moderate type. 60 patients were treated with Abraga Chendooram (Impcops, Madras) after a thorough clinical check-up and their detailed history was recorded. 200 mg of drug filled in an empty gelatine capsule was administered two times a day for 45 days. The total calorie intake for 24 hours is decided at the rate of 25 calories per kg of ideal body weight on the basis of the height and frame of the individual.

On observation, male sex predominate over females; age group was 41-60 years. 38 per cent were reported to have familial incidence. The results indicated that the drug has hypoglycaemic activity. Out of 60 patients 35 patients showed complete relief, twenty patients showed partial relief and five patients did not respond to the treatment. So far, no side effects of the drug has been observed.

REFERENCES

1. Chandola H.M., Tripathi S.N.: Diagnosis of 20 Subtypes of Prameha Based on Physical and Chemical Examination of Urine in Proved Cases of Diabetes Mellitus, *JRAS*: 1:2:1980.
2. Chandola H.M.,Tripathi S.N.:Clinical and Biochemical Correlation of Different Stages of Diabetes Mellitus with Different Doshic Types of Prameha: *JRAS*:1:2:1980.
3. Chandola H.N., Tripathi S.N., Udupa K.N.: Effect of C. tamala on Plasma Insulin vis-a-vis Blood Sugar in Patients of Diabetes Mellitus., *JRAS*:1:3:1980.
4. Gupta S.N., Mishra S.K., Singh G.: Correlations Between Blood Sugar Levels and Some Biochemical as Well as Ayurvedic Phenomena in the Patients of Madhumeha (Diabetes Mellitus):*JRAS*:II:1:1981.
5. Nande C.V., K ale P.M., Wagh S.Y., Antarkar D.S., Vaidya A.B.: Effect of Jambu Fruit Pulp (Eugenia jambolana Lam.) on Blood Sugar Levels in Healthy Volunteers and Diabetics: *JRAS*:IV:1-4:1983.
6. Sivaprakasam. K., Kalavathy K.Rao, Yashoda R., Veluchamy G.:Siddha Remedy for Diabetes Mellitus.*JRAS*:V:1-4:1984.
7. Ravi Shanker V., Aggarwal M.P.: Clinical Studies of Abraga (Mica) Chendooram in the Management of Diabetes /Mellitus (Neerazhivu) *JRAS*:IX:1-2:1988.
8. Shukla C.P.: Madhumeha—I and II: *JNIMA*:XXXVI:4 and 5: 1994.
9. Patil S.M. Kanase A.: Effect of Asanad on Blood Glucose in Diabetic Albino Rats: *JNIMA*:XXXVII:3:1995.
10. Biswas T.K., Reality about Hypoglycaemic Effect of Mesashrimgi (Gymnema sylvestre), *Ayurveda Samachar*: 14:1:1991.

4

NUTRITIONAL DISORDERS

THERAPEUTIC NUTRITION IN AYURVEDA

Introduction

Application of the science and art of human nutrition in helping people to select and obtain food for the primary purpose of nourishing their bodies in health or in disease throughout the life cycle is called Nutritional Care.[1]

Ayurveda is a science and art applicable to maintain the dynamic state of human living.[2] The state of living is a continuous reaction to the changing pattern of environmental stimuli.[3] Food is an important eco-factor having direct influence on structural and functional aspects of human body.

Food

Food is defined as that which is voluntarily degluted to nourish the tissues of the body.[4] The human body undergoes continuous depletion in order to generate energy needed to perform life activities.[5] The depleted body tissues are supplemented by food. Food has been equated to the fuel of sacred fire.[6] Being the source of energy for life activities food is said as life of living beings.[7] Food attributes the factors needed for a positive way of living. (Fig.4.1)

Food—Human Body and Disease

A man possessing the foregoing attributes of food can maintain positive health. In fact the human body is built by

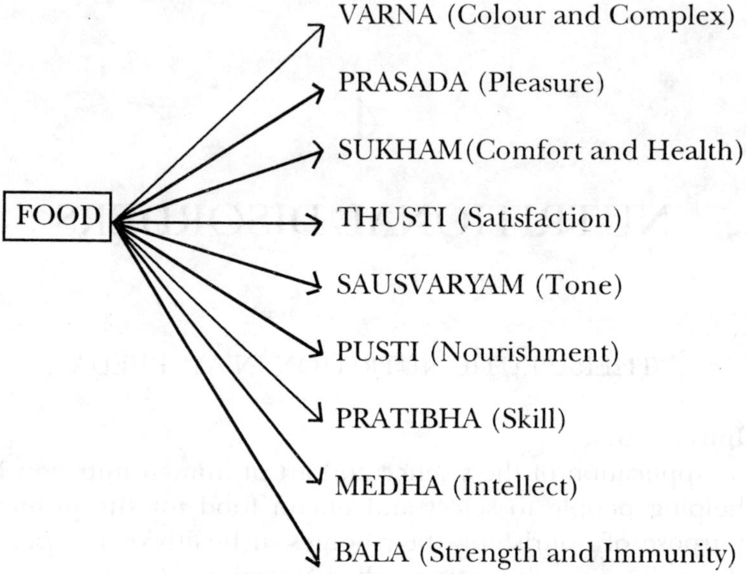

Fig. 4.1 Attributes of Food[8]

food. The balance among the constituents of human body is designated as health; the imbalance among them is disease.[9]

Either balance or imbalance among body constituents are depended on the diet consumed. Therefore it is evident that health and disease are caused by food. Briefing the procedings of a world congress in CHARAKA SAMHITA, it is said that human body and health or/and disease are sourced in food.[10]

Balancing Diet/Wholesome Diet (Hitaahara)[11]

The diet which maintains the balance among body elements/homestasis is called Balancing diet/Wholesome diet. Mere physically balanced diet may not achieve balance in all instances. Several factors are considered in Ayurveda as the determinants of Balancing diet (Fig. 4.2)

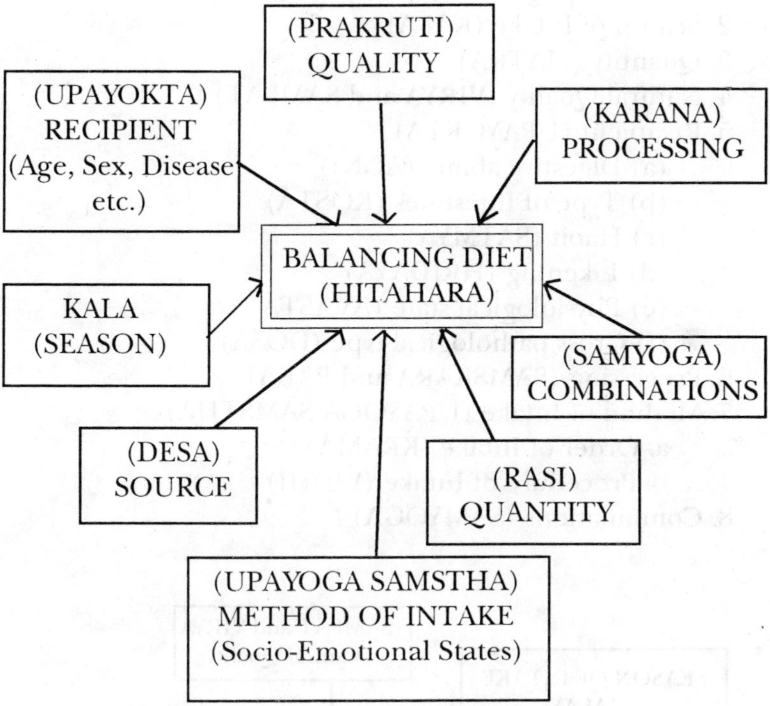

Fig. 4.2 Determinants of Balancing Diet[12]

The man who receives balancing diet determined by foregoing factors will be able to maintain health and prevent diseases.[13] He can live throughout his full span of life without any diseases.[14]

Unbalancing Diet (Ahita/Viruddha Ahara)

The diet which disturbs the balance among the body elements/homeostasis is called Unbalancing diet or Unwholesome diet. Certain times a physically balanced diet can also disturb the homeostasis. Unbalancing diet causes diseases on continuous indulgence.[15]

Factors Responsible for Unbalancing Diet[16]

The following factors turn a diet into Unbalancing and Unwholesome diet (Ahitahara/Viruddhahara)—(Fig. 4.3).

1. Place of living (DESA)
2. Season of Intake (KALA)
3. Quantity (MATRA)
4. Natural Quality (VIRYA and SAMPAT)
5. Recipient (UPAYOKTA)
    (a) Digestive ability (AGNI)
    (b) Type of Intestines (KOSTA)
    (c) Habit (SATMYA)
    (d) Likening (HRIDAYA)
    (e) Physiological state (AVASTA)
    (f) Gross pathological type (DOSA)
6. Processing (SAMSKARA and PAKA)
7. Method of Intake (UPAYOGA SAMSTHA)
    a. Order of Intake (KRAMA)
    b. Procedure of Intake (VIDHI)
8. Combinations (SAMYOGA)

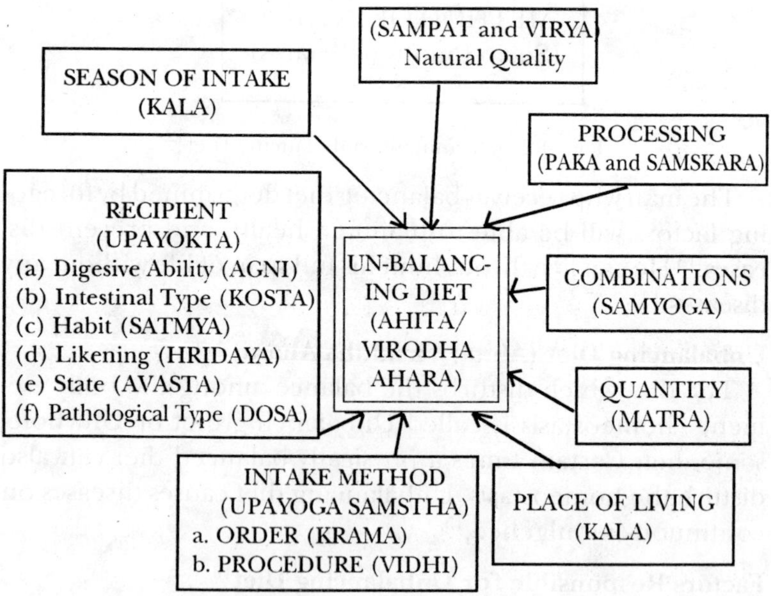

Fig. 4.3 Factors Responsible for Unbalancing Diet

Due to the foregoing factors a diet turns against to the body elements.[17] They excite certain body elements and will not allow body to expel, thus produce a persistent disturbance in the homeostasis.[18] A prolonged imbalance leads to disease.

The diet is divided into two types. 1. Balancing diet maintains health. 2. Unbalancing diet produces diseases. (Fig. 4.4)

(DIET) AHARA
- HITA (BALANCING) → AROGYAM (HEALTH)
- AHITA (UNBALANCING) → DISEASE (VYADHI)

Fig. 4.4 Impact of Diet on Health and Disease

Diet Treatment

Any effort to correct the imbalance among body elements and restore the equilibrium is called treatment.[19] Drugs; Foods and Regimen are tools of treatment and diagnosis.[20] Food has been given an equal share in treatment along with drugs. The perspective of diet in the treatment is evident with the following aspects of food and nutrition linked with treatment in Ayurveda.

Dietetic Etiology (Roga Karaka Ahara)[21]

The causative factors for all the diseases explained in Ayurveda essentially consist a list of unbalancing foods. They are specifically mentioned for each and every disease, in tune with the basic relation of foods and disease.

Dietary Prescriptions (Pathyam)[22]

The treatment of every disease ends with suitable dietary prescriptions. There will be an essential restriction on the diets which are the cause of the disease. The digestive capacity of the patient and state of the disease are considered to prescribe a Balancing diet. It has been mentioned that a patient who strictly adopts dietary prescriptions will be able to cure himself.

spontaneously. Medicines accelerate the process.[23] They are called as Pathyam. Pathyam is defined as the diet which is not harmful to the system involved in the pathology and liked by the patient.[24]

Medicated Diets (Ousadi Krita Ahara)[25]

In order to enhance the acceptability of the drugs prescribed in a disease various forms of diets have been considered as a media in Ayurveda. They are called as medicated diets.

Example: Kshira Paka (Medicated Milk)
Ghritam (Medicated Ghee)
Yusham (Medicated Soup)
Yavagu (Medicated Gruel)
Asava (Medicate Wines)
Lehya (Medicated Linctus)
Modaka (Medicated Condiment)
Panaka (Medicated Beverage)

Remedial Diets or Food Recipes[26]

Treatment for certain ailments has been given in the form of simple manipulated foods without including the drugs. Such preparations are in fact an unexplored corner of Ayurvedic therapeutic nutrition.

For Example *Wheat (Godhuma)*[27]

(a) Wheat flour dry fried and added with sugar controls gastric acidity instantly.
(b) Wheat flour fried in Ghee and cooked with milk and sugar promotes bone healing and provides nutrition to growing children.
(c) A bread or Chapati made with unshifted wheat flour helps free evacuation.

All the dietary items have been classified elaborately. Besides, their nutritional values, they are attributed with therapeutic benefits in the Ayurvedic Nighantus.

Dietetic Care of Pregnant Woman[28]

A specific monthwise dietary chart is given in Ayurveda for

the pregnant women.They are aimed at the control of problems during pregnancy, proper development of foetus and a trouble free and full time delivery.

Dietetic Management for Children[29]

Since infancy to the grown child, total dietary care has been explained in detail. The care helps for the child to shift gradually from breast milk to normal food, avoiding weaning problems and ensures complete physical and mental growth of the child.

Conclusion

The foregoing basics, and areas of clinical nutrition in Ayurveda evidently show the wider scope of the subject. Any treatment is successful only when the nutritional care is given due importance. In the light of growing awareness for the hazardous effects of synthetic drugs, it is high time to explore and propagate the Therapeutic nutritional aspects of Ayurveda for the betterment of human living.

REFERENCES

1. P.No. 6, Normal and Therapeutic Nutrition, 14th Ed. Corrine, H. Robinson; Oxford Publication Ltd., New Delhi, India, 1977.
2. Verse 42-Chapter 1: Charaka Samhita, Sutrasthana—Vidyotini Commentry, Kasinath Sastry et al. Chaukambha Bharathi Academy, Varanasi, India, 1983.
3. P.No.5 Environment Ecology, Eugene P. Odum, The University of Georgia, USA, Rinehard and Winston, Inc., USA, 1963.
4. P.P. 465 Charaka Samhita—Vadyotini commentary—Kasinath Sastry et-al., Chaukamba Bharati Academy, Varanasi, 1983.
5. Ibid.
6. Verse 375, Chapter 27th, Charaka Samhita, Sutrasthanam, Vidyotini commentary, Kasinatha Sastry et al., Chaukamba Bharati Academy, Varanasi, 1983.
7. Verse 349, Chapter 27th, Ibid.
8. Ibid.
9. Verse 41, Chapter 9th, Ibid.
10. Chapter 25th, Ibid
11. 7. Verse 31, Chapter 25th. Ibid.

12. Ibid.
13. Verse 13, Chapter 5th, Ibid.
14. Verse 348, Chapter 27th, Ibid.
15. Verse 31, Chapter 25th, Ibid.
16. Verse 85, Chapter 26th, Ibid.
17. Verse 81, Chapter 26th, Ibid.
18. Verse 85, Chapter 26th, Ibid.
19. Verse 53, Chapter Ist, Ibid.
20. Verse 10, Chapter Ist, Charaka Samhita Nidana Sthana, Ibid.
21. Nidana sections of Charaka; Sushruta and Vagbhata Samhitas and Madhava Nidanam by Madhavakara.
22. Chikitsa sections of Charaka, Sushruta and Vagbhata Samhitas and Chikitsa Granthas.
23. Vaidyajivanam by Lolamba Raju.
24. Verse 45, Chapter 28th, Charaka Samhita, Sutrasthana.
25. Charaka Samhita, Kalpastham and Sarangadhara Samhita.
26. "Mee arogyaniki ee aharam" by M. Paramkush Rao (Telugu), Live Long Publications, Tirupati, 1995.
27. Nighantu granthas of Ayurveda.
28. Chapter 8th, Charaka Samhita, Sareerasthana.
29. Kasyapa Samhita by Vriddajivaka.

Clinical Reports

Effect of Aswagandha (Withania somnifera Dunal) on the Process of Ageing in Human Volunteers—Kuppurajan K., Rajagopalan S.S., Sitaraman R., Rajagopalan V., Janaki K., Revathi R., Venkataraghavan S., *JRAS*: 1: 2: 1980.

A double blind clinical trial to study the effect of Aswagandha (Withania somnifera Dunal) on the prevention of process of ageing in 101 male health adults in the age group of 50-59 years has been completed. The results indicate that the increase in haemoglobin, Erythrocytes, hair melanin and seated stature in the treated group is statistically significant in comparison to the placebo. The decrease in serum cholesterol is more and in nail calcium it is less in the treated group as compared to the placebo and this difference is statistically significant. The decrease in Erythrocyte sedimentation rate is much higher in the treated group than in the Placebo and this difference is statistically significant.

Introduction

Aswagandha (Withania somnifera Dunal) has been mentioned in Ayurvedic classics as a Rasayana. In Ayurveda, it is stated that Rasayaya is the best profitable means of obtaining body tissues like Rasa, Raktha, Mamsa etc. (Charaka Samhita—Chikitsa Adl 1-Pada 1-Sloka 8). Aswagandha when taken with milk, ghee, oil or water for 1/2 a month (15 days) imparts strength for the emaciated body, as good rain does to a crop (Vagbhata, Asthanga Hridya–Uttarasthana Adh 39–Slo 158). Aswagandha gives lustre, virya and bala (strength). It is atisukrala, rasayanee, increases bala, relieves svitra, sotha, and kshaya (Bhavamisra; Bhavaprakasha–Poorvakhanda; Gudoochyadi varga. Slo 139-190). It is effective in the treatment of kshaya, anaemia, inflammation and cold. It is an aphrodisiac and appetiser.

On the basis of pharmacological studies, the drug has been shown to possess anti-inflammatory, diuretic, sedative activities and anti-bacterial activity against staphylococcus aureus.

In clinical studies, Aswagandha root powder has been found to be useful in cases of acute rheumatoid arthritis especially of recent onset and to some extent in the cases of acute exacerbations of chronic rheumatoid arthritis. It is proved to be a good analgesic in cases of vague aches and pains. No side effect of the drug has been observed so far.

In this paper, the results of a well planned implemented double blind clinical trial to study the effect of Aswagandha on prevention of the process of ageing, on normal healthy male adults in the age group of 50-59 years selecting the parameters suggested by Alex Comfort and Hollingworth are presented (Alex Comfort: Test Battery to Measure Ageing Rate in Man. Lancet, Vol. II, p. 1411-14).

Materials and Methods

331 persons were screened, out of which, 141 were found fit without any organic disease and included in the trial; whereas

the remaining 190 were rejected because of illness of varied aetiology.

Preparation of the Drug

The root of the plants, shade dried was powdered and tableted in the strength of 0.5 gm; Placebo of the same strength (0.5 gm) made out of starch was also tableted. Placebo and drug tablets were matched for colour, strength and appearance as far as possible. They were code named and administered. The dosage prescribed was two tablets 3 times daily (6 X 0.5 gm = 3 gms) with milk.

Duration of Treatment

One year. They were periodically followed up by social workers.

Out of 141 volunteers found fit and included in the trial, 101 volunteers completed the treatment period of one year.

The results were statistically analysed and tabulated.

Discussion

Alex Comfort suggests that a study to measure the process of ageing should be set for choice at the age of 50-55 years or 60—65 years where mortality will be significant and the rate of change in log measurables will be large. Hence in this study, the age group selected is 50-59 years. Alex Comfort statement that homeostasis declines 'across the board' with the advancement of age is also truly reflected in this finding that out of 331 volunteers screened, 190 had to be rejected due to various causes. He also suggested that 'the sample should be confined to males only to avoid further statistical breakdown,' and complications associated with the differences in the age of menopause which affects some variables.

In keeping with the above statement, only male volunteers of the stipulated age group have been included in this study.

The most promising anthrometric age measures (which give least error in assessment) are seated stature, trunk height and biacromical diameter. It is interesting to note that of the three parameters suggested above, in one parameter namely seated stature the change in the treated group as compared to the control group is in deisred direction and the difference is statistically significant.

In Hollingsworth's series of 17 tests, the highest age correlations were for characters like hair greying, skin elasticity which contribute most to the 'clinical impression' of age. In this study, hair melanin content has been taken as an index of estimating hair greying and it is worthwhile to recall that the drug increases the hair melanin content.

Serum cholesterol, serum albumin and vital capacity correlate with age in Libow's battery. In consistent with this, it has been shown in this study also that the decrease in serum cholesterol in the treated group is much higher than that in the control. The decline of serum albumin and vital capacity in the treated group is much less than in the control.

Aswagandha has been found to be an excellent haematinic in this study. Analysis for the total iron content by the dry ashing method gives a mean value of 68.94 mg per gram dry weight. A comparison of the value with the values of total iron content of a large number of roots reveals that the total iron content of Aswagandha is very high. While considering its haematinic activity, it is worth while to note that Aswagandha contains free aminoacids like valine, tyrosine, proline, alanine and glycine in abundance.

Aswagandha has been shown to reduce ESR significantly. It is interesting that the drug possesses anti-bacterial activity.

Aswagandha is more popular as an aphrodisiac agent. Perhaps this is due to its atisukrala property. In this study 71.4 per cent people have reported improvement in their capacity of sexual performance. Though it is a subjective clinical improvement, still the statement of majority of the volunteers testifying its aphrodisiac effect is worth noting.

Aswagandha is mentioned under Brihmaneeya by Charaka. It has been described under Rasayana by Vaghbhata. The increase in haemoglobin and RBC indicated its Brihmana (growth promoting and anabolic) effect while the same together with increase in hair melanin, seated stature and decrease in serum cholesterol and nail calcium indicates its Rasayana effect.

Aswagandha is described as Jwarahara, Vishahara, Vranahara, and Amavatahara. The decrease in ESR in our study only confirms these properties.

Ayurveda prescribes drugs and diet, taking the individual's constitution and temperament into consideration. Though Aswagandha is described as anti-vata and anti-kapha and therefore to be considered in vata dominant and kapha dominant prakritis, the effect of the drug was found to be more on kapha prakriti person than in pitta and vata, the significant levels being (P less than 0.1 and P less than 0.06 respectively). It may be used as anti-vata and anti-kapha drug in certain illnesses but as a rasayana drug for a prolonged period. It acts better in kapha dominant prakritis.

From the above, it may be evident that whenever a rasayana drug is to be prescribed in chronic diseases particularly of vata and kapha origin or during convalescence period after the treatment of any acute illness, Aswagandha deserves consideration.

The Comparative Effect of Milk Fortified with Aswagandha, Aswagandha and Punarnava in Children—A Double Blind Study—Venkataraghavan S., Seshadri C., Sundareshan T.P., Revati R., Rajagopalan V., and Janaki K.: *JRAS*: 1:3:1980.

Summary

A double blind trial to study the comparative effect of milk fortified with Aswagandha (Withania somnifera) and Punarnava (B. diffusa) and Aswagandha, Ferrous fumarate and Placebo, on haematinic, biochemical and anthropometric response in normal children of both sexes in the age group of 8-12 years residing in a nearby orphanage was undertaken. It was observed that Aswagandha increased body weight, total proteins and mean corpuscular haemoglobin and mean corpuscular haemoglobin concentration significantly while the combination of Punarnava and Aswagandha increased significantly haemoglobin concentration levels. The study throws light on the usefulness of these drugs as haematenics and growth promoters in the growing children. They deserve to be considered for fortifying milk for distribution particularly in children.

Introduction

Malnutrition is a very common nutritional disorder especially in developing countries like India. Milk is a complete food which has been universally acknowledged as the best nutritive substance available naturally to everybody—except for the deficiency of iron and vitamin C. For example, 100 gm of cow's milk contains 0.2 mg of iron only.

A number of rasayana drugs like Aswagandha (Withania somnifera), Punarnava (Boerhavia diffusa), Yashti (Glycorrhiza glabra) etc. are prescribed in the Ayurvedic texts to be administered with milk. The knowledge of the ancients regarding the utility of milk fortified with such rasayana drugs particularly to children deserves the attention of nutritionists. In one of the recent studies on arresting the process of ageing by some Rasayana drugs in this institute (Dr. A. Lakshmipathi Unit for Research in Indian Medicine (CCRAS), V.H.S. Medical Centre, Adyar, Madras-600020), it was found that Aswagandha when administered at a dose of 3 gm a day to 101 normal healthy male human voluntees in the age group of 50-59 years over a period of one year significantly increased haemoglobin and red blood cells. Pharmacognostically identified Nagori variety of Aswagandha contains 60 to 70 mg of iron per 100 gm dry weight of the sample, which is nearly twice the amount found in wild variety of Aswagandha (unpublished data). A comparison of this value with the other roots as given in the Bulletin of National Institute of Nutrition reveals that Aswagandha roots contain a large reserve of iron.

In Ayurvedic literature, it has been stated that Aswagandha when administered with milk to toddlers and growing children for 15 days nourished them as rain does to tender crops. Similarly, an earlier study conducted in this unit has revealed the haematinic and protein sparing effect of Punarnava (Rajagopal S.S. et al : Effect of Punarnava on Longevity, growth and Tissue Composition of Albino Rats. Nagarjun, Vol. XX, No. 10, p. 23).

In the light of the facts stated above, it was planned to study the comparative effect of cow's milk fortified with (i) Aswagandha, (ii) Aswagandha and Punarnava, (iii) Ferrous fumarate in two doses of 5 mg and 30 mg and, (iv) Placebo on normal children.

Materials and Methods

A total of 60 children who were thoroughly examined and fit for the study were selected (of which 58 children completed the trial successfully). All the children were dewormed with Mebendazole initially and again after 30 days. They were randomized into 5 groups. The first group received purified and powdered Nagori Aswagandha at the dose of 2 gm/day. The second group of children received 2 gm/day of a mixture of Aswagandha and Punarnava mixed in equal quantity. Commercially available Ferrous fumarate was mixed with lactose powder and administered at doses of 5 mg/day and 30 mg/day (in 2 g lactose) to the third and fourth group of children respectively. The fifth group received 2 g lactose powder which served as the Placebo. The drugs and Placebo treatments were given alongwith 100 cc of milk for a period of 60 days.

Results

The initial and final values of the haematinic, biochemical and anthropometric parameters have been statistically analysed and tabulated.

Group I: Aswagandha Group: There was a slight increase in Haemoglobin (Hb), Packed Cell Volume (PCV), serum iron body weight and Handgrip and a significant increase in Mean Corpuscular Haemoglobin (MCHb) and total proteins (P less than 0.01, P less than 0.01) respectively at the end of 60 days in the Aswagandha treated children as compared to their initial level and to the Placebo group. Out of the 13 children who received Aswagandha 11 showed increase in Haemoglobin (Hb). There was an increase in body weight in all the children.

Group II: Aswagandha and Punarnava: There was a significant increase in the level of Hb at the end of 30 days in this group as compared to the initial value and a marked increase in the level of Hb., PCV, Mean Corpuscular Volume (MCV), MCHb, Serum Iron, TIBC (Total Iron Binding Capacity), and Handgrip at the end of 60 days in the group as compared to their initial level. However when compared with the Placebo group only Hb at the end of 30 days and Handgrip showed significant results (P less than 0.05). The other parameters did not show any change. But it is worth mentioning here that out of the 15 children who received this treatment, 13 children showed increase in body weight, 10 children showed increase in Hb, PCV, and 11 children showed an increase in serum iron.

Group III and IV: Ferrous Fumarate 5 mg and 30 mg: There was a significant increase in Hb (P less than 0.01), MCHb (P less than 0.05), MCHbC (P less than 0.01), Serum Iron (P less than 0.05), and Handgrip (P less than 0.05) and a marked increase in PCV in children receiving 30 mg Ferrous fumarate as compared to the Placebo group. There was however no significant change in the children receiving Ferrous fumarate 5 mg/day.

Group V: Placebo Group: In the children who received Placebo, there was no significant or considerable change in any of the parameters studied.

Assessment of Prakriti

The results of the assessment of prakriti (constitution and temperament) indicate that ferrous fumarate has increased Hb in Kapha dominants. When Hb, body weight and handgrip were considered together, ferrous fumarate and Punarnava and Aswagandha compound caused better response than other treatments in the kapha dominants. Aswagandha was found to be better in Pitta, Vata, Kapha (PVK) and Vata, Kapha and Pitta (VKP) dominants.

Discussion

From the above findings it is evident that Aswagandha is a good growth promoter as observed from the increase in total proteins and a marked increase in body weight in the group of children receiving Aswagandha. The appreciable increase in PCV, and the significant rise in MCHb observed in this group after treatment is suggestive of its utility as a good haematinic and as an anti-anaemic drug. The significant increase in Hb and a marked increase in PCV observed in the second group indicate that the combination of Aswagandha and Punarnava has good haematinic potentialities. Out of the 15 children who were administered this combination, 13 children showed gain in body weight which was more than in the Placebo group. This observation together with the significant increase in the hand-grip observed in this group suggest that this combination of Punarnava and Aswagandha can be utilised for improving the growth and strength in the growing children. The haematinic effects of Aswagandha and a combination of Punarnava and Aswagandha noted in this study indicate that the iron present in Aswagandha has a better biological utility than the iron salts. The fact that 5 mg Ferrous fumarate did not evoke any haematinic response confirms that Aswangadha which contains the same amount of iron, possesses other growth promoting and other haematinic principles apart from its iron content.

In view of finding in group I (Aswagandha group), it is desirable to increase the quantity of Aswagandha in the IInd group to have optimum benefits noted in both the groups.

Effect of Chyavanaprasha on Malnutrition—Tersia T.L., Sridhar B.N., Pillai B.K.R.; Vijayan N.P., Namboodiri P.K.N.: *JRAS*:III: 3-4:1982.

Chyavanaprasha was taken to study its effect on malnourishment and disorders of the systems. Primary school going children in the age group of 5 to 12 years were selected for trial. 107 cases were selected and allotted to two groups. Group I was given trial medicine (Chyavanaprasha) and to Group II Placebo was given.

Chyavanaprasha increased body weight. It also increased the Hb per cent considerably. There was a marginal increase in chest measurement. Jwara was effectively controlled by Chyavanaprasha.

Malnutrition anaemia is still highly prevalent in India. Chyavanaprasha lehya was used by Chyavanarishi to get rid of the manifested signs and symptoms of old age.

In Ayurveda, Chyavanaprasha is used as a rasayana (Chemical compact) to promote and maintain good health. It is given to patients under convalescence in order to stimulate and increase their appetite and digestive powers. It is prescribed to the young and old patients to regain strength, memory power and courage. It is indicated in the treatment of Jwara, Kasa, Svasa, Shosha, and Hridroga. It has an anabolic effect. It raises the serum protein level and increases the body weight.

Material and Method

The Chyavanaprasha is a compound medicine consisting of Bilwa, Agnimanta, Shyonaka, Kashmari, Patala, Gokshura, Amlaki, Haritaka, Amruta, Bhruhatidwaya, Draksha, Jeevanti, Mustha, Punarnava, Tavaksheera, Pippali, Twak, Elam, Guda, Madhu, Taila, Ghee. It was prepared and supplied by Oushadi Pharmaceutical Corporation of Kerala State. 107 primary school going children in the age group of five to twelve years were selected for the trial. Detailed physical and clinical examinations were done before and after trial.

Selection of cases was done on the basis of following clinical features:

(i) Balakshaya (ii) Agnimandhya (iii) Kasasvasava, (iv) Jvara, (v) Atisara, (vi) Udarashoola, (vii) Asyapaka, (viii) Pandu.

Children appearing pale, dull, under built, under weight, malnourished and having nutritional edema were selected for trial. No case exhibited clear picture of marasmus or kwashiorkar.

The selected 107 cases were allotted into two groups. Group I 50 cases (6 dropped) (Trial group) and Group II 57 cases (like Placebo for comparison).

Group I was given the trial medicine Chyavanaprasha 10 gm twice daily. Students were advised to consume medicine once before breakfast and once after supper.

Group II was given Talisadi Choorna which was considered like Placebo for comparison. It was given in a dose of 20 gm daily. Medicine were supplied weekly for six weeks.

Assessment was done before and after the trial. Results were statistically analysed and tabulated.

Results

Body weight: Marginal increase in body weight was noted in the group which was given Chyavanaprasha, though increase was marginal; it was decidedly more while compared to Placebo group.

Haemoglobin level: Percentage of Hb increased considerably. The increase was highly significant statistically (P value 0.01 in Group I), but there was no significant increase in Group II.

Chest measurement: Marginal increase in the chest measurement was noted in the trial group. Though it was marginal, it was certainly more in comparison to Placebo group.

Intestinal parasites: Chyavanaprasha was found to have vermifuge action against pain and round worm during clinical investigation. 90 per cent cases got relief (13 out of 15 cases). In Placebo group, no effect was noticed.

Jwara: Chyavanaprasha was found effective in controlling fever. 100 per cent relief was noted in trial group (13 cases). In Placebo group, one got relief out of 8 cases. 13 cases had Atisara, which was controlled by the trial medicine, whereas, in Placebo group, one case got relief out of six cases recorded. Trial medicine and Placebo were found equally effective in controlling Kasa and Svasa. The Chyavanaprasha was found effective in controlling Udarashoola. Out of 22 cases recorded, 20 cases got relief. In Placebo group, out of 27 cases recorded only 3 cases got relief. Both the trial medicine and Placebo were found to be ineffective in cervical lymphadenitis and night blindness.

Discussion

Increase in body weight was noticed. It might be due to Amalaki, Pippali and Agnimantha; because they act as agnideepana and pachana. By this effect the digested food is well absorbed and assimilated to increase the body weight. Amalaki has anabolic effect; this might also be a reason behind the increase in body weight. There was significant raise in Hb level in blood. It might be due to Amalaki, Draksha and Guda (Guda contains small quantities of iron). Vermifuge action of the lehya might be due to Amalaki. The lehya was found effective in Jwara. It may be due to Amruta, Musta, and Amalaki. The lehya effectively controlled Atisara; this might be due to Bilwa and Amalaki. It relieved Udarashoola; it may be due to Guda and Amalaki.

Conclusion

Chyavanaprasha Avaleha was found effective in increasing the bodyweight alongwith considerable increase in Haemoglobin while a marginal increase in chest measurement was seen. No marked effect on the anthropometric parameters was observed.

DRUGS (DRAVYAS) AND THEIR EQUIVALENTS

SKIN DISEASES (KUSTHA)

Khadira— Acacia catechu
Apamarga— Achyranthes aspera
Chakramarda— Cassia tora
Kutki— Katuki; Picrorrhiza kurroa
Nimba— Azadirachta indica
Haridra— Curcuma longa
Bidanga—Embelia ribes
Chitraka— Plumbago indica
Bakuchi—Psoralia corylifolia
Aravadh—Aragvadha—Cassia fistula
Sariva—Sarsaparilla; Hemidesmus indicus
Karanja—Pongamia pinnata
Vasa—Adhatoda vasica
Patel—Patala—Stereospermum suaveolen
Triphala—Haritaki—Chebulic myrobalan; Bibhitaki-Beleric myrobalan; Amalaki-Emblic myrobalan.
Bringaraj—Eclipta prostrata
Amalta—sour gruel
Lelitaka—sulphur
Jati—Amlaki
Makshik dhatu—copper pyrite
Cow's urine
Rasa—mercury
Gandhak—sulphur
Silajatu—Asphalt-White-Gypsum
Swarna makshika—copper pyrites
Yogaraja—Balsmodendron mukul Comp.
Ela—Cardomum Matom
Kustha—Sausseria lappa
Darvi—Berberis aristata
Satapuspa—Anethum sowa
Rasanjana—extract of Berberis arista
Rock-salt—sodium chloride
Kapittha—Kapittha-Feronia lamonia
Lodhra—Symplocos racemosa
Karavira—Nerium indicum
Kutaja—Holarrhena antidysentrica
Daruharidra—see Darvi
Patala—Stereospermum suaveolens
Saptaparni—Alstonia scholaris
Arka—Calotropis gigantea
Tuttha—Copper sulphate
Mulaka—Raphnus sativus
Rohini—Picrorrhiza kurroa
Katuka— -do-
Utpala-Nymphaea—Water lily
Musta—Cyperus rotundus
Brihati—Solanum indicum
Loban—Styrax benzoin
Kampillaka—Mallotus philippinensis
Sarsapa—Brasica nigra
Sobhanjana—Moringa pterigosperma
Guduchi—Tinospora cordifolia
Devadaru—Cedrus deodara
Dhava—Eugenia hemispherica
Sariva-Sarsaparilla—Cryptolepis buchanani.
Sariva-Sarsaparilla—Ichnocarpus frutescens
Danti—Baliospermum axillare
Laksa—Laccifer lacca
Punarnava—Boerhavia diffusa
Trapu—Tin
Sisa—lead
Ayas—Iron
Hartal—Haritala; Yellow Orpiment; Ars. trisulphide

Kasis—Green vitreol; Ferrous sulphate
Bhallatak Gur—Semecarpus anacardium
Tamalpatra—Kokilaksa, Hygrophila spinosa
Maricha—Piper nigrum
Yabaskar—Yavaksara; Potassium carbonate
Kasamarda—Cassia occidentalis
Kanji—Gruel; Paya
Ghrita—Ghee
Jivanti—Leptadenia reticulata
Manjistha—Rubia cordifolia
Sarjarasa—Shorea robusta resin
Madhu chista—Bee's wax
Rai—Shorea robusta; see above
Saindhav lavana—sodium chloride; rocksalt
Guggul—Balsmodendron mukul resin
Gairik—Red ochre; Hydrous silicate of alumina
Sindur Rasa—Red oxide of mercury
Parad —Mercury
Sanka Bhasma—Xonchus pyrum; conch shell
Bakuchi—Psoralia cordifolia
Kanakapuspi (Svarnaksiri)
Avalguja—see Bakuchi
Suranjan—Colchicum luteum
Pippali—Piper longum
Kalaloha—Black iron
Gunjaphal—Abrus precatorius
Rakta Chitrak—Red Plumbago zeylanica
Vanga Bhasma—Stannum (Tin)
Haridra—Curcuma longa
Tuvaraka—Hydnocarpus castanea
Nimbadi Qwath
Nimba twak—bark of Azadirachta indica
Haridra—see above
Guduchi—see above
Hareetaki—Terminalia chebula
Vibheetaki—Bibhitaki; Terminalia belerica
Karpura—Cinnamomum camphora extract
Rasa (Parad—mercury)
Mahisha Mala Jala—Buffalo dung water
Sarkara—sugar
Dhanyaka Jala—Coriandrum sativum water
Dugdha—milk
Taila—oil
Suddha Gandhak—purified sulphur
Ghee—Ghrita
Kwath—decoction
Babbula—Acacia arabica
Badara—Zizypus jujuba
Kanksi—Alum
Tuttha—copper sulphate
Kusumanda rasa—Aloevera
Kadali svarasa—extraction of banana plant
Madanphal—Randia dumetorum
Draksha—Vitis Vinifera
Katuki—Picrorrhiza kurroa
Girisindura—Red oxide of mercury
Patolam—Trichosanthes cucumerina
Kadurohini—Picrorrhiza kurroa
Chandanum—Santalum album
Madhusravam—Chonemorpha macrophyla
Guduci—Tinospora cordifolia
Pata—Cyclea peltata
Durva—Gynodon dactylon
Sariba—Hemidesmus indicus
Usiram—Vetiveria zizaniodes
Madhuyasti—Glycorrhiza glabra
Nyagrodham—Ficus bengalensis
Plaksam—Ficus retusa
Bisam—Nelumbo nucifera
Ulpalam—Minochoria hastaefolia

Filariasis

Kiratakatiktaka—Swertia chirata
Saptachada—Alstonia scholaris
Katuki—Picrorrhiza kurroa
Kubeerakshibeeja—Caesalpinia bonducella
Shakotaka—Streblus asper Lour
Latakaranja—Kubeerakshibeeja
Amruta—Amra; Mangifera indica

Leprosy

Nirgund—Alectra parasitica var. chitrakutensis
Ghamra—Eclipta alba

Acne Vulgaris

Hirda—Terminalia chebula
Beheda—Terminalia belerica
Takan lahi—Borax pure
Sajjikshar—sodium chloride (salt)
Hing—Asafoetida

Alopecia Areata

Gunja—Abrus precatorius
Gokshuru—Tribulus terrestris
Jatiphala—Myristica fragrans

Vitiligo

Rasona—Rasna—Alpinia officinarum
Chakshushya—Cassis absus
Chakramarda—Cassia tora
Rajodumbra—Ficus carica
Yavatikta—Andrographis paniculata
Avalgujabeeja—Psoralia corylifolia
Harthala—Arsenic terculphurecticum
Dhatri Phala—fruits of Phyllanthus embelica

Psoriasis

Vetpalai—Wrightia tinctoria Linn.

II. NEUROLOGY AND RHEUMATOLOGY

Chopachini—Smilax china/S. glabra
Lasuna—Garlic; Allium sativum
Methi—Meyhika; Trigonella foenumgrae
Yastimadhu—Glycorrhiza glabra/cum

Rheumatoid Athritis

Sunthi—Zinzeber officinalis
Guggulu—purified resin of Commiphora mukul

Vatavyadhis

Bala—Sida cordifolia
Bilva—Aegle marmelos
Amlavetasa—Garcinia indica
Prishniparni—Uraria lagopoides
Eranda—Ricinus communis

Apasmara

Sankapuspi—Convolvulus pluricanlis Cholicy
Brahmi—Centella asiatica
Yashmi—see Yastimadhu
Jatamamsi—Nardostachya jatamamsi
Jyotismati—Celastrus paniculatus
Satavari—Asparagus racemosus
Arimeda—Acacia lengophola Willd.
Choraka—Angelia glauca Edgw.
Kakodumbara—Ficus hispida
Bharangi—Clerodendron sesratum
Pushkara mula—Inula racemosa
Kustha—Saussirea leppa
Vidari—Puerraria tuberosa
Sirisha—Albizzia lebbeck
Siddhardha—Brassica sps.
Mundi—Sphaeranthus indicus
Vandaka—Vanda roxburghie
Kushmanda—Benincasa urifera Savi
Musta—Cyperus rotundus

Tamra—Copper
Talaka—AS2S2
Manassila—AS2S3

Gridrasi

Ardraka—Zingiber officinale
Matulanga—Citrus medica
Trivrit—Operculina turpethum

Pakshaghata

Sarpagandha—Raulphina serpintina
Mandukaparni—Centella asiatica
Atibala—Abutilon indicum
Kapikachu—Mucuna pruriens

III. ENDOCRINOLOGY DIABETES MELLITUS

Yavagu—barley
Tagar—Valeriana wallichii
Arjuna—Terminalia arjuna
Khasa—Papaver somniferum
Neelkamal—Nilophar; Nymphaea stellata
Tejpatra—C. tamala
Jambu—Eugenia jambolanam

IV NUTRITIONAL DISORDERS

Ashwagandha—Withania somnifera
Punarnava—Boerhaavia diffusa
Agnimantha—Premna integrifolia
Shyonaka—Oroxylum indicum
Kashmari—Gmelina arboea; G. asiatica

Therapeutic Index

Summarised Data Basted on The Clinical Reports Presnted in the text

Disease	Treatment Internal	Treatment External	Success/ Duration
(1)	*(2)*	*(3)*	*(4)*
Ksudra Kushta —Pama, Dadru, Vicarcika	Gandhak Rasayan Vanga Bhasma Nimba	Nimba Argbadha Haridra —mixed churna	15 days
Sidhma Kushta	Nimba bark	Nimba oil	21 days
Vicarcika	Tuvaraka taila	—	20 days
Vicarcika	Nimbadi Quath	—	30 days
Vicarcika	Rasakarpura Dalchini	—	21 days
Ksudra Kushta	Panchakarma Therapy	—	Variable
Skin Infections	—	Aswatha Udumbara	Not useful
Dermatophytosis (FungalInfection)	—	Alcoholic Extract of Coconut shell	6 weeks
Dermatophytosis (Fungal Infection)	—	Rasottamadilepa	3 weeks
Skin Diseases	Patalokaturohinyadi Kwatham	Gopatmayadi Keram	30 days (better than Nimba, Argabadha)
Filariasis (Slipada, Elephantiasis)	Sakhotaka Ghana Vati	—	90 days
Filariasis	Sudarshan churna Kiratadi Compound (Ayush-64)	—	12 days

(1)	*(2)*	*(3)*	*(4)*
Filariasis (Slipad)	Ayush-64	Sarshapa lepa	100 days
Slipada	Sudarshan churna/ Sudarshan Ghan Vati Punarnavadyarishta	—	30 days
Filariasis (Acute)	Ayush-64	—	4 weeks
Slipada	Vata Slipada Caps. Slaishika Slipada Caps.	Sarshapa Haridra	40 days
Filariasis	Nityanand Ras Sudarshan Ghan Vati	—	2 weeks
Leprosy (Kushta)	Hydnocarpus Oil Extract	—	18 months
Leprosy	Nirgundi Bakuchi	Chitrak Nirgundi Bakuchi (mixture)	—
Acne (Tarunya Peedika)	Maha Manjishtadi Quath Sookshma Triphala	—	8 weeks
Alopecia (Khalitya)	—	Keedari Tailam	8 weeks
Vitiligo (Sweta Kushta)	—	Ayush-57	12 weeks
Vitiligo	Amlaki Khadira Avalgujabeeja	Avalgujabeeja Harathata	90 days
Vitiligo/ Leucoderma	Aletra parasitea. Psoralea	Aletra parasitea. Psoralea	—
Psoriasis	Panchakarma Therapy		Satisfactory
Psoriasis	Vetpalai Milk	Vetpalai Oil	5-15 weeks

(1)	(2)	(3)	(4)
	NEUROLOGY-RHEUMATOLOGY		
Rheumatoid Arthritis (Amavata)	1. Sunthi-Guduchi Quath/ 2. Yogaraja Guggulu Vatagajankush Ras Maharasnadi Ras Maharasnadi Quath (1 better than 2 combination)	Panchakarma Therapy	6-8 weeks
Amavata	Sunthi-Guggulu	—	6 weeks
Amavata	Rasonadi Quath For pain Pippalimoola churna Vishatundika vati	—	6 weeks
Epilepsy (Apasmara)	Medhyavati Saraswatarishta Aswagandha Churna	—	One Year
Sciatica (Gridhrasi)	Panchakarma Therapy		45 Days
Rheumatoid Arthritis (Amavata)	Dasamoolaarista Pippallyasava Vettumaran Gutika	—	90 days
Osteoarthritis (Sandhigatavata)	Trikushta Guggulu Paatra Pinda Sweda Therapy		60 days
Poliomyelitis (Baalapakshagata)	Panchakarma Therapy		Variable
Vaatavyadhis (General)	Hingutriguna Taila	Abhyanga with Ksheerabala Taila	4 weeks
Headache (Sirah-Shoola) Dyspeptic Headach	Shivkshar Pachan Samudrakvirechan Churna	—	—
After food-	Madanadi vaman Churna Eliyadiguti Samudrak virechan Churn.	—	—

(1)	*(2)*	*(3)*	*(4)*
Psychogenic-	Ksheerabala Oil (41 times)	Ksheerabala Oil -Abhyanga, Nasya	6 weeks
Hemiplegia (Paralysis) (Pakshagaata)	Panchakarma with Sneha, Sweda, Mrudu Virechana and Vasti-more effective than Drugs		60 days
Pakshagaata	Panchakarma Therapy Bhadradarvadi Kashaya Dhanvantari gutika Sahacharadi taila		15-60
Pakshagaata	Hingutriguna Taila	Abhyanga	6 weeks
Pakshagaata	Bhadradarvadi Taila Sahacharadi Taila	Abhyanga Matrabasti	30-90
Muscular Dystrophy (Pseudohypertrophic)	Panchakarma Therapy		10 weeks

ENDOCRINOLOGY

(1)	*(2)*	*(3)*	*(4)*
Obesity (Sthaulya)	Dasaanga Guggulu Trushanakya Lauha	—	30 days
Hypercholesterol-aemia	Arogyavardhani vati Ayush-55		3 months not useful
Diabetes Mellitus (Madhumeha)	Tej Patra Powder (C.tamala)	—	15 days
	Jambu (Eugenia jambola)	—	not useful
	Kadal Azhinil Churna Triphala (Combination)	—	6 months
	Abhrak Chandooram	—	45 days

(1)	(2)	(3)	(4)
	THERAPEUTIC NUTRITION		
Aging	Aswagandha Churna	—	one year
	Aswagandha and Punarnava	—	60 days
Malnutrition	Chyavanaprash Avaleha	—	6 weeks

Index

Aswatha 25
Ayush-64 42, 46
Acne vulgaris 55
Alopecia areata 57, 61
Ayush-57 69
Amavat 93, 105
Ankylosing spondylitis 121
Ardita 204
Ayush-55 317
Abraga (mica)
chandooram 375
Aswagandha 384
Ageing process 384
Apasnara 174

Bachache 199
Bala Pakshagata 223
Bhadradarvadi taila 284
Bell's Palsy 204

Coconut shell effect on fungi 25
Convulsive disorders 174
C. tamala 369
Chyvanaprasha 392

Dadru 12
Dermatophytosis 25, 28
Diabetes Mellitus 321, 329, 359

Epilepsy 174

Elephantiasis 34

Female genitalia, kustha 12
Filariasis 34
Fibromyalgia 122
Facial palsy 204

Gopatmajadi keram 30
Gridhrasi 191

Hingutriguna taila 166, 286
Headache 170
Hemiplegia 269
Hyperlipidema
and obesity 309, 311

Insulin 360

Kustha 1, 50
Ksudra kustha 6, 10, 12, 21
Khalitya 57
Kalanjaga Padai 76
(Psoriasis)
Ksheerabala taila 171
Katisula 199
Khanja 223, 291

Leprosy 50
Lepromatous L. 51
Leucoderma 63
Low backache 199

Mahakustha 8
Mahamanjisthadi Quath 56
Medhya Rasayan therapy 184
Masadiyoga 276
Muscular dystrophy 297
Malnutrition 392
Madhumeha 321, 329, 372

Nimba 14, 17
Neerazhivu
(Diabetes) 375
Nutritional disorders 377

Osteoarthritis 116
Obesity 304, 311

Pama 12
Patolakaturohinyadi Kwath 30
Puzuvethu 57
Psoriasis 76
Poliomyelitis 223
Pakshaghata 269
Panchakarma in Pakshagata 276
Pangu 291
Pseudohypertrophic Muscular dystrophy 297
Prameha 321, 341
Punarnava 388

Rasakarpoora 18
Rasottamadi lepa 28
Rheumatic diseases 90
Rheumatoid arthritis 103
Rasonadi quath 106

Skin diseases 1-89
Slipada 34
Shakhotaka ghana vati 37
Sooksham triphala 56
Svitra 63
Sunthi-guduchi 105
Sunthi-guggulu 109
Sandhigata vata 116
Sirah shoola 170
—psychogenic S. 171
Sciatica 191
Shodana in Gridhrasi 191, 200
Saisaveeya vata 223, 266
Sahacharadi taila 284
Sthaulya 304

Tuvaraka 15
Trikushta guggulu 118
Tej patra 369
Therapeutic nutrition 377

Udumbara 25

Vicarcika 12-21
Vitiligo 63
Vetpalai 84
(Psoriasis)
Vatavyadhis 122-174
Vatananatmaja vyadhi 147
Vataja sirah shoola 171
Vaman-Virechan in Kustha 21

Withania somnifera 384, 388
(Aswagandha)